B-Vitamins: Important Aspects in Nutrition and Health

B-Vitamins: Important Aspects in Nutrition and Health

Editor: Douglas Haywood

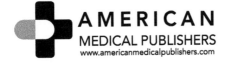
AMERICAN
MEDICAL PUBLISHERS
www.americanmedicalpublishers.com

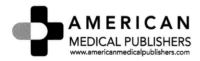

Cataloging-in-Publication Data

B-vitamins : important aspects in nutrition and health / edited by Douglas Haywood.
    p. cm.
Includes bibliographical references and index.
ISBN 978-1-63927-610-3
1. Vitamin B complex. 2. Vitamin B complex--Physiological effect. 3. Vitamin B in human nutrition.
4. Vitamin B complex--Therapeutic use. 5. Dietary supplements. 6. Nutrition. 7. Health. I. Haywood, Douglas.
QP772.V52 B563 2023
612.399--dc23

American Medical Publishers,
41 Flatbush Avenue,
1st Floor, New York,
NY 11217, USA

ISBN 978-1-63927-610-3 (Hardback)

Contents

Preface

This book aims to highlight the current researches and provides a platform to further the scope of innovations in this area. This book is a product of the combined efforts of many researchers and scientists, after going through thorough studies and analysis from different parts of the world. The objective of this book is to provide the readers with the latest information of the field.

B-vitamins are a group of water-soluble vitamins that play crucial roles in the synthesis of red blood cells and cell metabolism. There are eight types of B-vitamins, namely, B1 (thiamin), B2 (riboflavin), B3 (niacin), B5 (pantothenic acid), B6 (pyridoxine), B7 (biotin), B9 (folate), and B12 (cobalamin). These vitamins assist a number of enzymes in carrying out their functions. This includes releasing energy from fat and carbohydrates, breaking down amino acids, as well as facilitating transportation of oxygen and nutrients throughout the body. Sufficient levels of B-vitamins in the body are required for optimal neurological and physiological function. Dairy products, seafood, seeds, meat, poultry, legumes, eggs, leafy greens and fortified foods like nutritional yeast and breakfast cereal are best sources of B-vitamins. The deficiency effects of B-vitamins can cause beriberi, ariboflavinosis, pellagra, paresthesia and acne. This book explores all the important aspects of B-vitamins in nutrition and health. It presents researches and studies performed by experts across the globe. Those in search of information to further their knowledge will be greatly assisted by this book.

I would like to express my sincere thanks to the authors for their dedicated efforts in the completion of this book. I acknowledge the efforts of the publisher for providing constant support. Lastly, I would like to thank my family for their support in all academic endeavors.

Editor

One-Carbon Metabolism in Prostate Cancer: The Role of Androgen Signaling

Joshua M. Corbin [1] and Maria J. Ruiz-Echevarría [2,*]

[1] Department of Pathology, Oklahoma University Health Sciences Center, Oklahoma City, OK 73104, USA; Joshua-Corbin@ouhsc.edu
[2] Department of Pathology, Oklahoma University Health Sciences Center and Stephenson Cancer Center, Oklahoma City, OK 73104, USA
* Correspondence: Maria-RuizEchevarria@ouhsc.edu

Academic Editor: Li Yang

Abstract: Cancer cell metabolism differs significantly from the metabolism of non-transformed cells. This altered metabolic reprogramming mediates changes in the uptake and use of nutrients that permit high rates of proliferation, growth, and survival. The androgen receptor (AR) plays an essential role in the establishment and progression of prostate cancer (PCa), and in the metabolic adaptation that takes place during this progression. In its role as a transcription factor, the AR directly affects the expression of several effectors and regulators of essential catabolic and biosynthetic pathways. Indirectly, as a modulator of the one-carbon metabolism, the AR can affect epigenetic processes, DNA metabolism, and redox balance, all of which are important factors in tumorigenesis. In this review, we focus on the role of AR-signaling on one-carbon metabolism in tumorigenesis. Clinical implications of one-carbon metabolism and AR-targeted therapies for PCa are discussed in this context.

Keywords: one-carbon metabolism; androgen receptor; epigenetics; methylation; polyamine metabolism; transsufluration

1. Introduction

Prostate cancer (PCa) is the most frequently diagnosed non-skin cancer and the fifth leading cause of cancer death in men worldwide [1]. Clinically, PCa is a heterogeneous disease, ranging from an indolent disease, requiring no treatment, to highly aggressive PCa that develops into metastatic disease. Despite this heterogeneity, prostate tumor growth is, almost always, dependent upon the androgen receptor (AR) pathway [2–4], explaining the efficacy of androgen deprivation therapies (ADT) or anti-androgens for the treatment of hormone-naïve PCa [5,6]. However, most patients relapse following ADT and the disease progresses to castration-resistant prostate cancer (CRPC), which is lethal [7–9]. Central to the development of CRPC is the reactivation/adaptation of AR signaling to function under low androgen levels. Therefore, the AR and the processes downstream of the AR remain as targets for therapeutic intervention throughout the different stages of the disease. Recent results indicate that the AR drives a distinct transcriptional program in CRPC, and that changes in AR activity are critical to drive disease progression [10,11]. Efforts to identify clinically relevant, AR-modulated, transcriptional networks have established a link between the AR and cellular metabolism, consistent with the changes in metabolism that occur with disease progression [12,13]. Recent data indicate that expression of the constitutively active AR-V7 variant in CRPC has novel metabolic functions that may be specifically targeted [14].

In PCa, the one-carbon metabolism pathway is modulated by the AR. This pathway is comprised of several connected pathways that promote the folate-mediated transfer of one-carbon units necessary for essential cellular processes including DNA synthesis and repair and the maintenance of redox status. Because one-carbon metabolism is also the major source of methyl groups, as a modulator of this pathway, the AR also plays critical roles in histone and DNA methylation and in epigenetic mechanisms that are known to be relevant in oncogenesis [15–17]. Studies in PCa cell lines demonstrate AR-regulation of one-carbon metabolism enzymes, and altered cellular methylation potential in response to androgens [18–21]. In PCa clinical samples, accumulation of sarcosine, a methylated metabolite of the one-carbon pathway, correlates with disease progression [20]. Changes in several other metabolites also correlate with PCa risk [22]. These findings illustrate the role of the AR in PCa tumorigenesis by controlling metabolism, and the value of integrating metabolomic profiling and gene expression analysis for the identification of new biomarkers and therapeutic targets.

In this review, we will focus on the role of the AR on one-carbon metabolism and the implications for disease progression. The first two sections focus on the relevance of one-carbon metabolism and its link to cancer. The third section outlines how AR-signaling modulates the expression and activity of enzymes involved in one-carbon metabolism, and how it affects methylation-mediated epigenetic processes in PCa. The final section discusses targeting one-carbon metabolism in PCa, and the potential effects of current AR-targeting therapeutic modalities on one-carbon metabolism.

2. The One-Carbon Metabolism Network

One-carbon metabolism involves a complex network with two central cycles: (1) the folate cycle; and (2) the methionine cycle (Figure 1). In the folate cycle, tetrahydrofolate (THF) acts as a carbon carrier donor for the synthesis of purines and thymidilates, which are vital for DNA synthesis and repair. The transfer of methyl groups from 5-methylTHF to homocysteine to form methionine links the two cycles. Methionine is then converted to S-adenosyl-methionine (SAM), the universal methyl donor for protein and DNA methyltransferase reactions. By donating a methyl group, SAM is converted to S-adenosyl-homocysteine (SAH), and subsequently to homocysteine to close the cycle [17,23–25]. In addition to being recycled back to methionine, homocysteine can also be shunted to the transsulfuration pathway where it is converted into cystathionine, a precursor of glutathione, an important cofactor in oxidation/reduction (redox) reactions that regulate the cellular redox state. SAM can also contribute to the synthesis of polyamines, which are small organic cations that regulate multiple biological processes, including, translation and proliferation, linking the methionine cycle with polyamine synthesis [26,27]. Since one-carbon metabolism regulates essential processes including DNA synthesis and repair, epigenetic methylation reactions, redox homeostasis, and protein synthesis, the balanced flux through these four pathways (folate cycle, methionine cycle, transsulfuration pathway, polyamine synthesis) is essential for cellular homeostasis. In fact, disruptions in that balance contribute to the pathogenesis of many diseases, including cancer [28].

Balance within the one-carbon metabolism network is maintained in part by interactions involving substrates and enzymes from these pathways (Figure 2). SAM inhibits methylene-tetrahydrofolate reductase (MTHFR), the enzyme that catalyzes formation of 5-methylTHF, a necessary cofactor to regenerate methionine and, ultimately, SAM levels [17]. 5-methylTHF is an inhibitor of glycine N-methyltransferase (GNMT), the enzyme that catalyzes formation of sarcosine from glycine, which eventually donates methyl groups back to the THF in a reaction catalyzed by sarcosine dehydrogenase (SARDH) [29,30]. SAM also stimulates cystathionine beta-synthase (CBS), the enzyme that shuttles homocysteine into the transsulfuration pathway [31,32]. Additionally, folate regulates enzymes involved in polyamine metabolism [33,34]. These interactions maintain an exquisite balance between one-carbon metabolism and its associated pathways to maintain cellular homeostasis.

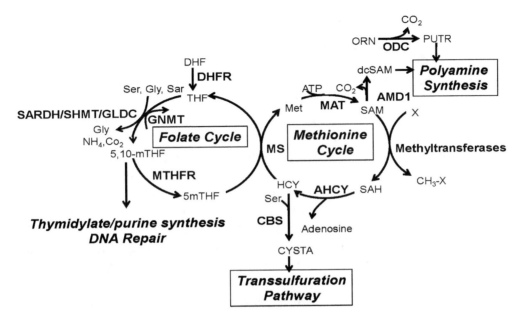

Figure 1. One-carbon metabolism and associated pathways. One-carbon metabolism involves the transfer of methyl groups to various substrates and cofactors within the folate and methionine cycles, and the polyamine biosynthetic and transsulfuration pathways. Methyl groups are utilized in the synthesis of nucleotides, and polyamines, as well as, DNA and protein methylation reactions. Enzymes are depicted in bold, while metabolites/substrates/cofactors are in regular font. Enzyme abbreviations are as follows: DHFR: Dihydrofolate reductase; SARDH: Sarcosine Dehydrogenase; SHMT: Serine hydroxymethyltransferase; GLDC: Glycine decarboxylase; GNMT: Glycine-*N*-methyltransferase; MTHFR: Methylene tetrahydrofolate reductase; MS: Methionine synthase; MAT: Methionine adenosyltransferase; AMD1: Adenosylmethionine decarboxylase; ODC: Ornithine decarboxylase; AHCY: S-adenosylhomocysteine hydrolase; CBS: Cystathionine beta-synthase.

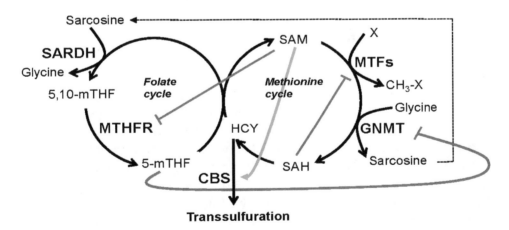

Figure 2. Regulation of the one-carbon metabolism maintains a balanced flux between the folate and methionine cycles and associated pathways. Metabolites produced within the folate and methionine pathways regulate the activity of the enzymes within the one-carbon metabolism network to maintain the balance of methyl groups and metabolites within the folate and methionine cycles and associated pathways and to allow for changes in response to cellular demands or growth conditions. See text for details. Enzymes are in bold, and substrates/cofactors are depicted in regular font. Black arrows indicate the directionality of reactions, red lines indicate inhibition, and the green arrow indicates activation. Enzyme abbreviations are as follows: SARDH: Sarcosine dehydrogenase; MTHFR: Methylene tetrahydrofolate reductase; CBS: Cystathionine beta-synthase; MTFs: Methyltransferases; GNMT: Glycine-*N*-methyltransferase.

Cancer creates a demand and dependency on one-carbon metabolism. Proliferation of tumor cells not only requires increased DNA synthesis, but can also result in increased levels of reactive radical oxygen species (ROS), which are cytotoxic unless neutralized [35,36]. Methyl group availability for methyltransferases that modulate gene expression via epigenetic mechanisms is influenced by flux within the folate cycle and methionine cycles [15,16]. In addition, synthesis of polyamines, which have been suggested to have oncogenic functions through regulating protein synthesis and proliferation [37,38], is SAM-dependent.

Several enzymes within the folate cycle are potentially oncogenic and are dysregulated in cancer. Serine hydroxymethyltransferase (SHMT) and glycine decarboxylase (GLDC) donate methyl groups to the folate pathway in sequential steps via the catabolism of serine and glycine, respectively [15]. SHMT, in concert with GLDC, drives tumorigenesis possibly by fueling the folate cycle and driving proliferation [39]. Thymidylate synthase (TS), another enzyme involved in the folate cycle, catalyzes the methylation of deoxyuracil-monophosphate to deoxythymidine-monophosphate, in a 5,10-methylene-THF-dependent reaction that is necessary for DNA synthesis and repair. The overexpression of TS is sufficient to induce a tumorigenic phenotype in NIH3T3 cells in vivo, and elevated TS expression correlates with a poor prognosis in multiple cancer types [40–46]. Furthermore, the TS inhibitor, 5-fluorouracil (5-FU), is used in the treatment of multiple cancers, especially colon cancer [47].

Paradoxically, although folate is necessary for cancer cell proliferation, multiple studies have reported a positive correlation between folate deficiency and disease risk for multiple cancers, especially breast and colon cancers [48–51]. Additionally, higher folate intake reduces the increased breast cancer risk associated with elevated alcohol consumption; this relationship may be due in part to the antagonistic effect of alcohol on folate absorption, metabolism and transport [51]. Aberrant uracil incorporation and chromosomal breaks can both be induced by folate deficiency, thus providing a potential mechanism by which folate deficiency can contribute to tumorigenesis [52,53]. Additionally, the MTHFR C677T polymorphism may be associated with increased breast cancer risk [49,54–58]. The C677T polymorphism reduces MTHFR activity, thus lowering 5-methyl-THF levels and decreasing methionine regeneration [59]. Not only can folate deficiency contribute to mutations during replication [53,60], but folate deficiency or MTHFR polymorphisms may also decrease methionine regeneration and SAM levels, thereby, reducing the ability of the cell to maintain DNA and histone methylation. Importantly, cancer cells often exhibit global DNA hypomethylation, a phenotype that may be linked to genomic instability [52,61,62].

In contrast, folate depletion blocked tumor progression in vivo and induced genetic instability in cells in vitro, in the Transgenic Adenocarcinoma of the Mouse Prostate (TRAMP) model for PCa [63,64]. Further, folate supplementation has been shown to drive tumor growth in some mouse and rat cancer models [65–67]. However, the timing of folate supplementation in disease progression is likely critical, as studies indicate that folate may be both protective against neoplastic lesion formation and a promoter of growth within established lesions [67–69]. These studies highlight a widely supported "double-edged sword" hypothesis for the role of the folate cycle in cancer: Folate depletion may contribute to initial transformation by inducing global DNA hypomethylation and subsequent genomic instability, while higher folate levels may promote the growth of transformed cells by enabling an increased rate of DNA synthesis [68,69].

Even in the presence of global DNA hypomethylation, many cancer cells contain gene specific hypermethylation, a silencing mechanism. The tumor suppressor Rb was the first gene found to be silenced by DNA hypermethylation during tumorigenesis [70]. Since then, numerous tumor suppressor genes have found to be silenced by DNA hypermethylation in cancer. Unlike DNA mutations, epigenetic aberrations—including DNA methylation—can be reversed by inhibiting the enzymes responsible for the epigenetic marks. This is one reason why targeting epigenetic enzymes has gained traction in cancer therapy [71].

Histone methylation is a SAM-dependent epigenetic process. Several methyl histone marks are dysregulated in many cancer types, and depending on the target residue, these methylated histones can contribute to gene activation or repression [72–77]. The enhancer of zeste homolog 2 (EZH2), DOT1L and mixed-lineage leukemia (MLL) methyltransferases are among the histone methyltransferases (HMTs) found to play important roles in driving a tumorigenic epigenome, which is similar to that of stem cells [78–86] HMTs use SAM as a methyl donor, and many HMTs are inhibited by SAH (Figure 2), a byproduct of methyltransferase reactions; therefore, one-carbon metabolism flux has a profound impact on the activity of these enzymes [87–89].

SAM not only serves as a cofactor for methyltransferases, but it is also shunted from one-carbon metabolism and utilized in polyamine synthesis. Polyamines have been implicated in cancer, and their oncogenic function may be linked to their roles in protein synthesis and cell cycle regulation [27,37,90]. Ornithine decarboxylase (ODC) catalyzes the formation of putrescine from ornithine, a rate-limiting step in the polyamine biosynthetic pathway. ODC is a MYC-regulated oncogene that is critical for cell cycle progression, in part by promoting MYC-induced p21 degradation [91,92].

Another shunt from the methionine cycle is the transsulfuration pathway, which is important for cellular redox homeostasis. The high intracellular oxygen levels required for aerobic respiration create an environment that produces highly reactive ROS. While physiological levels of ROS are essential for cell survival, an excess of ROS can have a wide range of detrimental effects, including DNA and protein damage. To prevent damage, the cell tightly regulates a series of antioxidant systems to restore redox homeostasis. One of the major antioxidants made within cells is glutathione, which is a product of the transsulfuration shunt of one-carbon metabolism. Reduced glutathione acts a cofactor for redox and conjugation reactions catalyzed by glutathione peroxidases and glutathione transferases to reduce hydrogen peroxide, a reactive product of initial superoxide neutralization, and neutralize toxins and carcinogens. Interestingly, in multiple cancers, glutathione peroxidases and glutathione transferases are silenced by DNA hypermethylation suggesting that the reduced activity of the enzymes drives tumorigenesis, likely through increased DNA damage [93–98]. However, the overexpression of glutathione peroxidases and glutathione transferases, along with elevated levels of reduced glutathione, has been observed to correlate with therapy resistance in multiple cancers [99–101]. This evidence suggests that the glutathione-dependent reduction and neutralization reactions may have complex pro-tumor and anti-tumor effects by improving survival and reducing DNA damage.

Interestingly, elevated homocysteine may promote oxidative stress by inhibiting the expression and activity of glutathione peroxidases. Elevated plasma homocysteine levels, a condition that may also be associated with folate deficiency, is often seen in the setting of malignancy [48,102–107]. In addition to being a metabolite that is utilized in glutathione synthesis, homocysteine regulates the activity of enzymes that use glutathione as a cofactor. By controlling glutathione synthesis and utilization, changes in one-carbon metabolism flux can have a profound impact on redox metabolism, and therefore, potentially tumorigenesis and cancer progression.

Taken together, alterations in one-carbon metabolism may contribute to tumorigenesis by fueling DNA synthesis, changing the DNA and histone methylomes, promoting protein translation, driving cell cycle progression and modulating redox balance. These changes can in turn promote sustained proliferation, induce tumorigenic gene expression changes, contribute to genomic instability, and promote survival—all important processes in tumorigenesis and cancer progression.

4. Androgen Signaling Modulates One-Carbon Metabolism and Epigenetics

In the prostate, androgens and the AR regulate the activity/expression of several enzymes involved in the one-carbon metabolism pathways, specifically enzymes involved in SAM homeostasis (GNMT and SARDH) and the entry into the transsulfuration (CBS) and polyamine synthesis (ODC) pathways (Figure 1 and Table 1). This suggests that the changes in the AR activity that occur during PCa progression may have profound effects on global one-carbon metabolism and the epigenetics of this disease. In this section, we review the role of androgens/AR signaling in these checkpoints of the one-carbon metabolism network, with an emphasis on the effect on gene expression and focusing on the best characterized genes. Based on the impact of the one-carbon metabolism in epigenetics, we will also discuss the effect of androgen signaling on the activity/expression of methyltransferases and epigenetic processes in PCa

Table 1. Androgen responsive genes of the one carbon metabolism network. * Data from the androgen responsive gene database (available online: http://argdb.fudan.edu.cn/index_info.php). MTHFD: methylenetetrahydrofolate dehydrogenase; SMS: spermine synthase; SAT: spermine/spermidine N1-acetyl transferase; CTH: cystathione gamma-lyase or gamma-cystathionase; GPX: glutathione peroxidase; GSR: glutathione reductase. Other names as in legend of Figures 1 and 2.

Androgen Responsive Genes *			
Folate	**Methionine**	**Polyamine**	**Transulfuration**
SHMT	MAT	ODC	CBS
SARDH	AHCY	SMS	CTH
GLDC		SAT	GPX
DHFR		AMD1	GSR
MTHFD			
MTHFR			
GNMT			

5. Androgen Signaling Regulates the Expression of Enzymes Involved in the One-Carbon Metabolism Network

The AR is a nuclear receptor that is essential for prostate differentiation and homeostasis and for PCa initiation and progression. Binding of androgen, its major ligand, triggers a conformational change that promotes AR homodimerization and translocation to the nucleus, where it binds to the regulatory regions of its target genes, affecting their transcription [108]. Studies directed to identify AR transcriptional networks in different models of PCa have demonstrated an involvement of the AR in global metabolism by directly targeting enzymes involved in several metabolic processes [12,13,109,110]. Below we focus on several specific AR targets involved in one-carbon metabolism and their role in PCa.

5.1. GNMT, SARDH and Sarcosine Metabolism

GNMT catalyzes the transfer of a methyl group from SAM to glycine to form SAH and sarcosine. The reverse reaction involves the oxidative demethylation of sarcosine into glycine, and it is catalyzed by mitochondrial SARDH or peroxisomal PIPOX [19,111]. It has been proposed that the "sarcosine cycle" and GNMT in particular regulate the SAM:SAH ratio, and therefore the methylation potential of the cell [111]. Methyltransferases are inhibited by SAH [87], GNMT is allosterically inhibited by 5-methylTHF [30], and SAM inhibits MTHFR and therefore formation of 5-methylTHF [111]. When SAM levels are low, this regulatory loop promotes release of the inhibition of MTHFR, resulting in de novo synthesis of 5-methylTHF and therefore ensuring inhibition of GNMT so that SAM will be saved for physiologically essential methylation reactions. High levels of SAM block formation of 5-methylTHF, releasing the inhibition of GNMT, which will convert excess SAM into sarcosine [111]. Because of the relevance of GNMT and the sarcosine cycle in methylation, changes in their expression or activity can have profound effects in essential cellular processes. The AR and the TMPRSS2-ERG fusion product (present in over 50% of localized PCa and whose expression is controlled by the AR) are known to coordinately regulate GNMT and SARDH expression [20,21]. Therefore, as expression/activity of these transcription factors changes with disease progression, so does the methylation potential of the cell. In fact, the role of GNMT and SARDH in PCa has gained recent interest, as both are dysregulated during tumorigenesis and control the metabolism of sarcosine. Sarcosine is a metabolite that increases during PCa progression to metastasis, and has been proposed as a potential non-invasive urine biomarker [20]. Using PCa cell lines, Sreekumar et al. [20] demonstrated that the enzymes involved in sarcosine metabolism act as regulators of cell invasion and are therefore potential therapeutic targets for prostate cancer. The addition of sarcosine or knockdown of SARDH in benign prostate epithelial cells enhanced their invasiveness. Recently, we demonstrated that sarcosine metabolism, not merely its concentration, and thus one-carbon availability, is responsible for the changes in invasion observed in PCa cells [18].

While controversy remains regarding whether the levels of GNMT in clinical PCa samples are downregulated [112] or upregulated [113], it is clear that dysregulation of GNMT may reflect changes in AR activity and ERG fusion status during PCa establishment and progression. Metabolomic analyses indicate that androgen supplementation results in elevated amino acid metabolism and increased methylation activity in PCa cells [114,115]. Interestingly, in breast cancer, the expression of sarcosine-related enzymes has been shown to vary according to cancer subtype [115]. A parallel with GNMT could be established with studies conducted on Nicotinamide N-methyltransferase (NNMT) [116]. NNMT, which catalyzes the transfer of a methyl group from SAM to nicotinamide to generate 1-methylnicotinamide (1-MNA) and SAH, and its products, are overexpressed in several aggressive cancer cell lines (e.g., ovarian, lung, and kidney) and in clinical samples [117]. Similar to sarcosine, 1-MNA does not have a known physiological role, but has been proposed to act as a sink for methyl groups, reducing the SAM:SAH ratio and the methylation potential of the cell [116]. The authors demonstrated that NNMT overexpression led to decreased methylation of proteins including histones, and associated changes in gene expression. It is possible that when GNMT is overexpressed and SARDH is underexpressed or its activity is decreased (as previously postulated for aggressive behavior in PCa; [20]), overproduction of sarcosine can exert a similar "methyl sink" effect. In this regard, we have previously demonstrated that the transmembrane protein with epidermal growth factor and two follistatin domains 2 (TMEFF2) is a tumor suppressor that cooperates with SARDH to modulate one-carbon metabolism in PCa cells [18,118] suggesting that additional factors may play a role in the activity of these enzymes. Metabolic changes in a TMEFF2 transgenic mouse model support this conclusion [119].

5.2. CBS and the Transsulfuration Pathway

As discussed above, homocysteine can enter the transsulfuration pathway in a reaction that involves condensation with serine, resulting in cystathionine. In mammals, this first and committed step of the pathway is catalyzed by CBS. The second step, the hydrolysis of cystathionine to cysteine, is catalyzed by the enzyme γ-cystathionase [120]. Cysteine is a limiting factor for glutathionine synthesis, but can also be catabolized via other routes, including a non-oxidative route that produces hydrogen sulfide (H2S). H2S plays a role in the regulation of many physiological processes, such as the cellular stress response, inflammation and energy metabolism [121–124], and it modulates AR activity [125]. Based on its roles in homocysteine homeostasis and H2S and glutathione generation, altered CBS activity/expression contributes to numerous diseases, including cancer [126–128].

The activity of CBS is stimulated by SAM binding [31,32,129], so that homocysteine metabolism can be directed towards remethylation when methionine/SAM levels are low, and towards the transsulfuration pathway when SAM levels are high. Studies using LNCaP, an androgen-dependent prostate cancer cell line, suggest that CBS expression may be downregulated by androgens via a currently unknown posttranscriptional mechanism and that this effect is accompanied by a decrease in glutathionine levels [130,131]. Reduced levels of CBS have also been reported in the metastatic PCa cell line PC3. However, this cell line does not express the AR, and the low levels of CBS did not seem to correlate with the cancer phenotype [132]. In addition, lower levels of plasma cysteine have been observed as a result of prostate tumor progression in mouse xenografts [133]. The above findings that suggest an impaired flux through the transsulfuration pathway in PCa are not supported by clinical metabolomic data. In a study analyzing metabolite levels in serum of patients who developed recurrent disease after primary treatment vs. patients that remained recurrence-free, the levels of homocysteine and cystathionine were significantly higher in the recurrent group than in the recurrence-free group [134]. Increased levels of homocysteine and methylated metabolites, with concomitant decrease in SAM, were observed in androgen-responsive PCa cells when compared with PCa cells that were non-responsive to androgens [114]. The levels of H2S are also significantly higher in patients with localized PCa than in patients with benign prostatic hyperplasia or healthy individuals [135]. These results suggest an androgen-mediated increase of methylation activity and an increased flux through the transsulfuration pathway in PCa and with the progression to aggressive disease. Reconciling these seemingly opposite results requires determining the role of transsulfuration metabolites in cancer, analyzing differences in methylation potential across individuals, and establishing the role of SAM and androgen signaling changes with disease progression in the one-carbon metabolism and transsulfuration pathways.

As we discussed earlier, the AR plays a role in regulation of GNMT. Thus, in modulating GNMT activity, the AR indirectly control homocysteine levels and the SAM:SAH ratio, critical to methylation reactions and to the level of CBS. H2S inhibits the activity of the AR [125] providing a feedback loop by which excess cysteine and, therefore H2S, modulates AR activity and the methylation and transsulfuration pathways. In hepatic and lymphocytic cells, androgens have been demonstrated to regulate expression of glutathione S-transferase Pi (GSTP), an enzyme with a role in detoxification, by catalyzing the conjugation of many compounds to reduced glutathione [136–138]. Consequently, the AR can play a role in detoxification not only by regulating CBS levels, and thus glutathione, but also by regulating/modulating the activity of enzymes that act downstream of glutathione. Changes in ROS are known to have a role in the etiology and progression of PCa [139].

5.3. ODC, SAM and Polyamine Synthesis

The relevance of polyamines to cellular physiology is illustrated by the fact that knockout of several enzymes of the pathway are embryonic lethal in the mouse [140] and dysregulation of polyamine metabolism leads to disease [141]. Increased levels of polyamine synthesis and ODC levels have been associated with cancer and other hyperproliferatives diseases [37,91,142–144]. ODC catalyzes the initial and rate limiting step in the biosynthesis of polyamines, a conversion of ornithine to putrescine. Sequential reactions catalyzed by spermidine and spermine synthase convert putrescine into spermidine and spermine, respectively. These reactions require dcSAM, which is obtained from the decarboxylation of SAM in a reaction catalyzed by SAM-decarboxylase (*AMD1*; Figure 1).

The prostate has exceptionally high levels of polyamines, which are synthesized in the epithelium for normal growth and for secretion into the seminal fluid [26,38,145–148]. The high level is due, in part, to the high expression of ODC and AMD1 [145,146,149–151]. Both enzymes, together with spermidine synthase, are induced transcriptionally by androgens/AR signaling in the prostate in a coordinated way [152–156]. Moreover, ODC is higher in PCa than in benign tissue, tissue from patients with benign prostate hyperplasia (BPH), or tissue from normal volunteers [149,157], indicating that changes that occur to the AR during PCa progression affect enzyme levels and polyamine synthesis. Providing further evidence for this notion, androgen-blocking therapies, inhibit production of spermine and spermidine [158,159].

The high polyamine requirements observed in the prostate, which are increased in PCa, sensitize the cells to folate levels [160]. Blocking polyamine synthesis by inhibiting AMD1 increases SAM levels and reduces the sensitivity to low levels of folate [160]. Interestingly, mild folate deficiency does not negatively impact polyamine levels, but does affect DNA methylation and cell growth, suggesting that maintaining polyamine pools is favored over maintaining SAM pools [63,160]. Due to the high demand for polyamines in the prostate and in PCa, changes in AR-mediated polyamine biosynthesis enzyme levels can create an imbalance in SAM levels and nucleotide pools, having profound effects on DNA damage, DNA methylation, and other epigenetic changes, leading to tumorigenesis and/or playing a role in disease progression (see below).

6. The Role of Androgen Signaling on Methyltransferases and the Epigenetics of PCa

DNA and histone methylation are important epigenetic mechanisms that contribute to initiation and progression of PCa [75,161–164]. Based on the link between these epigenetic mechanisms and one-carbon metabolism, in this section we briefly review the role of methylation in PCa and discuss how the AR modulates the epigenetics of PCa, indirectly controlling one-carbon metabolism and directly affecting the expression and activity of methyltransferases.

6.1. DNA and Histone Methyltransferases in PCa

In PCa, changes in DNA methylation are detected before the cancer becomes invasive and are maintained throughout disease progression [165,166]. These observations underscore the relevance of epigenetic mechanisms to PCa and suggest that epigenetic changes are early events that may even be responsible for PCa tumor initiation. The best-characterized epigenetic alteration in PCa is gene-specific DNA hypermethylation [167,168]. Aberrant hypermethylation of numerous genes including cell cycle control genes, detoxification and genes involved in apoptosis and DNA repair [166–176] and the AR itself [172,177–180] has been described. Correspondingly, expression and activity of DNA methyltransferase 1 (DNMT1), the methyltransferase that is primarily responsible for maintaining the DNA methylation pattern, is higher in localized, metastatic, and hormone-resistant PCa samples than in benign prostate hyperplasia (BPH) or normal tissue. DNMT1 level can predict disease recurrence after prostatectomy [167,168,175,180–183]. Changes in the level of DNMT1 with disease progression have also been reported in studies using the TRAMP mouse model [184]. Using this model, it was also demonstrated that inhibition of DNMT1 by 5-azacitidine treatment prevented tumorigenesis [185], underscoring the relevance of DNMT1 and hypermethylation to the establishment and progression of PCa. Expression of other enzymes involved in regulating DNA methylation (DNMT3, MBD4) is also increased in PCa and metastatic disease [74,186]. It is important to point out that global and gene specific hypomethylation changes are also associated with increased Gleason score and metastatic disease [161,187]. In Alzheimer's disease, demethylase activity is affected by one-carbon metabolism (SAM:SAH ratio) [188], however, to our knowledge, similar studies have not been conducted in PCa.

Histone methylation changes are also common in PCa. Studies using immunohistochemical methods have reported an overexpression of H3K27me3 global levels in metastatic prostate tumors compared with non-malignant prostate tissues [72]. Although other histone methylation changes have been reported in PCa, changes in H3K27 methylation are receiving more attention since EZH2, the histone methyltransferase responsible for H3K27 methylation, is overexpressed during prostate tumorigenesis and is associated with biochemical recurrence in patients with PCa [78,80,189–193]. Upregulation of EZH2 is associated with repression of tumor suppressor genes, high proliferation rates, and increased tumor aggressiveness in PCa [78]. It is also directly involved in DNA methylation through interaction with DNA methyltransferases [190,194], and can target genes for de novo methylation in cancer [195]. Although this review focusses on processes that are affected by one-carbon metabolism, changes in demethylases are also relevant to PCa. Several reviews have been recently published [196–198].

6.2. Androgen Signaling Regulates the Expression and Activity of Methyltransferases in PCa

DNA and histone methyltransferases utilize SAM as substrate leading to SAH production, an inhibitor of methyltransferases [199]. Therefore, methylation reactions are largely dictated by the SAM:SAH ratio and the level of expression of the methyltransferases. For in depth coverage of the effect of SAM levels on activity and specificity of methyltransferases, the reader is referred to an excellent review by Mentch and Locasale [16].

The AR and androgen signaling play a role in controlling methylation, modulating the expression of methyltransferases and/or their activity. As discussed above, the AR has important roles in regulating GNMT and the metabolism of sarcosine and the enzymes involved in the diversion of methyl groups into the transsulfuration and polyamine synthesis pathways. Increased GNMT expression leads to increased levels of the methyltransferase inhibitor SAH [200]. Therefore, changes in AR activity indirectly affect methyltransferase activity by modulating the SAM:SAH ratio. In clinical samples of PCa, increased GNMT expression significantly correlates with high Gleason score and reduced disease-free survival [113]. These effects could partly be due to inhibition of DNA and histone methylation. Global DNA hypomethylation has been correlated with high Gleason score and metastatic PCa [161,187]. In addition to this indirect effect, the AR has a direct effect on methyltransferase activity by binding to these enzymes and, in some cases, promoting their recruitment into specific regions on the chromatin. For example, the AR interacts with and recruits EHZ2, increasing H3K27 methylation and epigenetic silencing and leading to oncogenic transformation [201,202]. Similarly, using the protein Menin as a bridge, the AR recruits MLL, a SET-like H3K4 histone methyltransferase [84], promoting AR-mediated transcription [203]. Interaction of the AR with demethylases has also been described. For example, JHDM2A, a H3K9 demethylase, binds to and is recruited to AR target genes upon androgen stimulation, resulting in H3K9 demethylation and transcriptional activation [204]. Similarly, the AR can directly interact with LSD1 on many AR-repressed genes. LSD1 is a lysine demethylase that has a repressive function by demethylating H3K4me1 and H3K4me2 in response to androgen [205]. Interestingly, the AR is a target for LSD1. Since DNA/chromatin methylation influences AR activity, these examples illustrate the fact that by modulating methyltransferase/demethylase activity and/or expression, the AR can also control its own expression and/or activity (Figure 3).

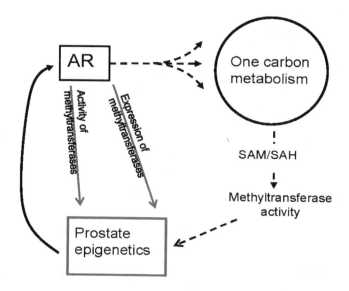

Figure 3. The impact of AR in prostate epigenetics. AR/androgen signaling can control the prostate epigenome: (1) indirectly by controlling expression of key enzymes involved in one-carbon metabolism and therefore the methylation potential of the cell (broken lines); or (2) directly by controlling the expression and activity of DNA and histone methyltransferases (solid lines).

Changes in the one-carbon metabolism affecting methyltransferases (SAM:SAH ratio) also modulate DNA and chromatin methylation affecting the activity and/or expression of the AR. In addition, direct post-translational modification of the AR and/or co-activators by methyltransferases also occurs. The AR is directly methylated by the histone methyltransferase SET9 on lysine K632 resulting in enhanced transcriptional activity [206]. Interestingly, in CRPC, EZH2 functions as a coactivator for transcription factors including the AR. The activating function of EZH2 requires the methyltransferase domain, and it has been suggested that it functions by altering the AR-associated lysine methylation [207].

Finally, AR signaling can regulate expression of enzymes involved in histone methylation. It has been reported that androgens modulate expression of EZH2 in a concentration-dependent manner (EZH2 is repressed at 1 nM or higher). This effect requires a functional AR and is mediated by the binding of retinoblastoma (RB) and p130-associated proteins to the EZH2 promoter. While both mechanisms seem to be synergistic, their androgen dependence varies. RB-E2F1 are themselves regulated by androgens in PCa cells. p130 and its partner proteins bind to the EZH2 promoter in androgen-treated, but not in control treated cells [208,209]. Finally, expression of EZH2 can be repressed by miRNA101, which is regulated by androgens [210,211].

In summary, AR/androgen signaling has an important role in PCa epigenetics, both indirectly by controlling expression of key enzymes involved in one-carbon metabolism and associated pathways, and directly by controlling the expression and activity of DNA and histone methyltransferases. These effects can ultimately affect AR expression, which is also epigenetically controlled by DNA and histone methylation, or activity. These observations emphasize the precise link between the AR and one-carbon metabolism, and the potential effects that changes in AR signaling, that can occur with disease progression, may have on essential cellular processes (Figure 3).

7. Therapeutic Approaches to Prostate Cancer: Targeting the One-Carbon Metabolism

The accelerated proliferation of cancer cells places a robust demand on one-carbon metabolism, which can be exploited for anticancer therapies. The antifolate, aminopterin, originally used by Sydney Farber to treat pediatric patients with acute lymphoblastic leukemia, was the first successful anticancer chemotherapeutic agent [212]. Today, multiple drugs targeting enzymes within the folate cycle are FDA-approved to treat a variety of cancer types [15]; however, these drugs have had mixed reports for the treatment of PCa. While early studies indicated that the antifolate, MTX, might have been beneficial in the treatment of CRPC, subsequent studies failed to support the original findings [213–215]. Because AR inhibition during ADT decreases polyamine synthesis, which may in turn increase methyl group availability in the folate cycle, it has been suggested that MTX may be more beneficial in the treatment of PCa at earlier stages of the disease [63,160].

Other branches of the one-carbon metabolism network have been explored as therapeutic targets. As we discussed previously, the natural polyamines, putrescine, spermine and spermidine are ubiquitous molecules; however, their requirements are particularly high in rapidly growing tissues during normal growth and development, and in tumors [37,216–218]. Several reports have described increased polyamine levels in the blood and/or urine of cancer patients [219–223] and elevated levels correlate with more advanced disease and worse prognosis [216,224–227]. Increased polyamine levels are associated with increased cell proliferation, decreased apoptosis and increased expression of genes affecting tumor invasion and metastasis [37,228]. More recently, it has been shown that increased polyamine levels indirectly lead to immunosuppressive conditions facilitating tumor spread [228].

Changes in polyamine levels have been reported in PCa [143,218,225,229–231]. Underscoring the clinical relevance of polyamines to prostate cancer, preclinical data suggest that inhibition of polyamine synthesis blocks the progression of the disease [232–237]. All together these observations validate the polyamine pathway as chemopreventive and chemotherapeutic for PCa. Several trials have focused on targeting the polyamine pathway as a strategy for chemoprevention in patients at risk for aggressive PCa using difluoromethylornithine (DFMO), an inhibitor of ODC [238,239]. The results of those trials indicated that DMFO treatment results in decreased levels of putrescine, decreased rate of prostate growth, and a trend towards decreased PSA doubling time. A recent clinical trial demonstrated that DFMO caused nearly complete depletion of putrescine (97.6%) but not of spermidine and spermine (73.6% and 50.8%, respectively) [150], and while very well tolerated [143], it seemed to be largely ineffective as a chemotherapeutic agent. The lack of effectiveness could be in part due to compensatory mechanisms such as increased polyamine uptake from circulation, or upregulation of other enzymes involved in the pathway. Supporting this, it was shown that polyamine reduced diet induced or maintained the quality of life of patients with CRPC [151]. In addition, studies in cell lines and xenografts indicate increased efficacy when using DMFO in combination with polyamine transport inhibitors [234]. Increased levels of SAM-dc [142] and spermine synthase [150] have been observed in patients with PCa. Other pathway inhibitors including polyamine analogs [142,143,240] or SAM-dc inhibitors [143] have been previously pursued in clinical trials; however, they have demonstrated high toxicity or only partial responses.

In addition to drugs targeting one-carbon metabolism itself, methyltransferase inhibitors are also used to treat a variety of cancers, and several inhibitors are currently being investigated for cancer therapy [241]. 5′Azacitidine is a DNA methyltransferase inhibitor that is commonly used to treat myelodysplastic syndromes [242]. Importantly, epigenetic alterations, including DNA methylation, have been found to play an important role in therapy resistance, and 5′Azacitidine, and other demethylating agents, have been shown to be effective in combination therapy to improve chemosensitivity in other cancer types [243–248]. In PCa, for example, 5′Azacitidine improved chemosensitivity to docetaxel in patients with metastatic CRPC in phase I/II clinical trials [248].

Histone methyltransferases are also prime targets in epigenetic cancer therapy. EZH2, MLL, and DOT1L are potentially attractive targets in PCa, as all three modulate the activity of the AR [203,207,249]. MI-503 (MLL inhibitor) inhibits AR activity, and both DZNeP and MI-503 inhibit CRPC growth in mouse xenograft models [203,250]. Because EZH2 is overexpressed in metastatic CRPC and it drives a transcriptional signature that is associated with this stage of the disease, the potential use of EZH2 inhibitors in the treatment of CRPC is of particular interest [207,251]. Furthermore, EZH2 seems to have a role in both AR positive and AR negative CRPC, making EZH2 a versatile potential target in advanced PCa [207,251]. It is possible that therapeutics targeting one-carbon metabolism could work synergistically with direct methyltransferase inhibition to block the oncogenic functions of EZH2 and/or other methyltransferases in CRPC; however, this hypothesis remains to be tested.

8. Summary and Conclusions

The one-carbon metabolism network integrates several pathways that, together, play central roles in the biosynthesis of nucleic acids and lipids, amino acid and vitamin metabolism, the maintenance of redox status, methylation reactions and polyamine biogenesis. Because of the relevance of these pathways to cell growth and proliferation, they are critical not only for cellular homeostasis but also for tumorigenesis, and are therefore significant therapeutic targets.

The tight dependency among the pathways of the one-carbon metabolism network imposes an exquisite regulation to allow rapid responses to changes in cellular demands. The AR and androgen signaling regulate key enzymes involved in these pathways, including the ones that control the methylation potential of the cell and the entrance into the glutathione and polyamine biosynthetic pathways. Therefore, changes that occur in the AR levels or activity will have profound effects on the activity and output of the one-carbon metabolism network and downstream processes (Figure 4). ADT designed to decrease the levels of circulating androgens, or AR-directed therapies, are the mainstay treatments against advanced PCa, and are also used as adjuvants for local treatment of high risk disease. Because of their effect on AR signaling, these therapies affect the balance of the one-carbon metabolism. For example, it has been described that neo-adjuvant androgen blockade using an LHRH agonist, together with an anti-androgen, leads to decreased spermine and spermidine levels of the normal glands [158]. While in some instances the ADT-mediated effect on one-carbon metabolism may be beneficial, i.e., lowering the high levels of polyamines observed in cancer cells may help decrease their proliferative capacity, it is conceivable that it may also have a detrimental outcome. For instance, the blockade of polyamine synthesis would alter the flux of methyl groups toward other branches of the one-carbon metabolism network including the folate cycle, which potentially may lead to reduced sensitivity to the anti-folate methotrexate as discussed previously [63,160]. In addition,

ADT or AR blockade would reduce the levels of GNMT, leading to increased SAM/SAH ratios and methyltransferase activity, a condition that maybe conducive to aggressive PCa (i.e., increased EZH2 levels in CRPC [78,191,193]). Finally, since the AR negatively regulates expression of CBS, an AR-signaling blockade would increase the flux towards the transsulfuration pathway, an effect that has been linked with increased therapeutic resistance [99–101]. Taken together these observations point to potential detrimental effects of ADT on one-carbon metabolism flux, and suggest that combination drug therapy in a precise order and timing may be helpful in the design of future clinical trials, and critical for successful treatment of PCa patients.

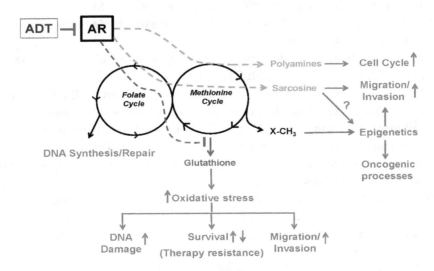

Figure 4. The AR impacts one-carbon metabolism and downstream processes by modulating the expression of specific associated enzymes. Green and red arrows/lines indicate reactions that are respectively activated and repressed by the AR via the modulation of enzyme expression. Enzymes include ODC1 (involved in polyamine synthesis), GNMT (catalyzes the conversion of glycine to sarcosine) and CBS (involved in glutathione synthesis). Metabolites increased and decreased by the AR in this manner are indicated in green and red, respectively. Black color depicts the one-carbon metabolism pathways and some other metabolites derived from it. Cellular processes potentially affected by AR-mediated one-carbon metabolism modulation are indicated in blue. By inhibiting AR, ADT (grey box) likely blocks many of these metabolic alterations in PCa cells, thus producing potentially beneficial and deleterious effects as discussed in the text.

Acknowledgments: The authors are thankful to Kathy J. Kyler for editing and reviewing this manuscript. We thank the Stephenson Cancer Center at the University of Oklahoma, Oklahoma City, OK for funding support. The authors wish to apologize to all the colleagues whose work has not been cited in this manuscript due to space limitations.

References

1. Torre, L.A.; Bray, F.; Siegel, R.L.; Ferlay, J.; Lortet-Tieulent, J.; Jemal, A. Global cancer statistics, 2012. *CA Cancer J. Clin.* **2015**, *65*, 87–108. [CrossRef] [PubMed]

2. De Winter, R.J.A.; Janssen, P.J.; Sleddens, H.M.; Verleun-Mooijman, M.C.; Trapman, J.; Brinkmann, A.O.; Santerse, A.B.; Schroder, F.H.; van der Kwast, T.H. Androgen receptor status in localized and locally progressive hormone refractory human prostate cancer. *Am. J. Pathol.* **1994**, *144*, 735–746.

3. Chodak, G.W.; Kranc, D.M.; Puy, L.A.; Takeda, H.; Johnson, K.; Chang, C. Nuclear localization of androgen receptor in heterogeneous samples of normal, hyperplastic and neoplastic human prostate. *J. Urol.* **1992**, *147,* 798–803. [PubMed]

4.   Sadi, M.V.; Walsh, P.C.; Barrack, E.R. Immunohistochemical study of androgen receptors in metastatic prostate cancer. Comparison of receptor content and response to hormonal therapy. *Cancer* **1991**, *67*, 3057–3064. [CrossRef]

5.   Hammerer, P.; Madersbacher, S. Landmarks in hormonal therapy for prostate cancer. *BJU Int.* **2012**, *110* (Suppl. 1), 23–29. [CrossRef] [PubMed]

6.   Scher, H.I.; Beer, T.M.; Higano, C.S.; Anand, A.; Taplin, M.E.; Efstathiou, E.; Rathkopf, D.; Shelkey, J.; Yu, E.Y.; Alumkal, J.; et al. Antitumour activity of MDV3100 in castration-resistant prostate cancer: A phase 1–2 study. *Lancet* **2010**, *375*, 1437–1446. [CrossRef]

7.   Albertsen, P.C.; Hanley, J.A.; Fine, J. 20-year outcomes following conservative management of clinically localized prostate cancer. *JAMA* **2005**, *293*, 2095–2101. [CrossRef] [PubMed]

8.   Merseburger, A.S.; Haas, G.P.; von Klot, C.A. An update on enzalutamide in the treatment of prostate cancer. *Ther. Adv. Urol.* **2015**, *7*, 9–21. [CrossRef] [PubMed]

9.   Pienta, K.J.; Bradley, D. Mechanisms underlying the development of androgen-independent prostate cancer. *Clin. Cancer Res.* **2006**, *12*, 1665–1671. [CrossRef] [PubMed]

10.   Sharma, N.L.; Massie, C.E.; Ramos-Montoya, A.; Zecchini, V.; Scott, H.E.; Lamb, A.D.; MacArthur, S.; Stark, R.; Warren, A.Y.; Mills, I.G.; et al. The androgen receptor induces a distinct transcriptional program in castration-resistant prostate cancer in man. *Cancer Cell* **2013**, *23*, 35–47. [CrossRef] [PubMed]

11.   Wang, Q.; Li, W.; Zhang, Y.; Yuan, X.; Xu, K.; Yu, J.; Chen, Z.; Beroukhim, R.; Wang, H.; Lupien, M.; et al. Androgen receptor regulates a distinct transcription program in androgen-independent prostate cancer. *Cell* **2009**, *138*, 245–256. [CrossRef] [PubMed]

12.   Barfeld, S.J.; Itkonen, H.M.; Urbanucci, A.; Mills, I.G. Androgen-regulated metabolism and biosynthesis in prostate cancer. *Endocr. Relat. Cancer* **2014**, *21*, T57–T66. [CrossRef] [PubMed]

13.   Massie, C.E.; Lynch, A.; Ramos-Montoya, A.; Boren, J.; Stark, R.; Fazli, L.; Warren, A.; Scott, H.; Madhu, B.; Sharma, N.; et al. The androgen receptor fuels prostate cancer by regulating central metabolism and biosynthesis. *EMBO J.* **2011**, *30*, 2719–2733. [CrossRef] [PubMed]

14.   Shafi, A.A.; Putluri, V.; Arnold, J.M.; Tsouko, E.; Maity, S.; Roberts, J.M.; Coarfa, C.; Frigo, D.E.; Putluri, N.; Sreekumar, A.; et al. Differential regulation of metabolic pathways by androgen receptor (AR) and its constitutively active splice variant, AR-V7, in prostate cancer cells. *Oncotarget* **2015**, *6*, 31997–32012. [PubMed]

15.   Locasale, J.W. Serine, glycine and one-carbon units: Cancer metabolism in full circle. *Nat. Rev. Cancer* **2013**, *13*, 572–583. [CrossRef] [PubMed]

16.   Mentch, S.J.; Locasale, J.W. One-carbon metabolism and epigenetics: Understanding the specificity. *Ann. N. Y. Acad. Sci.* **2016**, *1363*, 91–98. [CrossRef] [PubMed]

17.   Tibbetts, A.S.; Appling, D.R. Compartmentalization of mammalian folate-mediated one-carbon metabolism. *Annu. Rev. Nutr.* **2010**, *30*, 57–81. [CrossRef] [PubMed]

18.   Green, T.; Chen, X.; Ryan, S.; Asch, A.S.; Ruiz-Echevarria, M.J. TMEFF2 and SARDH cooperate to modulate one-carbon metabolism and invasion of prostate cancer cells. *Prostate* **2013**, *73*, 1561–1575. [CrossRef] [PubMed]

19.   Khan, A.P.; Rajendiran, T.M.; Ateeq, B.; Asangani, I.A.; Athanikar, J.N.; Yocum, A.K.; Mehra, R.; Siddiqui, J.; Palapattu, G.; Wei, J.T.; et al. The role of sarcosine metabolism in prostate cancer progression. *Neoplasia* **2013**, *15*, 491–501. [CrossRef] [PubMed]

20.   Sreekumar, A.; Poisson, L.M.; Rajendiran, T.M.; Khan, A.P.; Cao, Q.; Yu, J.; Laxman, B.; Mehra, R.; Lonigro, R.J.; Li, Y.; et al. Metabolomic profiles delineate potential role for sarcosine in prostate cancer progression. *Nature* **2009**, *457*, 910–914. [CrossRef] [PubMed]

21.   Ottaviani, S.; Brooke, G.N.; O'Hanlon-Brown, C.; Waxman, J.; Ali, S.; Buluwela, L. Characterisation of the androgen regulation of glycine N-methyltransferase in prostate cancer cells. *J. Mol. Endocrinol.* **2013**, *51*, 301–312. [CrossRef] [PubMed]

22.   Johansson, M.; van Guelpen, B.; Vollset, S.E.; Hultdin, J.; Bergh, A.; Key, T.; Midttun, O.; Hallmans, G.; Ueland, P.M.; Stattin, P. One-carbon metabolism and prostate cancer risk: Prospective investigation of seven circulating B vitamins and metabolites. *Cancer Epidemiol. Biomark. Prev.* **2009**, *18*, 1538–1543. [CrossRef] [PubMed]

23.   Appling, D.R. Compartmentation of folate-mediated one-carbon metabolism in eukaryotes. *FASEB J.* **1991**, *5*, 2645–2651. [PubMed]

24. Fox, J.T.; Stover, P.J. Folate-mediated one-carbon metabolism. *Vitam. Horm.* **2008**, *79*, 1–44. [PubMed]

25. Scotti, M.; Stella, L.; Shearer, E.J.; Stover, P.J. Modeling cellular compartmentation in one-carbon metabolism. *Wiley Interdiscip. Rev. Syst. Biol. Med.* **2013**, *5*, 343–365. [CrossRef] [PubMed]

26. Williams-Ashman, H.G.; Canellakis, Z.N. Polyamines in mammalian biology and medicine. *Perspect. Biol. Med.* **1979**, *22*, 421–453. [CrossRef] [PubMed]

27. Saini, P.; Eyler, D.E.; Green, R.; Dever, T.E. Hypusine-containing protein eIF5A promotes translation elongation. *Nature* **2009**, *459*, 118–121. [CrossRef] [PubMed]

28. Stover, P.J. One-carbon metabolism-genome interactions in folate-associated pathologies. *J. Nutr.* **2009**, *139*, 2402–2405. [CrossRef] [PubMed]

29. Luka, Z. Methyltetrahydrofolate in folate-binding protein glycine *N*-methyltransferase. *Vitam. Horm.* **2008**, *79*, 325–345. [PubMed]

30. Wagner, C.; Briggs, W.T.; Cook, R.J. Inhibition of glycine *N*-methyltransferase activity by folate derivatives: Implications for regulation of methyl group metabolism. *Biochem. Biophys. Res. Commun.* **1985**, *127*, 746–752. [CrossRef]

31. Prudova, A.; Bauman, Z.; Braun, A.; Vitvitsky, V.; Lu, S.C.; Banerjee, R. *S*-adenosylmethionine stabilizes cystathionine β-synthase and modulates redox capacity. *Proc. Natl. Acad. Sci. USA* **2006**, *103*, 6489–6494. [CrossRef] [PubMed]

32. Pey, A.L.; Majtan, T.; Sanchez-Ruiz, J.M.; Kraus, J.P. Human cystathionine β-synthase (CBS) contains two classes of binding sites for *S*-adenosylmethionine (SAM): Complex regulation of CBS activity and stability by SAM. *Biochem. J.* **2013**, *449*, 109–121. [CrossRef] [PubMed]

33. Bjelakovic, G.; Pavlovic, D.; Jevtovic, T.; Stojanovic, I.; Sokolovic, D.; Bjelakovic, G.B.; Nikolic, J.; Basic, J. Vitamin B-12 and folic acid effects on polyamine metabolism in rat liver. *Pteridines* **2006**, *17*, 90–94. [CrossRef]

34. Sun, D.; Wollin, A.; Stephen, A.M. Moderate folate deficiency influences polyamine synthesis in rats. *J. Nutr.* **2002**, *132*, 2632–2637. [PubMed]

35. Ott, M.; Gogvadze, V.; Orrenius, S.; Zhivotovsky, B. Mitochondria, oxidative stress and cell death. *Apoptosis* **2007**, *12*, 913–922. [CrossRef] [PubMed]

36. Ozben, T. Oxidative stress and apoptosis: Impact on cancer therapy. *J. Pharm. Sci.* **2007**, *96*, 2181–2196. [CrossRef] [PubMed]

37. Gerner, E.W.; Meyskens, F.L. Polyamines and cancer: Old molecules, new understanding. *Nat. Rev. Cancer* **2004**, *4*, 781–792. [CrossRef] [PubMed]

38. Heby, O. Role of polyamines in the control of cell proliferation and differentiation. *Differentiation* **1981**, *19*, 1–20. [CrossRef] [PubMed]

39. Zhang, W.C.; Shyh-Chang, N.; Yang, H.; Rai, A.; Umashankar, S.; Ma, S.; Soh, B.S.; Sun, L.L.; Tai, B.C.; Nga, M.E.; et al. Glycine decarboxylase activity drives non-small cell lung cancer tumor-initiating cells and tumorigenesis. *Cell* **2012**, *148*, 259–272. [CrossRef] [PubMed]

40. Rahman, L.; Voeller, D.; Rahman, M.; Lipkowitz, S.; Allegra, C.; Barrett, J.C.; Kaye, F.J.; Zajac-Kaye, M. Thymidylate synthase as an oncogene: A novel role for an essential DNA synthesis enzyme. *Cancer Cell* **2004**, *5*, 341–351. [CrossRef]

41. Suzuki, M.; Tsukagoshi, S.; Saga, Y.; Ohwada, M.; Sato, I. Enhanced expression of thymidylate synthase may be of prognostic importance in advanced cervical cancer. *Oncology* **1999**, *57*, 50–54. [CrossRef] [PubMed]

42. Shintani, Y.; Ohta, M.; Hirabayashi, H.; Tanaka, H.; Iuchi, K.; Nakagawa, K.; Maeda, H.; Kido, T.; Miyoshi, S.; Matsuda, H. New prognostic indicator for non-small-cell lung cancer, quantitation of thymidylate synthase by real-time reverse transcription polymerase chain reaction. *Int. J. Cancer* **2003**, *104*, 790–795. [CrossRef] [PubMed]

43. Pestalozzi, B.C.; Peterson, H.F.; Gelber, R.D.; Goldhirsch, A.; Gusterson, B.A.; Trihia, H.; Lindtner, J.; Cortes-Funes, H.; Simmoncini, E.; Byrne, M.J.; et al. Prognostic importance of thymidylate synthase expression in early breast cancer. *J. Clin. Oncol.* **1997**, *15*, 1923–1931. [PubMed]

44. Nomura, T.; Nakagawa, M.; Fujita, Y.; Hanada, T.; Mimata, H.; Nomura, Y. Clinical significance of thymidylate synthase expression in bladder cancer. *Int. J. Urol.* **2002**, *9*, 368–376. [CrossRef] [PubMed]

45. Mizutani, Y.; Wada, H.; Yoshida, O.; Fukushima, M.; Nonomura, M.; Nakao, M.; Miki, T. Significance of thymidylate synthase activity in renal cell carcinoma. *Clin. Cancer Res.* **2003**, *9*, 1453–1460. [PubMed]

46. Karlberg, M.; Ohrling, K.; Edler, D.; Hallstrom, M.; Ullen, H.; Ragnhammar, P. Prognostic and predictive value of thymidylate synthase expression in primary colorectal cancer. *Anticancer Res.* **2010**, *30*, 645–651. [PubMed]

47. Longley, D.B.; Harkin, D.P.; Johnston, P.G. 5-Fluorouracil: Mechanisms of action and clinical strategies. *Nat. Rev. Cancer* **2003**, *3*, 330–338. [CrossRef] [PubMed]

48. Zhang, D.; Wen, X.; Wu, W.; Guo, Y.; Cui, W. Elevated homocysteine level and folate deficiency associated with increased overall risk of carcinogenesis: Meta-analysis of 83 case-control studies involving 35,758 individuals. *PLoS ONE* **2015**, *10*, e0123423. [CrossRef] [PubMed]

49. Chen, J.; Gammon, M.D.; Chan, W.; Palomeque, C.; Wetmur, J.G.; Kabat, G.C.; Teitelbaum, S.L.; Britton, J.A.; Terry, M.B.; Neugut, A.I.; et al. One-carbon metabolism, MTHFR polymorphisms, and risk of breast cancer. *Cancer Res.* **2005**, *65*, 1606–1614. [CrossRef] [PubMed]

50. Giovannucci, E. Epidemiologic studies of folate and colorectal neoplasia: A review. *J. Nutr.* **2002**, *132*, 2350S–2355S. [PubMed]

51. Chen, P.; Li, C.; Li, X.; Li, J.; Chu, R.; Wang, H. Higher dietary folate intake reduces the breast cancer risk: A systematic review and meta-analysis. *Br. J. Cancer* **2014**, *110*, 2327–2338. [CrossRef] [PubMed]

52. Kim, Y.I.; Pogribny, I.P.; Basnakian, A.G.; Miller, J.W.; Selhub, J.; James, S.J.; Mason, J.B. Folate deficiency in rats induces DNA strand breaks and hypomethylation within the p53 tumor suppressor gene. *Am. J. Clin. Nutr.* **1997**, *65*, 46–52. [PubMed]

53. Blount, B.C.; Mack, M.M.; Wehr, C.M.; MacGregor, J.T.; Hiatt, R.A.; Wang, G.; Wickramasinghe, S.N.; Everson, R.B.; Ames, B.N. Folate deficiency causes uracil misincorporation into human DNA and chromosome breakage: Implications for cancer and neuronal damage. *Proc. Natl. Acad. Sci. USA* **1997**, *94*, 3290–3295. [CrossRef] [PubMed]

54. Ergul, E.; Sazci, A.; Utkan, Z.; Canturk, N.Z. Polymorphisms in the *MTHFR* gene are associated with breast cancer. *Tumour Biol. J. Int. Soc. Oncodev. Biol. Med.* **2003**, *24*, 286–290. [CrossRef]

55. Kumar, P.; Yadav, U.; Rai, V. Methylenetetrahydrofolate reductase gene c677t polymorphism and breast cancer risk: Evidence for genetic susceptibility. *Meta Gene* **2015**, *6*, 72–84. [CrossRef] [PubMed]

56. Lu, Q.; Jiang, K.; Li, Q.; Ji, Y.J.; Chen, W.L.; Xue, X.H. Polymorphisms in the *MTHFR* gene are associated with breast cancer risk and prognosis in a chinese population. *Tumour Biol. J. Int. Soc. Oncodev. Biol. Med.* **2015**, *36*, 3757–3762. [CrossRef] [PubMed]

57. Maruti, S.S.; Ulrich, C.M.; Jupe, E.R.; White, E. MTHFR C677T and postmenopausal breast cancer risk by intakes of one-carbon metabolism nutrients: A nested case-control study. *Breast Cancer Res.* **2009**, *11*, R91. [CrossRef] [PubMed]

58. Wang, Y.; Yang, H.; Duan, G. Mthfr gene a1298c polymorphisms are associated with breast cancer risk among chinese population: Evidence based on an updated cumulative meta-analysis. *Int. J. Clin. Exp. Med.* **2015**, *8*, 20146–20156. [PubMed]

59. Frosst, P.; Blom, H.J.; Milos, R.; Goyette, P.; Sheppard, C.A.; Matthews, R.G.; Boers, G.J.; den Heijer, M.; Kluijtmans, L.A.; van den Heuvel, L.P.; et al. A candidate genetic risk factor for vascular disease: A common mutation in methylenetetrahydrofolate reductase. *Nat. Genet.* **1995**, *10*, 111–113. [CrossRef] [PubMed]

60. Bester, A.C.; Roniger, M.; Oren, Y.S.; Im, M.M.; Sarni, D.; Chaoat, M.; Bensimon, A.; Zamir, G.; Shewach, D.S.; Kerem, B. Nucleotide deficiency promotes genomic instability in early stages of cancer development. *Cell* **2011**, *145*, 435–446. [CrossRef] [PubMed]

61. Ehrlich, M. DNA hypomethylation in cancer cells. *Epigenomics* **2009**, *1*, 239–259. [CrossRef] [PubMed]

62. Poirier, L.A. Methyl group deficiency in hepatocarcinogenesis. *Drug Metab. Rev.* **1994**, *26*, 185–199. [CrossRef] [PubMed]

63. Bistulfi, G.; Foster, B.A.; Karasik, E.; Gillard, B.; Miecznikowski, J.; Dhiman, V.K.; Smiraglia, D.J. Dietary folate deficiency blocks prostate cancer progression in the tramp model. *Cancer Prev. Res.* **2011**, *4*, 1825–1834. [CrossRef] [PubMed]

64. Bistulfi, G.; Vandette, E.; Matsui, S.; Smiraglia, D.J. Mild folate deficiency induces genetic and epigenetic instability and phenotype changes in prostate cancer cells. *BMC Biol.* **2010**, *8*, 6. [CrossRef] [PubMed]

65. Deghan Manshadi, S.; Ishiguro, L.; Sohn, K.J.; Medline, A.; Renlund, R.; Croxford, R.; Kim, Y.I. Folic acid supplementation promotes mammary tumor progression in a rat model. *PLoS ONE* **2014**, *9*, e84635.

66. Lindzon, G.M.; Medline, A.; Sohn, K.J.; Depeint, F.; Croxford, R.; Kim, Y.I. Effect of folic acid supplementation on the progression of colorectal aberrant crypt foci. *Carcinogenesis* **2009**, *30*, 1536–1543. [CrossRef] [PubMed]

67. Song, J.; Medline, A.; Mason, J.B.; Gallinger, S.; Kim, Y.I. Effects of dietary folate on intestinal tumorigenesis in the apcmin mouse. *Cancer Res.* **2000**, *60*, 5434–5440. [CrossRef]

68. Kim, Y.I. Folate: A magic bullet or a double edged sword for colorectal cancer prevention? *Gut* **2006**, *55*, 1387–1389. [CrossRef] [PubMed]

69. Ulrich, C.M.; Potter, J.D. Folate and cancer—Timing is everything. *JAMA* **2007**, *297*, 2408–2409. [CrossRef] [PubMed]

70. Greger, V.; Passarge, E.; Hopping, W.; Messmer, E.; Horsthemke, B. Epigenetic changes may contribute to the formation and spontaneous regression of retinoblastoma. *Hum. Genet.* **1989**, *83*, 155–158. [CrossRef] [PubMed]

71. Yoo, C.B.; Jones, P.A. Epigenetic therapy of cancer: Past, present and future. *Nat. Rev. Drug Discov.* **2006**, *5*, 37–50. [CrossRef] [PubMed]

72. Ellinger, J.; Kahl, P.; von der Gathen, J.; Heukamp, L.C.; Gütgemann, I.; Walter, B.; Hofstädter, F.; Bastian, P.J.; von Ruecker, A.; Müller, S.C.; et al. Global histone H3K27 methylation levels are different in localized and metastatic prostate cancer. *Cancer Investig.* **2012**, *30*, 92–97. [CrossRef] [PubMed]

73. Barlesi, F.; Giaccone, G.; Gallegos-Ruiz, M.I.; Loundou, A.; Span, S.W.; Lefesvre, P.; Kruyt, F.A.; Rodriguez, J.A. Global histone modifications predict prognosis of resected non small-cell lung cancer. *J. Clin. Oncol.* **2007**, *25*, 4358–4364. [CrossRef] [PubMed]

74. Bianco-Miotto, T.; Chiam, K.; Buchanan, G.; Jindal, S.; Day, T.K.; Thomas, M.; Pickering, M.A.; O'Loughlin, M.A.; Ryan, N.K.; Raymond, W.A.; et al. Global levels of specific histone modifications and an epigenetic gene signature predict prostate cancer progression and development. *Cancer Epidemiol. Biomark. Prev.* **2010**, *19*, 2611–2622. [CrossRef] [PubMed]

75. Ellinger, J.; Kahl, P.; von der Gathen, J.; Rogenhofer, S.; Heukamp, L.C.; Gutgemann, I.; Walter, B.; Hofstadter, F.; Buttner, R.; Muller, S.C.; et al. Global levels of histone modifications predict prostate cancer recurrence. *Prostate* **2010**, *70*, 61–69. [CrossRef] [PubMed]

76. Seligson, D.B.; Horvath, S.; McBrian, M.A.; Mah, V.; Yu, H.; Tze, S.; Wang, Q.; Chia, D.; Goodglick, L.; Kurdistani, S.K. Global levels of histone modifications predict prognosis in different cancers. *Am. J. Pathol.* **2009**, *174*, 1619–1628. [CrossRef] [PubMed]

77. Fraga, M.F.; Ballestar, E.; Villar-Garea, A.; Boix-Chornet, M.; Espada, J.; Schotta, G.; Bonaldi, T.; Haydon, C.; Ropero, S.; Petrie, K.; et al. Loss of acetylation at LYS16 and trimethylation at LYS20 of histone H4 is a common hallmark of human cancer. *Nat. Genet.* **2005**, *37*, 391–400. [CrossRef] [PubMed]

78. Bachmann, I.M.; Halvorsen, O.J.; Collett, K.; Stefansson, I.M.; Straume, O.; Haukaas, S.A.; Salvesen, H.B.; Otte, A.P.; Akslen, L.A. EZH2 expression is associated with high proliferation rate and aggressive tumor subgroups in cutaneous melanoma and cancers of the endometrium, prostate, and breast. *J. Clin. Oncol.* **2006**, *24*, 268–273. [CrossRef] [PubMed]

79. Simon, J.A.; Lange, C.A. Roles of the EZH2 histone methyltransferase in cancer epigenetics. *Mutat. Res.* **2008**, *647*, 21–29. [CrossRef] [PubMed]

80. Van Leenders, G.J.L.H.; Dukers, D.; Hessels, D.; van den Kieboom, S.W.M.; Hulsbergen, C.A.; Witjes, J.A.; Otte, A.P.; Meijer, C.J.; Raaphorst, F.M. Polycomb-group oncogenes EZH2, BMI1, and RING1 are overexpressed in prostate cancer with adverse pathologic and clinical features. *Eur. Urol.* **2007**, *52*, 455–463. [CrossRef] [PubMed]

81. Hyland, P.L.; McDade, S.S.; McCloskey, R.; Dickson, G.J.; Arthur, K.; McCance, D.J.; Patel, D. Evidence for alteration of EZH2, BMI1, and KDM6A and epigenetic reprogramming in human papillomavirus type 16 E6/E7-expressing keratinocytes. *J. Virol.* **2011**, *85*, 10999–11006. [CrossRef] [PubMed]

82. Lee, J.Y.; Kong, G. Dot1l: A new therapeutic target for aggressive breast cancer. *Oncotarget* **2015**, *6*, 30451–30452. [PubMed]

83. Wong, M.; Polly, P.; Liu, T. The histone methyltransferase DOT1L: Regulatory functions and a cancer therapy target. *Am. J. Cancer Res.* **2015**, *5*, 2823–2837. [PubMed]

84. Dou, Y.; Hess, J.L. Mechanisms of transcriptional regulation by MLL and its disruption in acute leukemia. *Int. J. Hematol.* **2008**, *87*, 10–18. [CrossRef] [PubMed]

85. Krivtsov, A.V.; Armstrong, S.A. MLL translocations, histone modifications and leukaemia stem-cell development. *Nat. Rev. Cancer* **2007**, *7*, 823–833. [CrossRef] [PubMed]

86.   Orzan, F.; Pellegatta, S.; Poliani, P.L.; Pisati, F.; Caldera, V.; Menghi, F.; Kapetis, D.; Marras, C.; Schiffer, D.; Finocchiaro, G. Enhancer of zeste 2 (EZH2) is up-regulated in malignant gliomas and in glioma stem-like cells. *Neuropathol. Appl. Neurobiol.* **2011**, *37*, 381–394. [CrossRef] [PubMed]

87.   Kerr, S.J. Competing methyltransferase systems. *J. Biol. Chem.* **1972**, *247*, 4248–4252. [PubMed]

88.   Shyh-Chang, N.; Locasale, J.W.; Lyssiotis, C.A.; Zheng, Y.; Teo, R.Y.; Ratanasirintrawoot, S.; Zhang, J.; Onder, T.; Unternaehrer, J.J.; Zhu, H.; et al. Influence of threonine metabolism on *S*-adenosylmethionine and histone methylation. *Science* **2013**, *339*, 222–226. [CrossRef] [PubMed]

89.   Huang, W.Y.; Yang, P.M.; Chang, Y.F.; Marquez, V.E.; Chen, C.C. Methotrexate induces apoptosis through p53/p21-dependent pathway and increases e-cadherin expression through downregulation of HDAC/EZH2. *Biochem. Pharmacol.* **2011**, *81*, 510–517. [CrossRef] [PubMed]

90.   Mandal, S.; Mandal, A.; Johansson, H.E.; Orjalo, A.V.; Park, M.H. Depletion of cellular polyamines, spermidine and spermine, causes a total arrest in translation and growth in mammalian cells. *Proc. Natl. Acad. Sci. USA* **2013**, *110*, 2169–2174. [CrossRef] [PubMed]

91.   O'Brien, T.G.; Megosh, L.C.; Gilliard, G.; Soler, A.P. Ornithine decarboxylase overexpression is a sufficient condition for tumor promotion in mouse skin. *Cancer Res.* **1997**, *57*, 2630–2637. [PubMed]

92.   Nilsson, J.A.; Keller, U.B.; Baudino, T.A.; Yang, C.; Norton, S.; Old, J.A.; Nilsson, L.M.; Neale, G.; Kramer, D.L.; Porter, C.W.; et al. Targeting ornithine decarboxylase in MYC-induced lymphomagenesis prevents tumor formation. *Cancer Cell* **2005**, *7*, 433–444. [CrossRef] [PubMed]

93.   Lee, O.J.; Schneider-Stock, R.; McChesney, P.A.; Kuester, D.; Roessner, A.; Vieth, M.; Moskaluk, C.A.; El-Rifai, W. Hypermethylation and loss of expression of glutathione peroxidase-3 in barrett's tumorigenesis. *Neoplasia* **2005**, *7*, 854–861. [CrossRef] [PubMed]

94.   Zhang, X.; Yang, J.J.; Kim, Y.S.; Kim, K.Y.; Ahn, W.S.; Yang, S. An 8-gene signature, including methylated and down-regulated glutathione peroxidase 3, of gastric cancer. *Int. J. Oncol.* **2010**, *36*, 405–414. [PubMed]

95.   Yu, Y.P.; Yu, G.; Tseng, G.; Cieply, K.; Nelson, J.; Defrances, M.; Zarnegar, R.; Michalopoulos, G.; Luo, J.H. Glutathione peroxidase 3, deleted or methylated in prostate cancer, suppresses prostate cancer growth and metastasis. *Cancer Res.* **2007**, *67*, 8043–8050. [CrossRef] [PubMed]

96.   Peng, D.F.; Razvi, M.; Chen, H.; Washington, K.; Roessner, A.; Schneider-Stock, R.; El-Rifai, W. DNA hypermethylation regulates the expression of members of the Mu-class glutathione *S*-transferases and glutathione peroxidases in barrett's adenocarcinoma. *Gut* **2009**, *58*, 5–15. [CrossRef] [PubMed]

97.   Jhaveri, M.S.; Morrow, C.S. Methylation-mediated regulation of the glutathione *S*-transferase p1 gene in human breast cancer cells. *Gene* **1998**, *210*, 1–7. [CrossRef]

98.   Lee, W.H.; Morton, R.A.; Epstein, J.I.; Brooks, J.D.; Campbell, P.A.; Bova, G.S.; Hsieh, W.S.; Isaacs, W.B.; Nelson, W.G. Cytidine methylation of regulatory sequences near the Pi-class glutathione *S*-transferase gene accompanies human prostatic carcinogenesis. *Proc. Natl. Acad. Sci. USA* **1994**, *91*, 11733–11737. [CrossRef] [PubMed]

99.   Townsend, D.M.; Tew, K.D. The role of glutathione-*S*-transferase in anti-cancer drug resistance. *Oncogene* **2003**, *22*, 7369–7375. [CrossRef] [PubMed]

100. Godwin, A.K.; Meister, A.; O'Dwyer, P.J.; Huang, C.S.; Hamilton, T.C.; Anderson, M.E. High resistance to cisplatin in human ovarian cancer cell lines is associated with marked increase of glutathione synthesis. *Proc. Natl. Acad. Sci. USA* **1992**, *89*, 3070–3074. [CrossRef] [PubMed]

101. Kramer, R.A.; Zakher, J.; Kim, G. Role of the glutathione redox cycle in acquired and de novo multidrug resistance. *Science* **1988**, *241*, 694–697. [CrossRef] [PubMed]

102. Chen, N.; Liu, Y.; Greiner, C.D.; Holtzman, J.L. Physiologic concentrations of homocysteine inhibit the human plasma gsh peroxidase that reduces organic hydroperoxides. *J. Lab. Clin. Med.* **2000**, *136*, 58–65. [CrossRef] [PubMed]

103. Durmaz, A.; Dikmen, N. Homocysteine effects on cellular glutathione peroxidase (GPX-1) activity under in vitro conditions. *J. Enzym. Inhib. Med. Chem.* **2007**, *22*, 733–738. [CrossRef] [PubMed]

104. Handy, D.E.; Zhang, Y.; Loscalzo, J. Homocysteine down-regulates cellular glutathione peroxidase (GPX1) by decreasing translation. *J. Biol. Chem.* **2005**, *280*, 15518–15525. [CrossRef] [PubMed]

105. Tastekin, D.; Erturk, K.; Bozbey, H.U.; Olmuscelik, O.; Kiziltan, H.; Tuna, S.; Tas, F. Plasma homocysteine, folate and vitamin B12 levels in patients with lung cancer. *Exp. Oncol.* **2015**, *37*, 218–222. [PubMed]

106. Lubos, E.; Loscalzo, J.; Handy, D.E. Homocysteine and glutathione peroxidase-1. *Antioxid. Redox Signal.* **2007**, *9*, 1923–1940. [CrossRef] [PubMed]

107. Lin, J.; Lee, I.M.; Song, Y.; Cook, N.R.; Selhub, J.; Manson, J.E.; Buring, J.E.; Zhang, S.M. Plasma homocysteine and cysteine and risk of breast cancer in women. *Cancer Res.* **2010**, *70*, 2397–2405. [CrossRef] [PubMed]

108. Matsumoto, T.; Sakari, M.; Okada, M.; Yokoyama, A.; Takahashi, S.; Kouzmenko, A.; Kato, S. The androgen receptor in health and disease. *Annu. Rev. Physiol.* **2013**, *75*, 201–224. [CrossRef] [PubMed]

109. Tsouko, E.; Khan, A.S.; White, M.A.; Han, J.J.; Shi, Y.; Merchant, F.A.; Sharpe, M.A.; Xin, L.; Frigo, D.E. Regulation of the pentose phosphate pathway by an androgen receptor-mtor-mediated mechanism and its role in prostate cancer cell growth. *Oncogenesis* **2014**, *3*, e103. [CrossRef] [PubMed]

110. Tennakoon, J.B.; Shi, Y.; Han, J.J.; Tsouko, E.; White, M.A.; Burns, A.R.; Zhang, A.; Xia, X.; Ilkayeva, O.R.; Xin, L.; et al. Androgens regulate prostate cancer cell growth via an AMPK-PGC-1α-mediated metabolic switch. *Oncogene* **2014**, *33*, 5251–5261. [CrossRef] [PubMed]

111. Luka, Z.; Mudd, S.H.; Wagner, C. Glycine N-methyltransferase and regulation of S-adenosylmethionine levels. *J. Biol. Chem.* **2009**, *284*, 22507–22511. [CrossRef] [PubMed]

112. Huang, Y.C.; Lee, C.M.; Chen, M.; Chung, M.Y.; Chang, Y.H.; Huang, W.J.; Ho, D.M.; Pan, C.C.; Wu, T.T.; Yang, S.; et al. Haplotypes, loss of heterozygosity, and expression levels of glycine N-methyltransferase in prostate cancer. *Clin. Cancer Res.* **2007**, *13*, 1412–1420. [CrossRef] [PubMed]

113. Song, Y.H.; Shiota, M.; Kuroiwa, K.; Naito, S.; Oda, Y. The important role of glycine N-methyltransferase in the carcinogenesis and progression of prostate cancer. *Mod. Pathol.* **2011**, *24*, 1272–1280. [CrossRef] [PubMed]

114. Putluri, N.; Shojaie, A.; Vasu, V.T.; Nalluri, S.; Vareed, S.K.; Putluri, V.; Vivekanandan-Giri, A.; Byun, J.; Pennathur, S.; Sana, T.R.; et al. Metabolomic profiling reveals a role for androgen in activating amino acid metabolism and methylation in prostate cancer cells. *PLoS ONE* **2011**, *6*, e21417. [CrossRef] [PubMed]

115. Yoon, J.K.; Kim, D.H.; Koo, J.S. Implications of differences in expression of sarcosine metabolism-related proteins according to the molecular subtype of breast cancer. *J. Transl. Med.* **2014**, *12*, 1–11. [CrossRef] [PubMed]

116. Ulanovskaya, O.A.; Zuhl, A.M.; Cravatt, B.F. NNMT promotes epigenetic remodeling in cancer by creating a metabolic methylation sink. *Nat. Chem. Biol.* **2013**, *9*, 300–306. [CrossRef] [PubMed]

117. Zhang, J.; Wang, Y.; Li, G.; Yu, H.; Xie, X. Down-regulation of nicotinamide N-methyltransferase induces apoptosis in human breast cancer cells via the mitochondria-mediated pathway. *PLoS ONE* **2014**, *9*, e89202. [CrossRef] [PubMed]

118. Chen, X.; Overcash, R.; Green, T.; Hoffman, D.; Asch, A.S.; Ruiz-Echevarria, M.J. The tumor suppressor activity of the transmembrane protein with epidermal growth factor and two follistatin motifs 2 (TMEFF2) correlates with its ability to modulate sarcosine levels. *J. Biol. Chem.* **2011**, *286*, 16091–16100. [CrossRef] [PubMed]

119. Corbin, J.M.; Overcash, R.F.; Wren, J.D.; Coburn, A.; Tipton, G.J.; Ezzell, J.A.; McNaughton, K.K.; Fung, K.M.; Kosanke, S.D.; Ruiz-Echevarria, M.J. Analysis of TMEFF2 allografts and transgenic mouse models reveals roles in prostate regeneration and cancer. *Prostate* **2016**, *76*, 97–113. [CrossRef] [PubMed]

120. Reed, M.C.; Thomas, R.L.; Pavisic, J.; James, S.J.; Ulrich, C.M.; Nijhout, H.F. A mathematical model of glutathione metabolism. *Theor. Biol. Med. Model.* **2008**, *5*, 1–16. [CrossRef] [PubMed]

121. Li, J.J.; Li, Q.; Du, H.P.; Wang, Y.L.; You, S.J.; Wang, F.; Xu, X.S.; Cheng, J.; Cao, Y.J.; Liu, C.F.; et al. Homocysteine triggers inflammatory responses in macrophages through inhibiting CSE-H2s signaling via DNA hypermethylation of CSE promoter. *Int. J. Mol. Sci.* **2015**, *16*, 12560–12577. [CrossRef] [PubMed]

122. Kabil, O.; Banerjee, R. Enzymology of h2s biogenesis, decay and signaling. *Antioxid. Redox Signal.* **2014**, *20*, 770–782. [CrossRef] [PubMed]

123. Kajimura, M.; Fukuda, R.; Bateman, R.M.; Yamamoto, T.; Suematsu, M. Interactions of multiple gas-transducing systems: Hallmarks and uncertainties of Co, No, and H_2S gas biology. *Antioxid. Redox Signal.* **2010**, *13*, 157–192. [CrossRef] [PubMed]

124. Mustafa, A.K.; Gadalla, M.M.; Snyder, S.H. Signaling by gasotransmitters. *Sci. Signal.* **2009**, *2*, re2. [CrossRef] [PubMed]

125. Zhao, K.; Li, S.; Wu, L.; Lai, C.; Yang, G. Hydrogen sulfide represses androgen receptor transactivation by targeting at the second zinc finger module. *J. Biol. Chem.* **2014**, *289*, 20824–20835. [CrossRef] [PubMed]

126. Schalinske, K.L.; Smazal, A.L. Homocysteine imbalance: A pathological metabolic marker. *Adv. Nutr.* **2012**, *3*, 755–762. [CrossRef] [PubMed]

127. Bhattacharyya, S.; Saha, S.; Giri, K.; Lanza, I.R.; Nair, K.S.; Jennings, N.B.; Rodriguez-Aguayo, C.; Lopez-Berestein, G.; Basal, E.; Weaver, A.L. Cystathionine β-synthase (CBS) contributes to advanced ovarian cancer progression and drug resistance. *PLoS ONE* **2013**, *8*, e79167. [CrossRef] [PubMed]

128. Szabo, C.; Coletta, C.; Chao, C.; Módis, K.; Szczesny, B.; Papapetropoulos, A.; Hellmich, M.R. Tumor-derived hydrogen sulfide, produced by cystathionine-β-synthase, stimulates bioenergetics, cell proliferation, and angiogenesis in colon cancer. *Proc. Natl. Acad. Sci. USA* **2013**, *110*, 12474–12479. [CrossRef] [PubMed]

129. Janošík, M.; Kery, V.; Gaustadnes, M.; Maclean, K.N.; Kraus, J.P. Regulation of human cystathionine β-synthase by S-adenosyl-L-methionine: Evidence for two catalytically active conformations involving an autoinhibitory domain in the C-terminal region. *Biochemistry* **2001**, *40*, 10625–10633. [CrossRef] [PubMed]

130. Prudova, A.; Albin, M.; Bauman, Z.; Lin, A.; Vitvitsky, V.; Banerjee, R. Testosterone regulation of homocysteine metabolism modulates redox status in human prostate cancer cells. *Antioxid. Redox Signal.* **2007**, *9*, 1875–1881. [CrossRef] [PubMed]

131. Guo, H.; Gai, J.-W.; Wang, Y.; Jin, H.-F.; Du, J.-B.; Jin, J. Characterization of hydrogen sulfide and its synthases, cystathionine β-synthase and cystathionine γ-lyase, in human prostatic tissue and cells. *Urology* **2012**, *79*, 483.e481–483.e485. [CrossRef] [PubMed]

132. Zhang, W.; Braun, A.; Bauman, Z.; Olteanu, H.; Madzelan, P.; Banerjee, R. Expression profiling of homocysteine junction enzymes in the nci60 panel of human cancer cell lines. *Cancer Res.* **2005**, *65*, 1554–1560. [CrossRef] [PubMed]

133. Al-Awadi, F.; Yang, M.; Tan, Y.; Han, Q.; Li, S.; Hoffman, R.M. Human tumor growth in nude mice is associated with decreased plasma cysteine and homocysteine. *Anticancer Res.* **2008**, *28*, 2541–2544. [PubMed]

134. Stabler, S.; Koyama, T.; Zhao, Z.; Martinez-Ferrer, M.; Allen, R.H.; Luka, Z.; Loukachevitch, L.V.; Clark, P.E.; Wagner, C.; Bhowmick, N.A. Serum methionine metabolites are risk factors for metastatic prostate cancer progression. *PLoS ONE* **2011**, *6*, e22486. [CrossRef] [PubMed]

135. Chwatko, G.; Forma, E.; Wilkosz, J.; Głowacki, R.; Jóźwiak, P.; Różański, W.; Bryś, M.; Krześlak, A. Thiosulfate in urine as a facilitator in the diagnosis of prostate cancer for patients with prostate-specific antigen less or equal 10 ng/mL. *Clin. Chem. Lab. Med.* **2013**, *51*, 1825–1831. [CrossRef] [PubMed]

136. Hatayama, I.; Satoh, K.; Sato, K. Developmental and hormonal regulation of the major form of hepatic glutathione s-transferase in male mice. *Biochem. Biophys. Res. Commun.* **1986**, *140*, 581–588. [CrossRef]

137. Ikeda, H.; Serria, M.S.; Kakizaki, I.; Hatayama, I.; Satoh, K.; Tsuchida, S.; Muramatsu, M.; Nishi, S.; Sakai, M. Activation of mouse pi-class glutathione S-transferase gene by Nrf2(Nf-E2-related factor 2) and androgen. *Biochem. J.* **2002**, *364*, 563–570. [CrossRef] [PubMed]

138. Imperlini, E.; Mancini, A.; Spaziani, S.; Martone, D.; Alfieri, A.; Gemei, M.; del Vecchio, L.; Buono, P.; Orru, S. Androgen receptor signaling induced by supraphysiological doses of dihydrotestosterone in human peripheral blood lymphocytes. *Proteomics* **2010**, *10*, 3165–3175. [CrossRef] [PubMed]

139. Khandrika, L.; Kumar, B.; Koul, S.; Maroni, P.; Koul, H.K. Oxidative stress in prostate cancer. *Cancer Lett.* **2009**, *282*, 125–136. [CrossRef] [PubMed]

140. Pendeville, H.; Carpino, N.; Marine, J.C.; Takahashi, Y.; Muller, M.; Martial, J.A.; Cleveland, J.L. The ornithine decarboxylase gene is essential for cell survival during early murine development. *Mol. Cell. Biol.* **2001**, *21*, 6549–6558. [CrossRef] [PubMed]

141. Casero, R.A.; Pegg, A.E. Polyamine catabolism and disease. *Biochem. J.* **2009**, *421*, 323–338. [CrossRef] [PubMed]

142. Nowotarski, S.L.; Woster, P.M.; Casero, R.A., Jr. Polyamines and cancer: Implications for chemotherapy and chemoprevention. *Expert Rev. Mol. Med.* **2013**, *15*, e3. [CrossRef] [PubMed]

143. Casero, R.A.; Marton, L.J. Targeting polyamine metabolism and function in cancer and other hyperproliferative diseases. *Nat. Rev. Drug Discov.* **2007**, *6*, 373–390. [CrossRef] [PubMed]

144. Giardiello, F.M.; Hamilton, S.R.; Hylind, L.M.; Yang, V.W.; Tamez, P.; Casero, R.A., Jr. Ornithine decarboxylase and polyamines in familial adenomatous polyposis. *Cancer Res.* **1997**, *57*, 199–201. [PubMed]

145. Pegg, A.E.; Lockwood, D.H.; Williams-Ashman, H.G. Concentrations of putrescine and polyamines and their enzymic synthesis during androgen-induced prostatic growth. *Biochem. J.* **1970**, *117*, 17–31. [CrossRef] [PubMed]

146. Blackshear, P.J.; Manzella, J.M.; Stumpo, D.J.; Wen, L.; Huang, J.K.; Oyen, O.; Young, W.S., 3rd. High level, cell-specific expression of ornithine decarboxylase transcripts in rat genitourinary tissues. *Mol. Endocrinol.* **1989**, *3*, 68–78. [CrossRef] [PubMed]

147. Pegg, A.E. Polyamine metabolism and its importance in neoplastic growth and a target for chemotherapy. *Cancer Res.* **1988**, *48*, 759–774. [PubMed]

148. Janne, J.; Alhonen, L.; Leinonen, P. Polyamines: From molecular biology to clinical applications. *Ann. Med.* **1991**, *23*, 241–259. [CrossRef] [PubMed]

149. Mohan, R.R.; Challa, A.; Gupta, S.; Bostwick, D.G.; Ahmad, N.; Agarwal, R.; Marengo, S.R.; Amini, S.B.; Paras, F.; MacLennan, G.T.; et al. Overexpression of ornithine decarboxylase in prostate cancer and prostatic fluid in humans. *Clin. Cancer Res.* **1999**, *5*, 143–147. [PubMed]

150. Rhodes, D.R.; Barrette, T.R.; Rubin, M.A.; Ghosh, D.; Chinnaiyan, A.M. Meta-analysis of microarrays: Interstudy validation of gene expression profiles reveals pathway dysregulation in prostate cancer. *Cancer Res.* **2002**, *62*, 4427–4433. [PubMed]

151. Cipolla, B.G.; Havouis, R.; Moulinoux, J.P. Polyamine reduced diet (PRD) nutrition therapy in hormone refractory prostate cancer patients. *Biomed. Pharmacother.* **2010**, *64*, 363–368. [CrossRef] [PubMed]

152. Janne, O.A.; Crozat, A.; Palvimo, J.; Eisenberg, L.M. Androgen-regulation of ornithine decarboxylase and S-adenosylmethionine decarboxylase genes. *J. Steroid Biochem. Mol. Biol.* **1991**, *40*, 307–315. [CrossRef]

153. Fjosne, H.E.; Strand, H.; Sunde, A. Dose-dependent induction of ornithine decarboxylase and S-adenosyl-methionine decarboxylase activity by testosterone in the accessory sex organs of male rats. *Prostate* **1992**, *21*, 239–245. [CrossRef] [PubMed]

154. Cyriac, J.; Haleem, R.; Cai, X.; Wang, Z. Androgen regulation of spermidine synthase expression in the rat prostate. *Prostate* **2002**, *50*, 252–261. [CrossRef] [PubMed]

155. Crozat, A.; Palvimo, J.J.; Julkunen, M.; Janne, O.A. Comparison of androgen regulation of ornithine decarboxylase and S-adenosylmethionine decarboxylase gene expression in rodent kidney and accessory sex organs. *Endocrinology* **1992**, *130*, 1131–1144. [PubMed]

156. Fjosne, H.E.; Strand, H.; Ostensen, M.A.; Sunde, A. Ornithine decarboxylase and S-adenosylmethionine decarboxylase activity in the accessory sex organs of intact, castrated, and androgen-stimulated castrated rats. *Prostate* **1988**, *12*, 309–320. [CrossRef] [PubMed]

157. Bai, G.; Kasper, S.; Matusik, R.J.; Rennie, P.S.; Moshier, J.A.; Krongrad, A. Androgen regulation of the human ornithine decarboxylase promoter in prostate cancer cells. *J. Androl.* **1998**, *19*, 127–135. [PubMed]

158. Cohen, R.J.; Fujiwara, K.; Holland, J.W.; McNeal, J.E. Polyamines in prostatic epithelial cells and adenocarcinoma: The effects of androgen blockade. *Prostate* **2001**, *49*, 278–284. [CrossRef] [PubMed]

159. Lloyd, S.M.; Arnold, J.; Sreekumar, A. Metabolomic profiling of hormone-dependent cancers: A bird's eye view. *Trends Endocrinol. Metab.* **2015**, *26*, 477–485. [CrossRef] [PubMed]

160. Bistulfi, G.; Diegelman, P.; Foster, B.A.; Kramer, D.L.; Porter, C.W.; Smiraglia, D.J. Polyamine biosynthesis impacts cellular folate requirements necessary to maintain S-adenosylmethionine and nucleotide pools. *FASEB J.* **2009**, *23*, 2888–2897. [CrossRef] [PubMed]

161. Yegnasubramanian, S.; Haffner, M.C.; Zhang, Y.; Gurel, B.; Cornish, T.C.; Wu, Z.; Irizarry, R.A.; Morgan, J.; Hicks, J.; DeWeese, T.L.; et al. DNA hypomethylation arises later in prostate cancer progression than CPG island hypermethylation and contributes to metastatic tumor heterogeneity. *Cancer Res.* **2008**, *68*, 8954–8967. [CrossRef] [PubMed]

162. Jerónimo, C.; Bastian, P.J.; Bjartell, A.; Carbone, G.M.; Catto, J.W.F.; Clark, S.J.; Henrique, R.; Nelson, W.G.; Shariat, S.F. Epigenetics in prostate cancer: Biologic and clinical relevance. *Eur. Urol.* **2011**, *60*, 753–766. [CrossRef] [PubMed]

163. Labbe, D.P.; Zadra, G.; Ebot, E.M.; Mucci, L.A.; Kantoff, P.W.; Loda, M.; Brown, M. Role of diet in prostate cancer: The epigenetic link. *Oncogene* **2015**, *34*, 4683–4691. [CrossRef] [PubMed]

164. Seligson, D.B.; Horvath, S.; Shi, T.; Yu, H.; Tze, S.; Grunstein, M.; Kurdistani, S.K. Global histone modification patterns predict risk of prostate cancer recurrence. *Nature* **2005**, *435*, 1262–1266. [CrossRef] [PubMed]

165. Perry, A.S.; Watson, R.W.; Lawler, M.; Hollywood, D. The epigenome as a therapeutic target in prostate cancer. *Nat. Rev. Urol.* **2010**, *7*, 668–680. [CrossRef] [PubMed]

166. Nelson, W.G.; de Marzo, A.M.; Yegnasubramanian, S. Epigenetic alterations in human prostate cancers. *Endocrinology* **2009**, *150*, 3991–4002. [CrossRef] [PubMed]

167. Yegnasubramanian, S.; Kowalski, J.; Gonzalgo, M.L.; Zahurak, M.; Piantadosi, S.; Walsh, P.C.; Bova, G.S.; de Marzo, A.M.; Isaacs, W.B.; Nelson, W.G. Hypermethylation of CPG islands in primary and metastatic human prostate cancer. *Cancer Res.* **2004**, *64*, 1975–1986. [CrossRef] [PubMed]

168. Jeronimo, C.; Henrique, R.; Hoque, M.O.; Mambo, E.; Ribeiro, F.R.; Varzim, G.; Oliveira, J.; Teixeira, M.R.; Lopes, C.; Sidransky, D. A quantitative promoter methylation profile of prostate cancer. *Clin. Cancer Res.* **2004**, *10*, 8472–8478. [CrossRef] [PubMed]

169. Maruyama, R.; Toyooka, S.; Toyooka, K.O.; Virmani, A.K.; Zöchbauer-Müller, S.; Farinas, A.J.; Minna, J.D.; McConnell, J.; Frenkel, E.P.; Gazdar, A.F. Aberrant promoter methylation profile of prostate cancers and its relationship to clinicopathological features. *Clin. Cancer Res.* **2002**, *8*, 514–519. [PubMed]

170. Florl, A.R.; Steinhoff, C.; Müller, M.; Seifert, H.H.; Hader, C.; Engers, R.; Ackermann, R.; Schulz, W.A. Coordinate hypermethylation at specific genes in prostate carcinoma precedes line-1 hypomethylation. *Br. J. Cancer* **2004**, *91*, 985–994. [CrossRef] [PubMed]

171. Padar, A.; Sathyanarayana, U.G.; Suzuki, M.; Maruyama, R.; Hsieh, J.T.; Frenkel, E.P.; Minna, J.D.; Gazdar, A.F. Inactivation of cyclin D2 gene in prostate cancers by aberrant promoter methylation. *Clin. Cancer Res.* **2003**, *9*, 4730–4734. [PubMed]

172. Yamanaka, M.; Watanabe, M.; Yamada, Y.; Takagi, A.; Murata, T.; Takahashi, H.; Suzuki, H.; Ito, H.; Tsukino, H.; Katoh, T.; et al. Altered methylation of multiple genes in carcinogenesis of the prostate. *Int. J. Cancer* **2003**, *106*, 382–387. [CrossRef] [PubMed]

173. Ellinger, J.; Bastian, P.J.; Jurgan, T.; Biermann, K.; Kahl, P.; Heukamp, L.C.; Wernert, N.; Müller, S.C.; von Ruecker, A. Cpg island hypermethylation at multiple gene sites in diagnosis and prognosis of prostate cancer. *Urology* **2008**, *71*, 161–167. [CrossRef] [PubMed]

174. Lodygin, D.; Epanchintsev, A.; Menssen, A.; Diebold, J.; Hermeking, H. Functional epigenomics identifies genes frequently silenced in prostate cancer. *Cancer Res.* **2005**, *65*, 4218–4227. [CrossRef] [PubMed]

175. Perry, A.S.; Foley, R.; Woodson, K.; Lawler, M. The emerging roles of DNA methylation in the clinical management of prostate cancer. *Endocr. Relat. Cancer* **2006**, *13*, 357–377. [CrossRef] [PubMed]

176. Li, L.C. Epigenetics of prostate cancer. *Front. Biosci. J. Virtual Libr.* **2007**, *12*, 3377–3397. [CrossRef]

177. Sasaki, M.; Tanaka, Y.; Perinchery, G.; Dharia, A.; Kotcherguina, I.; Fujimoto, S.; Dahiya, R. Methylation and inactivation of estrogen, progesterone, and androgen receptors in prostate cancer. *J. Natl. Cancer Inst.* **2002**, *94*, 384–390. [CrossRef] [PubMed]

178. Reibenwein, J.; Pils, D.; Horak, P.; Tomicek, B.; Goldner, G.; Worel, N.; Elandt, K.; Krainer, M. Promoter hypermethylation of GSTP1, AR, and 14-3-3σ in serum of prostate cancer patients and its clinical relevance. *Prostate* **2007**, *67*, 427–432. [CrossRef] [PubMed]

179. Chen, M.F.; Chen, W.C.; Chang, Y.J.; Wu, C.F.; Wu, C.T. Role of DNA methyltransferase 1 in hormone-resistant prostate cancer. *J. Mol. Med.* **2010**, *88*, 953–962. [CrossRef] [PubMed]

180. Patra, S.K.; Patra, A.; Zhao, H.; Dahiya, R. DNA methyltransferase and demethylase in human prostate cancer. *Mol. Carcinog.* **2002**, *33*, 163–171. [CrossRef] [PubMed]

181. Zhang, W.; Jiao, H.; Zhang, X.; Zhao, R.; Wang, F.; He, W.; Zong, H.; Fan, Q.; Wang, L. Correlation between the expression of DNMT1, and GSTP1 and APC, and the methylation status of GSTP1 and APC in association with their clinical significance in prostate cancer. *Mol. Med. Rep.* **2015**, *12*, 141–146. [CrossRef] [PubMed]

182. Valdez, C.D.; Kunju, L.; Daignault, S.; Wojno, K.J.; Day, M.L. The e2f1/dnmt1 axis is associated with the development of ar negative castration resistant prostate cancer. *Prostate* **2013**, *73*, 1776–1785. [CrossRef] [PubMed]

183. Zhang, Q.; Chen, L.; Helfand, B.T.; Jang, T.L.; Sharma, V.; Kozlowski, J.; Kuzel, T.M.; Zhu, L.J.; Yang, X.J.; Javonovic, B.; et al. Tgf-beta regulates DNA methyltransferase expression in prostate cancer, correlates with aggressive capabilities, and predicts disease recurrence. *PLoS ONE* **2011**, *6*, e25168.

184. Kinney, S.R.; Moser, M.T.; Pascual, M.; Greally, J.M.; Foster, B.A.; Karpf, A.R. Opposing roles of DNMT1 in early- and late-stage murine prostate cancer. *Mol. Cell. Biol.* **2010**, *30*, 4159–4174. [CrossRef] [PubMed]

185. McCabe, M.T.; Low, J.A.; Daignault, S.; Imperiale, M.J.; Wojno, K.J.; Day, M.L. Inhibition of DNA methyltransferase activity prevents tumorigenesis in a mouse model of prostate cancer. *Cancer Res.* **2006**, *66*, 385–392. [CrossRef] [PubMed]

186. Kobayashi, Y.; Absher, D.M.; Gulzar, Z.G.; Young, S.R.; McKenney, J.K.; Peehl, D.M.; Brooks, J.D.; Myers, R.M.; Sherlock, G. DNA methylation profiling reveals novel biomarkers and important roles for DNA methyltransferases in prostate cancer. *Genome Res.* **2011**, *21*, 1017–1027. [CrossRef] [PubMed]

187. Brothman, A.R.; Swanson, G.; Maxwell, T.M.; Cui, J.; Murphy, K.J.; Herrick, J.; Speights, V.O.; Isaac, J.; Rohr, L.R. Global hypomethylation is common in prostate cancer cells: A quantitative predictor for clinical outcome? *Cancer Gen. Cytogenet.* **2005**, *156*, 31–36. [CrossRef] [PubMed]

188. Fuso, A.; Nicolia, V.; Cavallaro, R.A.; Scarpa, S. DNA methylase and demethylase activities are modulated by one-carbon metabolism in Alzheimer's disease models. *J. Nut. Biochem.* **2011**, *22*, 242–251. [CrossRef] [PubMed]

189. Rhodes, D.R.; Sanda, M.G.; Otte, A.P.; Chinnaiyan, A.M.; Rubin, M.A. Multiplex biomarker approach for determining risk of prostate-specific antigen-defined recurrence of prostate cancer. *J. Natl. Cancer Inst.* **2003**, *95*, 661–668. [CrossRef] [PubMed]

190. Hoffmann, M.J.; Engers, R.; Florl, A.R.; Otte, A.P.; Müller, M.; Schulz, W.A. Expression changes in EZH2, but not in BMI-1, SIRT1, DNMT1 or DNMT3b, are associated with DNA methylation changes in prostate cancer. *Cancer Biol. Ther.* **2007**, *6*, 1403–1412. [CrossRef] [PubMed]

191. Varambally, S.; Dhanasekaran, S.M.; Zhou, M.; Barrette, T.R.; Kumar-Sinha, C.; Sanda, M.G.; Ghosh, D.; Pienta, K.J.; Sewalt, R.G.A.B.; Otte, A.P.; et al. The polycomb group protein EZH2 is involved in progression of prostate cancer. *Nature* **2002**, *419*, 624–629. [CrossRef] [PubMed]

192. Laitinen, S.; Martikainen, P.M.; Tolonen, T.; Isola, J.; Tammela, T.L.J.; Visakorpi, T. EZH2, Ki-67 and MCM7 are prognostic markers in prostatectomy treated patients. *Int. J. Cancer* **2008**, *122*, 595–602. [CrossRef] [PubMed]

193. Yu, J.; Rhodes, D.R.; Tomlins, S.A.; Cao, X.; Chen, G.; Mehra, R.; Wang, X.; Ghosh, D.; Shah, R.B. A polycomb repression signature in metastatic prostate cancer predicts cancer outcome. *Cancer Res.* **2007**, *67*, 10657–10663. [CrossRef] [PubMed]

194. Viré, E.; Brenner, C.; Deplus, R.; Blanchon, L.; Fraga, M.; Didelot, C.; Morey, L.; van Eynde, A.; Bernard, D.; Vanderwinden, J.M.; et al. The polycomb group protein EZH2 directly controls DNA methylation. *Nature* **2006**, *439*, 871–874. [CrossRef] [PubMed]

195. Schlesinger, Y.; Straussman, R.; Keshet, I.; Farkash, S.; Hecht, M.; Zimmerman, J.; Eden, E.; Yakhini, Z.; Ben-Shushan, E.; Reubinoff, B.E.; et al. Polycomb-mediated methylation on LYS27 of histone H3 pre-marks genes for de novo methylation in cancer. *Nat. Genet.* **2007**, *39*, 232–236. [CrossRef] [PubMed]

196. Crea, F.; Sun, L.; Mai, A.; Chiang, Y.T.; Farrar, W.L.; Danesi, R.; Helgason, C.D. The emerging role of histone lysine demethylases in prostate cancer. *Mol. Cancer* **2012**, *11*, 1–10. [CrossRef] [PubMed]

197. Berry, W.L.; Janknecht, R. KDM4/JMJD2 histone demethylases: Epigenetic regulators in cancer cells. *Cancer Res.* **2013**, *73*, 2936–2942. [CrossRef] [PubMed]

198. Franci, G.; Ciotta, A.; Altucci, L. The Jumonji family: Past, present and future of histone demethylases in cancer. *Biomol. Concepts* **2014**, *5*, 209–224. [CrossRef] [PubMed]

199. Deguchi, T.; Barchas, J. Inhibition of transmethylations of biogenic amines by *S*-adenosylhomocysteine. Enhancement of transmethylation by adenosylhomocysteinase. *J. Biol. Chem.* **1971**, *246*, 3175–3181. [PubMed]

200. Wang, Y.-C.; Tang, F.-Y.; Chen, S.-Y.; Chen, Y.-M.; Chiang, E.-P.I. Glycine-N methyltransferase expression in HepG2 cells is involved in methyl group homeostasis by regulating transmethylation kinetics and DNA methylation. *J. Nutr.* **2011**, *141*, 777–782. [CrossRef] [PubMed]

201. Zhao, J.C.; Yu, J.; Runkle, C.; Wu, L.; Hu, M.; Wu, D.; Liu, J.S.; Wang, Q.; Qin, Z.S.; Yu, J. Cooperation between polycomb and androgen receptor during oncogenic transformation. *Genome Res.* **2012**, *22*, 322–331. [CrossRef] [PubMed]

202. Chng, K.R.; Chang, C.W.; Tan, S.K.; Yang, C.; Hong, S.Z.; Sng, N.Y.; Cheung, E. A transcriptional repressor co-regulatory network governing androgen response in prostate cancers. *EMBO J.* **2012**, *31*, 2810–2823. [CrossRef] [PubMed]

203. Malik, R.; Khan, A.P.; Asangani, I.A.; Cieślik, M.; Prensner, J.R.; Wang, X.; Iyer, M.K.; Jiang, X.; Borkin, D.; Escara-Wilke, J.; et al. Targeting the MLL complex in castration resistant prostate cancer. *Nat. Med.* **2015**, *21*, 344–352. [CrossRef] [PubMed]

204. Yamane, K.; Toumazou, C.; Tsukada, Y.; Erdjument-Bromage, H.; Tempst, P.; Wong, J.; Zhang, Y. JHDM2A, a JMJC-containing H3K9 demethylase, facilitates transcription activation by androgen receptor. *Cell* **2006**, *125*, 483–495. [CrossRef] [PubMed]

205. Cai, C.; He, H.H.; Chen, S.; Coleman, I.; Wang, H.; Fang, Z.; Chen, S.; Nelson, P.S.; Liu, X.S.; Brown, M.; et al. Androgen receptor gene expression in prostate cancer is directly suppressed by the androgen receptor through recruitment of lysine-specific demethylase 1. *Cancer Cell* **2011**, *20*, 457–471. [CrossRef] [PubMed]

206. Gaughan, L.; Stockley, J.; Wang, N.; McCracken, S.R.C.; Treumann, A.; Armstrong, K.; Shaheen, F.; Watt, K.; McEwan, I.J.; Wang, C.; et al. Regulation of the androgen receptor by set9-mediated methylation. *Nucleic Acids Res.* **2011**, *39*, 1266–1279. [CrossRef] [PubMed]

24 B-Vitamins: Important Aspects in Nutrition and Health

207. Xu, K.; Wu, Z.J.; Groner, A.C.; He, H.H.; Cai, C.; Lis, R.T.; Wu, X.; Stack, E.C.; Loda, M.; Liu, T.; et al. Ezh2 oncogenic activity in castration-resistant prostate cancer cells is polycomb-independent. *Science* **2012**, *338*, 1465–1469. [CrossRef] [PubMed]

208. Bohrer, L.R.; Chen, S.; Hallstrom, T.C.; Huang, H. Androgens suppress ezh2 expression via retinoblastoma (RB) and p130-dependent pathways: A potential mechanism of androgen-refractory progression of prostate cancer. *Endocrinology* **2010**, *151*, 5136–5145. [CrossRef] [PubMed]

209. Hofman, K.; Swinnen, J.V.; Verhoeven, G.; Heyns, W. E2f activity is biphasically regulated by androgens in lncap cells. *Biochem. Biophys. Res. Commun.* **2001**, *283*, 97–101. [CrossRef] [PubMed]

210. Cao, P.; Deng, Z.; Wan, M.; Huang, W.; Cramer, S.D.; Xu, J.; Lei, M.; Sui, G. MicroRNA-101 negatively regulates EZH2 and its expression is modulated by androgen receptor and HIF-1α/HIF-1β. *Mol. Cancer* **2010**, *9*, 108. [CrossRef] [PubMed]

211. Varambally, S.; Cao, Q.; Mani, R.S.; Shankar, S.; Wang, X.; Ateeq, B.; Laxman, B.; Cao, X.; Jing, X.; Ramnarayanan, K.; et al. Genomic loss of microRNA-101 leads to overexpression of histone methyltransferase EZH2 in cancer. *Science* **2008**, *322*, 1695–1699. [CrossRef] [PubMed]

212. Farber, S.; Diamond, L.K. Temporary remissions in acute leukemia in children produced by folic acid antagonist, 4-aminopteroyl-glutamic acid. *N. Engl. J. Med.* **1948**, *238*, 787–793. [CrossRef] [PubMed]

213. Loening, S.A.; Beckley, S.; Brady, M.F.; Chu, T.M.; deKernion, J.B.; Dhabuwala, C.; Gaeta, J.F.; Gibbons, R.P.; McKiel, C.F.; McLeod, D.G.; et al. Comparison of estramustine phosphate, methotrexate and cis-platinum in patients with advanced, hormone refractory prostate cancer. *J. Urol.* **1983**, *129*, 1001–1006. [PubMed]

214. Saxman, S.; Ansari, R.; Drasga, R.; Miller, M.; Wheeler, B.; McClean, J.; Einhorn, L. Phase III trial of cyclophosphamide versus cyclophosphamide, doxorubicin, and methotrexate in hormone-refractory prostatic cancer. A hoosier oncology group study. *Cancer* **1992**, *70*, 2488–2492. [CrossRef]

215. Jones, W.G.; Fossa, S.D.; Verbaeys, A.C.; Droz, J.P.; Klijn, J.G.; Boven, E.; de Pauw, M.; Sylvester, R. Low-dose fortnightly methotrexate in advanced prostate cancer. The eortc genito-urinary tract cancer cooperative group. *Eur. J. Cancer* **1990**, *26*, 646. [CrossRef]

216. Linsalata, M.; Caruso, M.G.; Leo, S.; Guerra, V.; D'Attoma, B.; di Leo, A. Prognostic value of tissue polyamine levels in human colorectal carcinoma. *Anticancer Res.* **2002**, *22*, 2465–2469. [PubMed]

217. Canizares, F.; Salinas, J.; de las Heras, M.; Diaz, J.; Tovar, I.; Martinez, P.; Penafiel, R. Prognostic value of ornithine decarboxylase and polyamines in human breast cancer: Correlation with clinicopathologic parameters. *Clin. Cancer Res.* **1999**, *5*, 2035–2041. [PubMed]

218. Heston, W.D. Prostatic polyamines and polyamine targeting as a new approach to therapy of prostatic cancer. *Cancer Surv.* **1991**, *11*, 217–238. [PubMed]

219. Durie, B.G.; Salmon, S.E.; Russell, D.H. Polyamines as markers of response and disease activity in cancer chemotherapy. *Cancer Res.* **1977**, *37*, 214–221. [PubMed]

220. Kubota, S.; Okada, M.; Yoshimoto, M.; Murata, N.; Yamasaki, Z.; Wada, T.; Imahori, K.; Ohsawa, N.; Takaku, F. Urinary polyamines as a tumor marker. *Cancer Detect. Prev.* **1985**, *8*, 189–192. [PubMed]

221. Russell, D.H. Clinical relevance of polyamines. *Crit. Rev. Clin. Lab. Sci.* **1983**, *18*, 261–311. [CrossRef] [PubMed]

222. Sakai, S.; Ito, Y.; Koide, T.; Tei, K.; Hara, A.; Sawada, H. Detection of urinary polyamine by a new enzymatic differential assay. (III). Studies on urinary polyamines in patients with malignant genitourinary diseases. *Hinyokika Kiyo* **1986**, *32*, 343–350. [PubMed]

223. Chatel, M.; Darcel, F.; Quemener, V.; Hercouet, H.; Moulinoux, J.P. Red blood cell polyamines as biochemical markers of supratentorial malignant gliomas. *Anticancer Res.* **1987**, *7*, 33–38. [PubMed]

224. Cipolla, B.; Guille, F.; Moulinoux, J.P.; Bansard, J.Y.; Roth, S.; Staerman, F.; Corbel, L.; Quemener, V.; Lobel, B. Erythrocyte polyamines and prognosis in stage D2 prostatic carcinoma patients. *J. Urol.* **1994**, *151*, 629–633. [PubMed]

225. Cipolla, B.; Guille, F.; Moulinoux, J.P.; Quemener, V.; Staerman, F.; Corbel, L.; Lobel, B. Polyamines and prostatic carcinoma: Clinical and therapeutic implications. *Eur. Urol.* **1993**, *24*, 124–131. [PubMed]

226. Weiss, T.S.; Bernhardt, G.; Buschauer, A.; Thasler, W.E.; Dolgner, D.; Zirngibl, H.; Jauch, K.W. Polyamine levels of human colorectal adenocarcinomas are correlated with tumor stage and grade. *Int. J. Colorectal Dis.* **2002**, *17*, 381–387. [CrossRef] [PubMed]

227. Bergeron, C.; Bansard, J.Y.; Le Moine, P.; Bouet, F.; Goasguen, J.E.; Moulinoux, J.P.; Le Gall, E.; Catros-Quemener, V. Erythrocyte spermine levels: A prognostic parameter in childhood common acute lymphoblastic leukemia. *Leukemia* **1997**, *11*, 31–36. [CrossRef] [PubMed]

228. Soda, K. The mechanisms by which polyamines accelerate tumor spread. *J. Exp. Clin. Cancer Res.* **2011**, *30*, 1–9. [CrossRef] [PubMed]

229. Cipolla, B.; Moulinoux, J.P.; Quemener, V.; Havouis, R.; Martin, L.A.; Guille, F.; Lobel, B. Erythrocyte polyamine levels in human prostatic carcinoma. *J. Urol.* **1990**, *144*, 1164–1166. [PubMed]

230. Cheng, L.L.; Wu, C.-L.; Smith, M.R.; Gonzalez, R.G. Non-destructive quantitation of spermine in human prostate tissue samples using HRMAS 1 H NMR spectroscopy at 9.4 T. *FEBS Lett.* **2001**, *494*, 112–116. [CrossRef]

231. McDunn, J.E.; Li, Z.; Adam, K.P.; Neri, B.P.; Wolfert, R.L.; Milburn, M.V.; Lotan, Y.; Wheeler, T.M. Metabolomic signatures of aggressive prostate cancer. *Prostate* **2013**, *73*, 1547–1560. [CrossRef] [PubMed]

232. Gupta, S.; Ahmad, N.; Marengo, S.R.; MacLennan, G.T.; Greenberg, N.M.; Mukhtar, H. Chemoprevention of prostate carcinogenesis by α-difluoromethylornithine in tramp mice. *Cancer Res.* **2000**, *60*, 5125–5133. [PubMed]

233. Kee, K.; Foster, B.A.; Merali, S.; Kramer, D.L.; Hensen, M.L.; Diegelman, P.; Kisiel, N.; Vujcic, S.; Mazurchuk, R.V.; Porter, C.W. Activated polyamine catabolism depletes acetyl-coa pools and suppresses prostate tumor growth in tramp mice. *J. Biol. Chem.* **2004**, *279*, 40076–40083. [CrossRef] [PubMed]

234. Devens, B.H.; Weeks, R.S.; Burns, M.R.; Carlson, C.L.; Brawer, M.K. Polyamine depletion therapy in prostate cancer. *Prostate Cancer Prostatic Dis.* **2000**, *3*, 275–279. [CrossRef] [PubMed]

235. Kadmon, D. Chemoprevention in prostate cancer: The role of difluoromethylornithine (DFMO). *J. Cell. Biochem. Suppl.* **1992**, *16H*, 122–127. [CrossRef] [PubMed]

236. Moulinoux, J.P.; Quemener, V.; Cipolla, B.; Guille, F.; Havouis, R.; Martin, C.; Lobel, B.; Seiler, N. The growth of MAT-LyLu rat prostatic adenocarcinoma can be prevented in vivo by polyamine deprivation. *J. Urol.* **1991**, *146*, 1408–1412. [PubMed]

237. Danzin, C.; Jung, M.J.; Grove, J.; Bey, P. Effect of alpha-difluoromethylornithine, an enzyme-activated irreversible inhibitor of ornithine decarboxylase, on polyamine levels in rat tissues. *Life Sci.* **1979**, *24*, 519–524. [CrossRef]

238. Meyskens, F.L., Jr.; Simoneau, A.R.; Gerner, E.W. Chemoprevention of prostate cancer with the polyamine synthesis inhibitor difluoromethylornithine. *Recent Results Cancer Res.* **2014**, *202*, 115–120. [PubMed]

239. Simoneau, A.R.; Gerner, E.W.; Nagle, R.; Ziogas, A.; Fujikawa-Brooks, S.; Yerushalmi, H.; Ahlering, T.E.; Lieberman, R.; McLaren, C.E.; Anton-Culver, H.; et al. The effect of difluoromethylornithine on decreasing prostate size and polyamines in men: Results of a year-long phase IIB randomized placebo-controlled chemoprevention trial. *Cancer Epidemiol. Biomarkers Prev.* **2008**, *17*, 292–299. [CrossRef] [PubMed]

240. Streiff, R.R.; Bender, J.F. Phase I study of N1-N11-diethylnorspermine (DENSPM) administered TID for 6 days in patients with advanced malignancies. *Investig. New Drugs* **2001**, *19*, 29–39. [CrossRef]

241. Wagner, T.; Jung, M. New lysine methyltransferase drug targets in cancer. *Nat. Biotechnol.* **2012**, *30*, 622–623. [CrossRef] [PubMed]

242. Kaminskas, E.; Farrell, A.; Abraham, S.; Baird, A.; Hsieh, L.S.; Lee, S.L.; Leighton, J.K.; Patel, H.; Rahman, A.; Sridhara, R.; et al. Approval summary: Azacitidine for treatment of myelodysplastic syndrome subtypes. *Clin. Cancer Res.* **2005**, *11*, 3604–3608. [CrossRef] [PubMed]

243. Fu, S.; Hu, W.; Iyer, R.; Kavanagh, J.J.; Coleman, R.L.; Levenback, C.F.; Sood, A.K.; Wolf, J.K.; Gershenson, D.M.; Markman, M.; et al. Phase 1b–2a study to reverse platinum resistance through use of a hypomethylating agent, azacitidine, in patients with platinum-resistant or platinum-refractory epithelial ovarian cancer. *Cancer* **2011**, *117*, 1661–1669. [CrossRef] [PubMed]

244. Iwata, H.; Sato, H.; Suzuki, R.; Yamada, R.; Ichinomiya, S.; Yanagihara, M.; Okabe, H.; Sekine, Y.; Yano, T.; Ueno, K. A demethylating agent enhances chemosensitivity to vinblastine in a xenograft model of renal cell carcinoma. *Int. J. Oncol.* **2011**, *38*, 1653–1661. [CrossRef] [PubMed]

245. Kiziltepe, T.; Hideshima, T.; Catley, L.; Raje, N.; Yasui, H.; Shiraishi, N.; Okawa, Y.; Ikeda, H.; Vallet, S.; Pozzi, S.; et al. 5-Azacytidine, a DNA methyltransferase inhibitor, induces ATR-mediated DNA double-strand break responses, apoptosis, and synergistic cytotoxicity with doxorubicin and bortezomib against multiple myeloma cells. *Mol. Cancer Ther.* **2007**, *6*, 1718–1727. [CrossRef] [PubMed]

246. Mao, M.; Tian, F.; Mariadason, J.M.; Tsao, C.C.; Lemos, R., Jr.; Dayyani, F.; Gopal, Y.N.; Jiang, Z.Q.; Wistuba, II; Tang, X.M.; et al. Resistance to braf inhibition in braf-mutant colon cancer can be overcome with pi3k inhibition or demethylating agents. *Clin. Cancer Res.* **2013**, *19*, 657–667. [CrossRef] [PubMed]

247. Ramachandran, K.; Gordian, E.; Singal, R. 5-Azacytidine reverses drug resistance in bladder cancer cells. *Anticancer Res.* **2011**, *31*, 3757–3766. [PubMed]

248. Singal, R.; Ramachandran, K.; Gordian, E.; Quintero, C.; Zhao, W.; Reis, I.M. Phase I/II study of azacitidine, docetaxel, and prednisone in patients with metastatic castration-resistant prostate cancer previously treated with docetaxel-based therapy. *Clin. Genitourin. Cancer* **2015**, *13*, 22–31. [CrossRef] [PubMed]

249. Yang, L.; Lin, C.; Jin, C.; Yang, J.C.; Tanasa, B.; Li, W.; Merkurjev, D.; Ohgi, K.A.; Meng, D.; Zhang, J.; et al. Lncrna-dependent mechanisms of androgen-receptor-regulated gene activation programs. *Nature* **2013**, *500*, 598–602. [CrossRef] [PubMed]

250. Wee, Z.N.; Li, Z.; Lee, P.L.; Lee, S.T.; Lim, Y.P.; Yu, Q. EZH2-mediated inactivation of IFN-γ-JAK-STAT1 signaling is an effective therapeutic target in MYC-driven prostate cancer. *Cell Rep.* **2014**, *8*, 204–216. [CrossRef] [PubMed]

251. Beltran, H.; Prandi, D.; Mosquera, J.M.; Benelli, M.; Puca, L.; Cyrta, J.; Marotz, C.; Giannopoulou, E.; Chakravarthi, B.V.; Varambally, S.; et al. Divergent clonal evolution of castration-resistant neuroendocrine prostate cancer. *Nat. Med.* **2016**, *22*, 298–305. [CrossRef] [PubMed]

The Antioxidant Role of One-Carbon Metabolism on Stroke

Kassidy Burgess [1,2,†], Calli Bennett [2,3,†], Hannah Mosnier [4,5], Neha Kwatra [2,5] (ID),
Forrest Bethel [2,3] and Nafisa M. Jadavji [1,2,6,*] (ID)

1   College of Veterinary Medicine, Midwestern University, Glendale, AZ 85308, USA;
    kburgess99@midwestern.edu
2   Biomedical Sciences Program, Midwestern University, Glendale, AZ 85308, USA;
    cbennett83@midwestern.edu (C.B.); nkwatra46@midwestern.edu (N.K.); fbethel37@midwestern.edu (F.B.)
3   College of Osteopathic Medicine, Midwestern University, Glendale, AZ 85308, USA
4   School of Medicine, National University of Ireland Galway, H91 TK33, Ireland; H.Mosnier1@nuigalway.ie
5   College of Dental Medicine, Midwestern University, Glendale, AZ 85308, USA
6   Department of Neuroscience, Carleton University, Ottawa, ON K1S 5B6, Canada
*   Correspondence: njadav@midwestern.edu
†   These authors contributed equally to this work.

Abstract: One-carbon (1C) metabolism is a metabolic network that is centered on folate, a B vitamin; it integrates nutritional signals with biosynthesis, redox homeostasis, and epigenetics. This metabolic pathway also reduces levels of homocysteine, a non-protein amino acid. High levels of homocysteine are linked to increased risk of hypoxic events, such as stroke. Several preclinical studies have suggested that 1C metabolism can impact stroke outcome, but the clinical data are unclear. The objective of this paper was to review preclinical and clinical research to determine whether 1C metabolism has an antioxidant role on stroke. To accomplish the objective, we searched for publications using the following medical subject headings (MeSH) keywords: antioxidants, hypoxia, stroke, homocysteine, one-carbon metabolism, folate, methionine, and dietary supplementation of one-carbon metabolism. Both pre-clinical and clinical studies were retrieved and reviewed. Our review of the literature suggests that deficiencies in 1C play an important role in the onset and outcome of stroke. Dietary supplementation of 1C provides beneficial effects on stroke outcome. For stroke-affected patients or individuals at high risk for stroke, the data suggest that nutritional modifications in addition to other therapies could be incorporated into a treatment plan.

Keywords: hypoxia; antioxidant; stroke; one-carbon metabolism; methionine; transsulfuration

1. Introduction

One-carbon (1C) metabolism is a metabolic network that integrates nutritional signals with biosynthesis, redox homeostasis, and epigenetics, as summarized in Figure 1. It plays an essential role in the regulation of cell proliferation, stress resistance, and embryonic development [1]. The natural form of the B vitamin, folate, is central in 1C, as well as the synthetic form of the vitamin referred to as folic acid. Other vitamins involved in 1C include vitamin B12 and the nutrient choline. In the brain, choline is involved in acetylcholine synthesis and lipid metabolism. Folate and choline metabolism are tightly linked. Choline can act as a 1C donor, especially when there is a deficiency in folate. In the cell, 1C plays an essential role in nucleotide synthesis of purines, removal of uracil from DNA, and methylation, through the metabolism of homocysteine and generation of *S*-adenosylmethionine. Homocysteine can also be metabolized by being pulled into the transsulfuration pathway to generate glutathione.

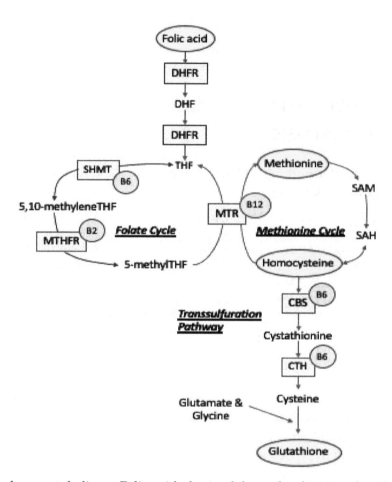

Figure 1. One-carbon metabolism. Folic acid obtained from the diet is reduced to dihydrofolate (DHF) and tetrahydrofolate (THF) by dihydrofolate reductase (DHFR). A methyl group is then transferred to THF by serine hydroxymethyltransferase (SHMT), forming 5,10-methyleneTHF. Vitamin B6 is a cofactor for SHMT. 5,10-methyleneTHF can be reduced by 5,10-methylene tetrahydrofolate reductase (MTHFR) to 5-methylTHF. The methyl group of 5-methyl-THF is transferred to homocysteine by methionine synthase (MTR), generating methionine and regenerating THF. Vitamin B12 is a cofactor for MTR. Methionine is then activated to form S-adenosylmethionine (SAM), which is converted to S-adenosylhomocysteine (SAH) after donating its methyl group. SAH is subsequently hydrolyzed to generate homocysteine. Homocysteine is then used either to regenerate methionine, or homocysteine can be converted to cystathionine by cystathionine beta-synthase (CBS) and further to cysteine by cystathionine gamma-lyase (CTH), using vitamin B6 as cofactor and glutathione, via the transsulfuration pathway.

Several clinical studies have shown that elevations in plasma homocysteine are associated with an increased risk of atherosclerosis and hypoxic events, such as stroke [2–4]. The hypothesis that homocysteine may lead to hypoxia was first recognized in 1969 in homocystinuric children with vascular disease [5]. Since this discovery, several studies have demonstrated that homocysteine levels are significantly higher in individuals with multiple stenotic sites within their vasculature [6,7]. Additionally, a prospective study of 5661 men in the UK found that total homocysteine (tHcy) was predictive of increased stroke risk [8]. Many other investigations have observed similar results and found moderate levels of tHcy (9–15 μmol/L) to be associated with ischemic stroke risk independent of sex, ethnicity, and various risk factors associated with stroke [3,9,10]. A 25% decrease in the usual tHcy level has been associated with a 19% lower stroke risk [11]. In mice that were deficient in low-density lipoprotein, increased homocysteine stimulated the dedifferentiation of vascular smooth muscle cells, causing the state of atherosclerosis [12].

Endothelial injury and dysfunction are the leading mechanisms contributing to the development of hypoxia observed in hyperhomocysteinemia. Homocysteine-induced depletion of bioactive nitric oxide (NO), the endothelium-derived factor responsible for vasodilation, has been suggested for the endothelial dysfunction leading to hypoxia [13]. As shown in microvasculature from murine hearts, homocysteine inhibits dimethylarginine dimethylaminohydrolase activity, resulting in the accumulation of the e-NOS (nitric oxide synthase) inhibitor preventing the production of NO [14,15]. Studies using bovine aortic endothelial cells have shown that homocysteine impairs the transportation of L-arginine, a precursor of NO, into endothelial cells, leading to the enzymatic uncoupling of endothelial nitric oxide synthase (e-NOS) [16,17]. The uncoupling of e-NOS causes it to produce superoxide, which can then react with any remaining NO, producing peroxynitrite. A model using murine aortas showed peroxynitrite depletes the cofactor of the e-NOS domain, diverting it from a NO-producing enzyme to a producer of reactive oxygen species (ROS), which could, in turn, trigger a vicious cycle of further e-NOS uncoupling [18–20]. A study performed on the cerebral cortex of rats showed additional superoxide can be generated from copper-catalyzed oxidation of homocysteine's thiol group, inhibiting NO-related cerebrovascular responses [21].

The autoxidation of homocysteine can also produce ROS, and this can induce endothelial damage via oxidative stress, which is considered to be the first step of atherogenesis [22,23]. In addition to increased production of ROS, homocysteine has been shown in bovine aortic endothelial cells (BAECs) in vitro to reduce the intracellular antioxidant enzyme, glutathione peroxidase, thereby potentiating endothelial damage and the inactivation of NO by ROS [24]. As shown in cultured human and bovine endothelial cells, the ROS can directly damage the vessel endothelium, activating the coagulation cascade in an already prothrombotic environment due to enhanced coagulation and impaired fibrinolysis induced by hyperhomocysteinemia [25–27]. Furthermore, ROS have been reported to initiate lipid peroxidation of low-density lipoproteins, inducing platelet activation in vitro and exerting an atherogenic effect [28,29]. In addition, excess homocysteine leads to the generation of homocysteine-thiolactone, which can impair the structure and function of proteins, potentially triggering ER stress-related endothelial detachment and apoptosis [30–32]. It is worthwhile to note that the concentrations of homocysteine used in some model system studies are far higher than those reported in human plasma (5 to 15 μM) [33].

The remethylation of homocysteine leads to the generation of methionine and then S-adenosylmethionine, a global methyl donor. Elevated levels of homocysteine have been shown to target DNA methylation patterns, altering gene expression and creating endothelial cells that are more vulnerable to damage and have an altered response to hypoxia [4,34,35]. In addition, these alterations in gene expression are believed to contribute to atherogenesis [36]. Homocysteine also inhibited DNA synthesis in human vascular endothelial cells and arrested their growth [37]. In contrast, studies using murine cerebral arterioles found that homocysteine promotes hypertrophy vascular smooth muscle cells, creating a smaller lumen within the vessels [38,39]. In summary, deficiencies in 1C metabolism impact vasculature in the body.

The objective of this paper is to review preclinical and clinical research to determine whether one-carbon metabolism has an antioxidant impact on stroke. We searched for publications using the following medical subject headings (MeSH) keywords; antioxidants, hypoxia, stroke, homocysteine, one-carbon metabolism, folate, methionine, and dietary supplementation of one-carbon metabolism. We have reviewed four components of 1C, and these areas include folates/folic acid, dietary supplementation of 1C, methionine, and transsulfuration. Each section includes a review of clinical and preclinical studies. The main findings from all preclinical studies reviewed are summarized in Table 1.

2. Folates

A diet deficient in folate can directly cause various biological complications related to the deficiency itself, but can additionally cause indirect damage due to increased homocysteine concentrations [40].

Due to its role in the progression of atherosclerosis, a low folate status can exacerbate the effects of a hypoxic event, such as ischemic stroke. Data collected from ischemic and hemorrhagic stroke patients were used to determine whether stroke risk was affected by folate status. One study reported that increased folate concentrations reduced the risk of hemorrhagic stroke, but the results for ischemic stroke were unclear. The study suggested that, while a low folate status is associated with negative implications related to ischemic stroke, an adequate folate status was not found to be protective against ischemic stroke [41].

After a period of hypoxia, folate concentration can play a role in recovery. A study using rats investigated the mechanisms of folic acid deficiency-induced neuronal injury and found that folate deficiency can promote and aggravate neuronal cell damage after ischemia [42]. The mechanism of this damage was shown to be overactivation of autophagy that was triggered by the deficiency and may also involve oxidative injury [42]. Another study using a gerbil model system reported that a folic acid deficiency can induce early and significant neuronal death through oxidative DNA damage. This demonstrates that folic acid deficiency influences and potentiates the pathological processes that are activated by ischemia [40].

Due to the myriad negative health outcomes that can occur when there is a deficiency in folate, many studies have focused on methods by which to reduce folate deficiencies. It is widely acknowledged that under-provision of folate can be attributed to the poor bioavailability of folate in natural food sources [43]. While naturally occurring folate is labile, its synthetic form, folic acid, is fully oxidized and much more stable. Many factors contribute to the absorption of folate, such as incomplete hydrolysis and destruction of folate in the gastrointestinal tract. However, these factors are mitigated when ingesting the synthetic form because it is more stable and does not require the same cellular machinery to convert it into an active form [44].

While it is understood that folate has a reduced bioavailability (Figure 1), the extent to which it is reduced is controversial [43]. Several studies have demonstrated that folate bioavailability is modulated by factors such as genetic variation and ethnicity/race. For example, the methyl tetrahydrofolate reductase (*MTHFR*) gene, which codes for an essential enzyme in folate metabolism, has a common mutation (*MTHFR* C→T) that has variable occurrence according to location and ethnicity [45]. Even when the *MTHFR* C→T mutation is controlled for, African American women display much lower levels of folate following a diet-controlled study [46]. Due ot these many factors affecting folate bioavailability, folic acid is the preferred compound for supplementation.

3. Dietary Supplementation of 1C

1C supplementation, including B vitamins and choline, is an effective method to reduce levels of homocysteine. Since elevated levels of homocysteine lead to increased ROS, downstream oxidative damage has been suggested as a potential mechanism behind homocysteine as a risk factor. Therefore, antioxidant supplementation has been proposed as a method to attenuate stroke risk and improve recovery. In a mouse model study, B vitamin supplementation, along with choline and riboflavin, was demonstrated to increase nuclear factor erythroid 2-related factor 2 (Nrf2) and super oxide dismutase 2 (SOD2), markers of antioxidant activity, after ischemic stroke in a mouse model system [47]. Furthermore, model studies have indicated that supplementation of B vitamins improves functional recovery following an ischemic stroke [47,48]. In addition to functional improvement, folic acid supplementation increased Notch signaling and neurogenesis in the hippocampus [48]. Another model study demonstrated folic acid supplementation leads to increased angiogenesis and neuroprotection after an ischemic event [49]. Additionally, folic acid stabilizes hypoxia inducible factor 1 alpha (HIF-1α), a transcription factor that facilitates cellular adaptation to hypoxia and ischemia [49]. Many model studies have produced promising results, however, benefits become less clear when translated into clinical trials.

Several large-scale clinical trials have evaluated supplementation with folic acid and other B vitamins with supplementation to varying results; we will highlight a few. The Vitamins to Prevent

Stroke (VITATOPS) study was a multi-country study investigating potential benefits of folic acid supplementation. A secondary analysis of the study demonstrated that although supplementation reduced levels of homocysteine, it did not have an impact on incidence of cognitive impairment [50]. Additionally, a study conducted in France suggested that B vitamin, omega-3 fatty acid supplementation, or a combination of the two have no significant impact on the prevention of cardiovascular disease for individuals with a history of ischemic heart disease or ischemic stroke [51]. In contrast, the China Stroke Primary Prevention Trial (CSPPT) indicated that folic acid supplementation leads to a significant decrease in incidence of stroke in hypertensive patients when combined with enalapril, an angiotensin-converting enzyme (ACE) inhibitor [52,53]. The CSPPT study indicated that folic acid supplementation is reliable in decreasing the incident of stroke in populations with little to no folic acid fortification programs [54]. However, several meta-data analyses have presented similarly conflicting results [55–57].

There could be several possibilities as to why there is a disconnect between the model system and clinical literature. First, it is important to consider where these studies are taking place, and if folic acid fortification is common in those countries or regions. Second, underlying concomitant health factors and drug use of subjects could be significant. A sub-analysis of the CSPPT suggested the effects of folic acid supplementation can be modified based on the patients' cholesterol levels, with the most significant risk reduction in individuals with high cholesterol [58]. Along a similar vein, statin use has been shown to decrease the effect of folic acid supplementation on stroke risk [54]. A second sub-analysis of the CSPPT data indicated a greatly attenuated impact of folic acid supplementation when patients demonstrated low platelet counts [59]. Additionally, a post hoc analysis of the VITATOPs data indicated that folic acid therapy was modified by anti-platelet therapy [60]. With the conflicting data on the role of 1C supplementation and the myriad factors by which it can be modified, further focused studies are required.

In a clinical setting, folic acid supplementation has been demonstrated to significantly increase the total antioxidant capacity [61]. Additionally, a double-blind placebo-controlled trial on diabetic patients indicated similar effects of folic acid supplementation on total antioxidant capacity [62]. Significantly, higher total antioxidant capacity has been associated with decreased mortality following ischemic stroke [63]. Therefore, it would be logical to assume that with folic acid supplementation leading to increased total antioxidant capacity and increased total antioxidant capacity leading to decreased ischemic stroke mortality, folic acid supplementation would lead to decreased mortality following ischemic stroke.

In model systems studying the impact of reduced levels of dietary folates, it is demonstrated that choline metabolism is also affected [64]. Similar to folates, choline bioavailability is dependent on several factors. It is modulated by the diet and genome via the microbiota of individuals [65]. Additionally, the bioavailability is affected by the structure of the choline source [66]. Further, and also similar to folic acid, several model studies have indicated that choline supplementation following an ischemic event provides neuroprotection. This neuroprotection is especially evident in the hippocampus, including the CA1 pyramidal cells [47,67], and increases cortical sparing following a traumatic brain injury [68]. Components of choline metabolism, including citicoline, have also been examined as potential treatments following an ischemic event. In model studies, citicoline has been demonstrated to restore phospholipid membranes and mitigate oxidative stress following an ischemic event [69]. Additionally, chronic supplementation of citicoline following an ischemic event increased neuroplasticity and functional recovery [70].

4. Methionine

Once homocysteine has been remethylated, it will be activated to form methionine (Figure 1) [71]. Methionine is an amino acid that is essential in all animal species for protein [72] and cysteine synthesis [73]. It is involved in 1C through the transmethylation reaction to produce S-adenosylmethionine (SAM) [73]. Several research reports suggest that methionine also plays an important role in the brain during and after hypoxia [74–76]. Interestingly, methionine and related derivatives have been shown to protect the brain from the detrimental effects of hypoxia [74–76]. The bioavailability of methionine in humans is not well characterized, due to the invasive nature of such studies. There is a study suggesting that the DL-isomer is used at ~30% [73].

Using model systems, researchers studied whether methionine oxidation increases NF-kB (nuclear factor kappa-light-chain-enhancer of activated B) activation, thereby contributing to cerebral ischemia reperfusion injury [74]. In order to have a protective role, methionine must inhibit the NF-kB pathway, since it promotes inflammation. This is because inhibition of this pathway protects against cerebral ischemia reperfusion injury, notably post-ischemic neurovascular inflammation. It was found that the derivative of methionine referred to as methionine sulfoxide reductase (MsrA) protects against hypoxic injury by inhibiting the NF-kB pathway HIV-LTR/Luciferase (HLL) in transgenic male mice. MsrA decreases protein methionine oxidation of calcium/calmodulin-dependent protein kinase II (CaMKII), which partially controls the redox regulation of the NF-kB pathway. Therefore, inhibition of CaMKII results in inhibition of the NF-kB pathway, ultimately mediating brain injury due to hypoxia and reperfusion [74]. For this study, only male mice were used, so it remains unknown what the impact of MsrA is in female mice [74]. Similar results were found regarding the protective effects of MsrA in another study [76]. The focus of this study was to determine whether overexpression of MsrA protects neuronal cells against hypoxia reoxygenation injury. The main findings of this study were that brief hypoxia and reoxygenation cause significant and quick changes in ROS levels in the cells. This increase in ROS causes a depolarization of the mitochondrial membrane of the cells, thereby facilitating cell death and increasing apoptosis. MsrA is an antioxidant that promotes the reduction of met-O in proteins to methionine and, when overexpressed, was found to protect against cellular injuries caused by hypoxia reoxygenation. Overexpression of MsrA lowered the ROS levels in cells caused by hypoxia and reoxygenation, therefore playing a protective role against oxidative stress and promoting cell survival [76]. A strength of this study is that each of the outcomes assessed was a clear indicator of cell death or injury, which allowed researchers to confidently infer the effect of MsrA in protecting against hypoxia and reoxygenation injury. However, this study focused on the effects of hypoxia/reoxygenation only in rat PC12 cells and liver cells. The results of hypoxia and reoxygenation on oxidative status as well as the protective effects of MsrA may be different in other types of cells and in vivo [76].

In another study, researchers looked at the protective effects of methionine sulfoximine (MSO) in middle cerebral artery occlusion as an animal model for stroke [75]. The main findings were that intraperitoneal injection of MSO twenty-four hours before middle cerebral artery occlusion prevented significant infarct volume in the rat cerebral cortex, but not in the basal ganglia. The infarct size of the cerebral cortex was significantly decreased, whereas that in the basal ganglia was not [75]. A strength of this study is that the infarct volume in both the cortex and basal ganglia were measured, instead of only the cortex. This shows that the protective effects of MSO cannot be generalized to all regions of the brain. The study did not determine the specific cause of MSO's protective effects. This will have to be investigated in future research. In addition, a limitation of this study is that only male Sprague-Dawley rats were used. Therefore, results may differ in female rats [75].

5. Transsulfuration

Through the transsulfration pathway, cystathionine β-synthase (CBS) is an enzyme that functions to remove excess homocysteine via direct conversion to cystathionine (Figure 1). CBS acts as the rate-limiting enzyme in the conversion of homocysteine to cystathionine, which is then converted to cysteine, a component of the antioxidant glutathione. Some estimate that upwards of 50% of the cysteine produced in this systemic pathway will be utilized in hepatic glutathione synthesis [77]. There is an increase in glutathione during oxidative stress as shown in mouse cerebral brain tissue. Glutathione can exert its antioxidant abilities, namely the reduction of hydrogen peroxide and lipid peroxides, catalyzed by the enzyme glutathione peroxidase (GPx).

5.1. Cystathionine β-synthase (CBS)

An association with CBS expression and hypoxia has been established; when researchers subjected an in vitro model of U87-MG human glioblastoma cells and PC12 pheochromocytoma cells to hypoxic conditions, they reported increased transcription of CBS mRNA and protein synthesis. Application of hypoxia-induced factor (HIF) inhibitors blocked the increases in CBS mRNA and protein synthesis found under hypoxic conditions. The same increases in CBS mRNA and protein synthesis were observed in vivo using Sprague-Dawley rats who were then exposed to hypobaric hypoxia. These results were found to be attenuated by treatment with digoxin, an HIF inhibitor clinically prescribed as an anti-arrhythmic, concurrent with hypobaric hypoxia conditions [78].

More recently, changes of CBS promoter methylation levels in hypertensive and stroke patients as compared to a healthy population. In doing so, promotor methylation was determined to be an independent risk factor for both hypertension and stroke, however, results were only significant in men, and it remains unclear why females did not exhibit the same results. Notably, the study is limited in its population, having only studied participants native to Shenzhen, China [79]. Following the found association of CBS deficiency and vascular thromboembolism, researchers sought to compare proteome alterations in CBS-deficient individuals to those with various subtypes of ischemic stroke (e.g., cardioembolic, lacunar, and large-vessel stroke). The authors concluded that common mechanisms exist between individuals with CBS deficiency and ischemic stroke, particularly cardioembolic stroke, as a result of proteome alterations in molecular networks possessing strong interactions with NFκB. This was found to be particularly affected in acute-phase proteins and blood coagulation. However, results may be influenced by the fact that some of the tested CBS-deficient individuals had a prior history of stroke and thus proteome alterations may have already occurred as a result of the prior ischemia [80].

It is still not fully conclusive whether upregulation of CBS during ischemia is either protective or beneficial to recovery. For example, in a population of 75 patients presenting with premature occlusive arterial disease or occlusive cerebrovascular disease, they were found to have increased levels of homocysteine compared to a normal population. Thus, the authors suppose that CBS deficiency predisposes individuals to occlusive arterial disorders [81]. However, even though its CBS deficiency may be related, its role in the development of stroke is unclear. Interestingly, CBS, via its product cystathionine, has actually been positively associated with risk of stroke. Patients with suspected angina pectoris were followed for a median of 7.3 years. In that time, a linear positive trend was found between plasma cystathionine and stroke risk [82]. Thus, more direct research into the levels of CBS products or enzymatic activity itself is warranted for in vivo research.

Several additional experiments come to the conclusion that either CBS or its downstream products may in fact be negative contributors for risk of ischemic stroke. For example, researchers set out to investigate the association of cysteine, a downstream product of the CBS pathway and upstream substrate of H_2S production, and its association with impaired outcomes in situations of ischemia and stroke. First, authors analyzed excitotoxic amino acid concentrations (e.g., cysteine, methionine, glutamate, aspartate, and glycine) in 36 patients immediately following clinical diagnosis of stroke by a neurologist. Patients were then stratified into two groups, good outcome or poor outcome, after reassessment at 90 days using the Rankin scale. Plasma cysteine levels provided the most significant association with lower levels resulting in better patient outcomes. The researchers further investigated possible mechanisms using male Wistar rats that were subjected to a middle cerebral artery occlusion (MCAO) concurrent with cysteine administration. Forebrain sections were analyzed for extent of infarct volume. It was found in a dose-dependent manner that cysteine levels were positively correlated with infarct volume. Intraperitoneal administration of aminooxyacetic acid (AOAA), a CBS inhibitor, abolished the cysteine-induced increase in infarct volume. More investigation is necessary since, as the authors point out, rat models demonstrate increased sensitivity to cysteine neurotoxicity and thus infarct volume may be influenced by this factor alone [83]. However, given the efficacy of AOAA in diminishing cysteine induced infarct volume, it necessitates further investigation into CBS and its role in ischemia. More investigation into CBS, its regulation, and downstream products is necessary. The evidence for the positive direct correlation with CBS activity is becoming clear, however the results warrant more research.

5.2. Glutathione

Glutathione is rapidly oxidized in periods of oxidative stress in order to prevent cellular damage as a result of the production of ROS. Rodent [84] and clinical studies [85] have shown that glutathione concentrations are increased after supplementation. In rodents, the increase is seen in thirty minutes, whereas in humans it takes up to one month. Thus, all enzymes related to the synthesis of glutathione pose liabilities in the conditions of ischemia and resulting oxidative stress. As an example of its importance in periods of oxidative stress, researchers found that when male Sprague-Dawley rats were placed in hypoxic conditions with subsequent reoxygenation, significant reductions in glutathione and superoxide dismutase (SOD) were observed [86]. Additionally, as another example of the importance of glutathione, the effects of glutathione peroxidase deficiency under conditions of hyperhomocysteinemia were studied. Investigators found that mice heterozygote for glutathione peroxidase (Gpx$^{+/-}$) fed a high-methionine diet, to recreate conditions of hyperhomocysteinemia, were found to be particularly susceptible to endothelial dysfunction with specific impairment in endothelium-dependent vasodilator function. Moreover, in Gpx$^{+/-}$ mice fed high-methionine diets, acetylcholine aortic ring relaxation was found to be impaired when compared to wild-type mice. Hyperhomocysteinemia was suspected of contributing to this impairment through a peroxide-dependent oxidative mechanism, and GPx deficiency did not impair vascular responses with administration of endothelium-independent vasodilators in either the presence or absence of hyperhomocysteinemia [87]. Thus, GPx reduced susceptibility of endothelial dysfunction during hyperhomocysteinemia conditions through its effects on peroxide oxidative mechanisms.

Glutathione has also been shown to play an important role in periods of ischemia and recovery. Male Sprague-Dawley rats were subjected to transient middle cerebral artery occlusion with or without injection of glutathione 10 min following reperfusion. After 24 h, rats were then analyzed for both brain tissue edema and infarct volume. The experimental control exhibited increased brain tissue edema and infarct volume by 2-fold compared to those with glutathione administration. The glutathione-treated group had more healthy cells in the cortex and striatum compared to control animals. Additionally, analysis of claudin-5, a protein important in the formation of the blood–brain barrier (BBB), revealed a potential role in the protective nature of glutathione following cerebral ischemia. Specifically, models administered glutathione treatment showed increased claudin-5 expression compared to controls. Murine brain endothelial cells were placed in an anaerobic chamber and then administered glutathione or saline. Glutathione resulted in decreased ROS production, as well as increased viability following hypoxia/reperfusion injury. Through Western blot and RT-PCR, the underlying mechanism was found to be associated with increased PI3K/Akt activation as well as forkhead box O3 (FOXO3) inactivation [88]. (See Table 1).

Table 1. Summary of main findings of model system studies.

Reference	Model System and Sex Used	Design	Major Findings
[42]	Sprague-Dawley rats (male)	Using focal cerebral ischemia model and folic acid deficiency to investigate neuronal autophagy in neuronal cells.	Autophagy was induced in rats subjected to ischemic insults. Further autophagy activation in cortex neurons caused by folic acid deficiency was confirmed by the increase in the LC3II/LC3I ratio and beclin 1 expression. The increased formation of autophagosomes. results suggest that cerebral cortex cell injury by folic acid deficiency in ischemic brains is partially mediated by the activation of autophagy. Oxidative injury seems to be involved in excessive activation of autophagy caused by folic acid deficiency.
[40]	Mongolian gerbils (male)	Examined whether folic acid deficiency and transient forebrain ischemia enhances neuronal damage and gliosis via oxidative stress in the gerbil hippocampus.	After transient cerebral ischemia Folic acid deficiency increases delayed neuronal death, DNA damage, platelet endothelial cell adhesion molecule 1 immunoreactivity, and gliosis in the hippocampus.
[47]	C57BL/6J mice (male)	Investigated the impact of dietary deficiency of folic acid and supplementation after with folic acid, vitmain B12, riboflavin and choline promoted recovery after photothrombosis ischemic damage.	Combination of B-vitamins, including folic acid, riboflavin and vitamin B12 with choline supplementation promotes some degree of functional improvement following ischemic damage. Additionally, study shows increased neuroplasticity markers deltaFosB and brain derived neurotrophic factor (BDNF), as well as increased levels of nuclear factor erythroid 2-related factor 2 (Nrf2) and superoxide dismutase 2 (SOD2), indicators of anti-oxidant activity
[67]	Wistar Hannover rats (male)	The impact of choline supplementation on the survival of hippocampal neurons following transient forebrain ischemia	There was no difference between choline treated rats up to 200 mg/kg/day and controls (vehicle-treated animals). Choline administered at 400 mg/kg/day provided a significant neuroprotection to ischemic animals at the dose.
[68]	Sprague-Dawley rats (male)	The aim of this study was to determine whether the low-potency and elective alpha-7 neuronal nicotinic cholinergic receptor (nAChR) agonist choline could be a useful treatment for improvement of neurological outcome in a rat model of traumatic brain injury (TBI).	Choline supplemented animals show improved memory retention tests; dietary choline supplementation was associated with cortical tissue preservation; choline supplementation attenuates TBI-induced decreases in cortical levels of alpha-7 nAChR.

Table 1. *Cont.*

Reference	Model System and Sex Used	Design	Major Findings
[69]	Gerbils (male)	Examined changes and effects of citocoline on pholipids and glutathione synthesis after transient ischemia and reperfusion. Citocline is a precursor to choline, which can be metabolized to methionine (1C metabolism), which may be further converted to glutathione, which is one of the primary endogenous antioxidant defense systems in the brain.	The study demonstrated that citicoline supplementation improved phospholipid membrane short-term, while the neuroprotective factors (demonstrated by glutathione) were more significant 3+ days post infarct.
[70]	Sprague-Dawley rats (male)	Investigated whether a chronic treatment with CDP-choline starting 24 h after is middle cerebral artery occlusion in the rat.	Increased neuronal plasticity and contribution to sensorimotor function recovery when chronically treated with CDP-choline.
[74]	C57BL/6J mice (male) and human umbical vein endothelial cells	Study tried to determine if NF-kB (nuclear factor kappa-light-chain-enhancer of activated B) activation is increased by methionine oxidation after ischemic stroke.	The main findings are that using the oxidation of methionine and of CaMMKII Met281/282, reactive oxygen species (ROS) promote the NF-kB pathway in endothelial cells in vitro and in vivo. Furthermore, NF-kB pathway activation and cerebral ischemia/reperfusion injury can be prevented by MsrA, through the expression of MsrA in nonhematopoietic cells. Finally, mice deficient in methionine sulfoxide reductase A (MsrA-/-) have decreased outcome after stroke, but outcome can be protected against by inhibition of the NF-kB pathway or CaMKII.
[75]	Sprague-Dawley rats (male)	The focus of this study was to look at the protective effects of methionine sulfoximine (MSO) in middle cerebral artery occlusion, which was used as an animal model for stroke.	The main findings of this study are that intraperitoneal MSO injection prevented significant infarct volume in the rat cerebral cortex but not the basal ganglia after middle cerebral artery occlusion. MSO administration was found to increase cortical glycogen by 81% 24hours after administration, but did not change glucose levels significantly. Methionine sulfoximine might be changing the presynaptic cells by interrupting the astrocyte-neuron glutamate shuttle and impairing neuronal glutamine synthetase.

Table 1. *Cont.*

Reference	Model System and Sex Used	Design	Major Findings
[76]	PC12 Cells	To determine whether overexpression of methionine sulfoxide reductase A (MSRA) impacts protection in cells after hypoxia and reoxygenation injury.	The main findings of this study are that brief hypoxia and reoxygenation cause significant and quick changes in reactive oxygen species (ROS) levels in the cells. This increase in ROS causes a depolarization of the mitochondrial membrane of the cells, thereby facilitating cell death, as well as an increase in apoptosis of cells due to the ROS. Methionine sulfoxide reductase type A (MSRA) is an antioxidant that promotes the reduction of met-O in proteins to methionine and, when overexpressed, was found to protect against these cellular injuries caused by hypoxia/reoxygenation. MSRA was found to lower the ROS levels in cells caused by hypoxia/reoxygenation therefore playing a protective role against oxidative stress causing cell injury.
[78]	Cells: U87-MG, PC12, human lung microvascular and aortic endothelial cells, and primary vascular smooth muscle Sprague-Dawley Wistar rats cell cultures	Study examined the relationship of hypoxia and expression of cystathionine beta synthase (CBS).	mRNA and protein expression of CBS were increased after hypoxia. The increase may be mediated by hypoxia-inducible factors (HIFs) in the cell models.
[86]	Sprague-Dawley rats (male)	The study evaluate the effects of exposition to acute severe repiratory hypoxia followed by reoxygenation in brain injury.	After hypoxia and reoxygenation, oxidative stress and apoptosis were increased.
[88]	Sprague-Dawley rats (male) and endothelial cells	The study examined whether glutathione reduces cerebral infarct size after middle cerebral artery occlusion	In vivo GSH-deficiency resulted in increased cerebral infarction volume. GSH reduced brain infarct volume. the expression of claudin-5 associated with brain infarct formation. We also examined activation of the PI3K/Akt pathway, inactivation of FOXO3, and expression of Bcl2 to assess the role of GSH in promoting cell survival in response to ischemic injury.

6. Conclusions

The in vivo model system studies reviewed in this manuscript used males, therefore the impact of deficiencies in 1C metabolism on stroke in females remains relatively unknown. Women are affected by cardiovascular disease [89], therefore model system studies need to include both sexes in future studies.

1C metabolism is far reaching and impacts several processes in the cell. It plays an important role in metabolizing homocysteine, which is a known risk factor for hypoxic events, such as stroke. Increasing dietary components of 1C has been shown to reduce oxidative stress in animal models. However, more work investigating the clinical applicability is required in order to determine benefits for stroke outcome in patients. Since combinational therapies have been shown to be effective for stroke patients [90], it may be worthwhile to consider incorporating nutrition into a therapeutic plan.

Author Contributions: Conceptualization, N.M.J.; writing—original draft preparation, K.B., C.B., H.M., N.K., F.B., N.M.J.; writing—review and editing, K.B., C.B., H.M., N.K., F.B., N.M.J.; visualization, K.B., N.M.J.; supervision, N.M.J. All authors have read and agreed to the published version of the manuscript.

References

1. Murray, L.; Emmerson, J.; Jadavji, N.M. Roles of Folate in Neurological Function. In *Folic Acid: Sources, Health Effects and Role in Disease*; Nova Publishers Science Inc.: Hauppauge, NY, USA, 2017.

2. Ashjazadeh, N.; Fathi, M.; Shariat, A. Evaluation of homocysteine level as a risk factor among patients with ischemic stroke and its subtypes. *Iran. J. Med. Sci.* **2013**, *38*, 233–239. [PubMed]

3. Han, L.; Wu, Q.; Wang, C.; Hao, Y.; Zhao, J.; Zhang, L.; Fan, R.; Liu, Y.; Li, R.; Chen, Z.; et al. Homocysteine, Ischemic Stroke, and Coronary Heart Disease in Hypertensive Patients: A Population-Based, Prospective Cohort Study. *Stroke* **2015**, *46*, 17777–17786. [CrossRef] [PubMed]

4. Castro, R.; Rivera, I.; Blom, H.J.; Jakobs, C.; Tavares de Almeida, I. Homocysteine metabolism, hyperhomocysteinaemia and vascular disease: An overview. *J. Inherit. Metab. Dis.* **2006**, *29*, 3–20. [CrossRef] [PubMed]

5. McCully, K.S. Vascular pathology of homocysteinemia: Implications for the pathogenesis of arteriosclerosis. *Am. J. Pathol.* **1969**, *56*, 111–128.

6. Yoo, J.H.; Chung, C.S.; Kang, S.S. Relation of plasma homocyst(e)ine to cerebral infarction and cerebral atherosclerosis. *Stroke* **1998**, *29*, 2478–2483. [CrossRef]

7. Sasaki, T.; Watanabe, M.; Nagai, Y.; Hoshi, T.; Takasawa, M.; Nukata, M.; Taguchi, A.; Kitagawa, K.; Kinoshita, N.; Matsumoto, M. Association of plasma homocysteine concentration with atherosclerotic carotid plaques and lacunar infarction. *Stroke* **2002**, *33*, 1493–1496. [CrossRef]

8. Perry, I.J.; Morris, R.W.; Ebrahim, S.B.; Shaper, A.G.; Refsum, H.; Ueland, P.M. Prospective study of serum total homocysteine concentration and risk of stroke in middle-aged British men. *Lancet* **1995**, *346*, 1395–1398. [CrossRef]

9. Kittner, S.J.; Giles, W.H.; Macko, R.F.; Hebel, J.R.; Wozniak, M.A.; Wityk, R.J.; Stolley, P.D.; Stern, B.J.; Sloan, M.A.; Sherwin, R.; et al. Homocyst(e)ine and Risk of Cerebral Infarction in a Biracial Population: The Stroke Prevention in Young Women Study. *Stroke* **1999**, *30*, 1554–1560. [CrossRef]

10. Wang, C.; Han, L.; Wu, Q.; Zhuo, R.; Liu, K.; Zhao, J.; Zhang, L.; Hao, Y.; Fan, R.; Liu, Y.; et al. Association between homocysteine and incidence of ischemic stroke in subjects with essential hypertension: A matched case-control study. *Clin. Exp. Hypertens.* **2015**, *37*, 557–562. [CrossRef]

11. The Homocysteine Studies Collaboration Homocysteine and Risk of Ischemic Heart Disease and Stroke. *Am. Med. Assoc.* **2002**, *288*, 2015–2023. [CrossRef]

12. Pan, S.; Liu, H.; Gao, F.; Luo, H.; Lin, H.; Meng, L.; Jiang, C.; Guo, Y.; Chi, J.; Guo, H. Folic acid delays development of atherosclerosis in low-density lipoprotein receptor-deficient mice. *J. Cell. Mol. Med.* **2018**, *22*, 3183–3191. [CrossRef]

13. Loscalzo, J. The oxidant stress of hyperhomocyst(e)inemia. *J. Clin. Investig.* **1996**, *98*, 5–7. [CrossRef] [PubMed]

14. Stühlinger, M.C.; Tsao, P.S.; Her, J.H.; Kimoto, M.; Balint, R.F.; Cooke, J.P. Homocysteine impairs the nitric oxide synthase pathway role of asymmetric dimethylarginine. *Circulation* **2001**, *104*, 2569–2575. [CrossRef] [PubMed]

15. Tyagi, N.; Sedoris, K.C.; Steed, M.; Ovechkin, A.V.; Moshal, K.S.; Tyagi, S.C. Mechanisms of homocysteine-induced oxidative stress. *Am. J. Physiol. Heart Circ. Physiol.* **2005**, *289*, H2649–H2656. [CrossRef] [PubMed]

16. Tyagi, S.C.; Lominadze, D.; Roberts, A.M. Homocysteine in microvascular endothelial cell barrier permeability. *Cell Biochem. Biophys.* **2005**, *43*, 37–44. [CrossRef]

17. Jin, L.; Caldwell, R.B.; Li-Masters, T.; Caldwell, R.W. Homocysteine induces endothelial dysfunction via inhibition of arginine transport. *J. Physiol. Pharmacol.* **2007**, *58*, 191–206. [PubMed]

18. Laursen, J.B.; Somers, M.; Kurz, S.; Mccann, L.; Warnholtz, A.; Freeman, B.A.; Tarpey, M.; Fukai, T.; Harrison, D.G. Implications for Interactions Between Peroxynitrite. *Circulation* **2001**, *103*, 1282–1289. [CrossRef]

19. Förstermann, U.; Münzel, T. Endothelial nitric oxide synthase in vascular disease: From marvel to menace. *Circulation* **2006**, *113*, 1708–1714. [CrossRef]

20. Milstien, S.; Katusic, Z. Oxidation of tetrahydrobiopterin by peroxynitrite: Implications for vascular endothelial function. *Biochem. Biophys. Res. Commun.* **1999**, *263*, 681–684. [CrossRef]

21. Zhang, F.; Slungaard, A.; Gregory, M.; Vercellotti; Iadecola, C. Superoxide-dependent cerebrovascular effects of homocysteine. *Am. J. Physiol. Regul. Integr. Comp. Physiol.* **1998**, *274*, R1704–R1711. [CrossRef]

22. Outinen, P.A.; Sood, S.K.; Liaw, P.C.Y.; Sarge, K.D.; Maeda, N.; Hirsh, J.; Ribau, J.; Podor, T.J.; Weitz, J.I.; Austin, R.C. Characterization of the stress-inducing effects of homocysteine. *Biochem. J.* **1998**, *332*, 213–221. [CrossRef] [PubMed]

23. Welch, G.N.; Upchurch, G.R.; Loscalzo, J. Homocysteine, oxidative stress, and vascular disease. *Hosp. Pract.* **1997**, *32*, 81–92. [CrossRef] [PubMed]

24. Upchurch, G.R.; Welche, G.N.; Fabian, A.J.; Freedman, J.E.; Johnson, J.L.; Keaney, J.F.; Loscalzo, J. Homocyst(e)ine decreases bioavailable nitric oxide by a mechanism involving glutathione peroxidase. *J. Biol. Chem.* **1997**, *272*, 17012–17017. [CrossRef] [PubMed]

25. Dayal, S.; Wilson, K.M.; Leo, L.; Arning, E.; Bottiglieri, T.; Lentz, S.R. Enhanced susceptibility to arterial thrombosis in a murine model of hyperhomocysteinemia. *Blood* **2006**, *108*, 2237–2243. [CrossRef] [PubMed]

26. Starkebaum, G.; Harlan, J.M. Endothelial cell injury due to copper-catalyzed hydrogen peroxide generation from homocysteine. *J. Clin. Investig.* **1986**, *77*, 1370–1376. [CrossRef] [PubMed]

27. Sauls, D.L.; Lockhart, E.; Warren, M.E.; Lenkowski, A.; Wilhelm, S.E.; Hoffman, M. Modification of fibrinogen by homocysteine thiolactone increases resistance to fibrinolysis: A potential mechanism of the thrombotic tendency in hyperhomocysteinemia. *Biochemistry* **2006**, *45*, 2480–2487. [CrossRef]

28. Magwenzi, S.; Woodward, C.; Wraith, K.S.; Aburima, A.; Raslan, Z.; Jones, H.; McNeil, C.; Wheatcroft, S.; Yuldasheva, N.; Febbraio, M.; et al. Oxidized LDL activates blood platelets through CD36/NOX2-mediated inhibition of the cGMP/protein kinase G signaling cascade. *Blood* **2015**, *125*, 2693–2703. [CrossRef] [PubMed]

29. Ardlie, N.G.; Selley, M.L.; Simons, L.A. Platelet activation by oxidatively modified low density lipoproteins. *Atherosclerosis* **1989**, *76*, 117–124. [CrossRef]

30. Austin, R.C.; Lentz, S.R.; Werstuck, G.H. Role of hyperhomocysteinemia in endothelial dysfunction and atherothrombotic disease. *Cell Death Differ.* **2004**, *11* (Suppl. 1), S56–S64. [CrossRef]

31. Lai, W.K.C.; Kan, M.Y. Homocysteine-induced endothelial dysfunction. *Ann. Nutr. Metab.* **2015**, *67*, 1–12. [CrossRef]

32. Jakubowski, H.; Zhang, L.; Bardeguez, A.; Aviv, A. Homocysteine Thiolactone and Protein Homocysteinylation in Human Endothelial Cells. *Circ. Res.* **2000**, *87*, 45–51. [CrossRef] [PubMed]

33. MacCoss, M.J.; Fukagawa, N.K.; Matthews, D.E. Measurement of homocysteine concentrations and stable isotope tracer enrichments in human plasma. *Anal. Chem.* **1999**, *71*, 4527–4533. [CrossRef] [PubMed]

34. Perna, A.F.; Ingrosso, D.; De Santo, N.G. Homocysteine and oxidative stress. *Amino Acids* **2003**, *25*, 409–417. [CrossRef]

35. James, S.J.; Melnyk, S.; Pogribna, M.; Pogribny, I.P.; Caudill, M.A. Elevation in S-Adenosylhomocysteine and DNA Hypomethylation: Potential Epigenetic Mechanism for Homocysteine-Related Pathology. *J. Nutr.* **2002**, 2361–2366. [CrossRef] [PubMed]

36. Dong, C.; Yoon, W.; Goldschmidt-Clermont, P.J. DNA methylation and athersclerosis. *J. Nutr.* **2002**, *131*, 2406S–2409S. [CrossRef]

37. Wang, H.; Yoshizumi, M.; Lai, K.; Tsai, J.-C.C.; Perrella, M.A.; Haber, E.; Lee, M.-E.E. Inhibition of growth and p21ras methylation in vascular endothelial cells by homocysteine but not cysteine. *J. Biol. Chem.* **1997**, *272*, 25380–25385. [CrossRef] [PubMed]

38. Walsh, B.H.; Broadhurst, D.I.; Mandal, R.; Wishart, D.S.; Boylan, G.B.; Kenny, L.C.; Murray, D.M. The Metabolomic Profile of Umbilical Cord Blood in Neonatal Hypoxic Ischaemic Encephalopathy. *PLoS ONE* **2012**, *7*, e50520. [CrossRef]

39. Tsai, J.C.; Perrella, M.A.; Yoshizumi, M.; Hsieh, C.M.; Haber, E.; Schlegel, R.; Lee, M.E. Promotion of vascular smooth muscle cell growth by homocysteine: A link to atherosclerosis. *Proc. Natl. Acad. Sci. USA* **1994**, *91*, 6369–6373. [CrossRef]

40. Hwang, I.K.; Yoo, K.-Y.; Suh, H.-W.; Kim, Y.S.; Kwon, D.Y.; Kwon, Y.-G.; Yoo, J.-H.; Won, M.-H. Folic acid deficiency increases delayed neuronal death, DNA damage, platelet endothelial cell adhesion molecule-1 immunoreactivity, and gliosis in the hippocampus after transient cerebral ischemia. *J. Neurosci. Res.* **2008**, *86*, 2003–2015. [CrossRef]

41. Van Guelpen, B.; Hultdin, J.; Johansson, I.; Stegmayr, B.; Hallmans, G.; Nilsson, T.K.; Weinehall, L.; Witthöft, C.; Palmqvist, R.; Winkvist, A. Folate, vitamin B12, and risk of ischemic and hemorrhagic stroke: A prospective, nested case-referent study of plasma concentrations and dietary intake. *Stroke* **2005**, *36*, 1426–1431. [CrossRef]

42. Zhao, Y.; Huang, G.; Chen, S.; Gou, Y.; Dong, Z.; Zhang, X. Folic acid deficiency increases brain cell injury via autophagy enhancement after focal cerebral ischemia. *J. Nutr. Biochem.* **2016**, *38*, 41–49. [CrossRef] [PubMed]

43. McNulty, H.; Pentieva, K. Folate bioavailability. *Folate Health Dis. Second Ed.* **2004**, *63*, 25–47. [CrossRef] [PubMed]

44. Caudill, M.A. Folate bioavailability: Implications for establishing dietary recommendations and optimizing status. *Am. J. Clin. Nutr.* **2010**, *91*, 1455S. [CrossRef] [PubMed]

45. Liew, S.C.; Gupta, E. Das Methylenetetrahydrofolate reductase (MTHFR) C677T polymorphism: Epidemiology, metabolism and the associated diseases. *Eur. J. Med. Genet.* **2015**, *58*, 1–10. [CrossRef] [PubMed]

46. Perry, C.A.; Renna, S.A.; Khitun, E.; Ortiz, M.; Moriarty, D.J.; Caudill, M.A. Ethnicity and race influence the folate status response to controlled folate intakes in young women. *J. Nutr.* **2004**, *134*, 1786–1792. [CrossRef]

47. Jadavji, N.M.; Emmerson, J.; Willmore, W.G.; MacFarlane, A.J.; Smith, P. B-vitamin and choline supplementation increases neuroplasticity and recovery after stroke. *Neurobiol. Dis.* **2017**, *103*, 89–100. [CrossRef]

48. Zhang, X.; Huang, G.; Liu, H.; Chang, H.; Wilson, J.X. Folic acid enhances Notch signaling, hippocampal neurogenesis, and cognitive function in a rat model of cerebral ischemia. *Nutr. Neurosci.* **2012**, *15*, 55–61. [CrossRef]

49. Davis, C.K.; Nampoothiri, S.S.; Rajanikant, G.K. Folic Acid Exerts Post-Ischemic Neuroprotection In Vitro Through HIF-1α Stabilization. *Mol. Neurobiol.* **2018**, *55*, 8328–8345. [CrossRef]

50. Hankey, G.J.; Ford, A.H.; Yi, Q.; Eikelboom, J.W.; Lees, K.R.; Chen, C.; Xavier, D.; Navarro, J.C.; Ranawaka, U.K.; Uddin, W.; et al. Effect of B vitamins and lowering homocysteine on cognitive impairment in patients with previous stroke or transient ischemic attack: A prespecified secondary analysis of a randomized, placebo-controlled trial and meta-analysis. *Stroke* **2013**, *44*, 2232–2239. [CrossRef]

51. Galan, P.; Kesse-Guyot, E.; Czernichow, S.; Briancon, S.; Blacher, J.; Hercberg, S. Effects of B vitamins and omega 3 fatty acids on cardiovascular diseases: A randomised placebo controlled trial. *BMJ* **2011**, *342*, 36. [CrossRef]

52. Huang, X.; Li, Y.; Li, P.; Li, J.; Bao, H.; Zhang, Y.; Wang, B.; Sun, N.; Wang, J.; He, M.; et al. Association between percent decline in serum total homocysteine and risk of first stroke. *Neurology* **2017**, *89*, 2101–2107. [CrossRef] [PubMed]

53. Huo, Y.; Li, J.; Qin, X.; Huang, Y.; Wang, X.; Gottesman, R.F.; Tang, G.; Wang, B.; Chen, D.; He, M.; et al. Efficacy of folic acid therapy in primary prevention of stroke among adults with hypertension in China: The CSPPT randomized clinical trial. *JAMA J. Am. Med. Assoc.* **2015**, *313*, 1325–1335. [CrossRef] [PubMed]

54. Huo, Y.; Qin, X.; Wang, J.; Sun, N.; Zeng, Q.; Xu, X.; Liu, L.; Xu, X.; Wang, X. Efficacy of folic acid supplementation in stroke prevention: New insight from a meta-analysis. *Int. J. Clin. Pract.* **2012**, *66*, 544–551. [CrossRef] [PubMed]

55. Zhang, C.; Chi, F.L.; Xie, T.H.; Zhou, Y.H. Effect of B-vitamin supplementation on stroke: A meta-analysis of randomized controlled trials. *PLoS ONE* **2013**, *8*, e81577. [CrossRef]

56. Tian, T.; Yang, K.-Q.; Cui, J.-G.; Zhou, L.-L.; Zhou, X.-L. Folic Acid Supplementation for Stroke Prevention in Patients with Cardiovascular Disease. *Am. J. Med. Sci.* **2017**, *354*, 379–387. [CrossRef]

57. Zeng, R.; Xu, C.H.; Xu, Y.N.; Wang, Y.L.; Wang, M. The effect of folate fortification on folic acid-based homocysteine-lowering intervention and stroke risk: A meta-analysis. *Public Health Nutr.* **2015**, *18*, 1514–1521. [CrossRef]

58. Qin, X.; Li, J.; Spence, J.D.; Zhang, Y.; Li, Y.; Wang, X.; Wang, B.; Sun, N.; Chen, F.; Guo, J.; et al. Folic Acid Therapy Reduces the First Stroke Risk Associated with Hypercholesterolemia Among Hypertensive Patients. *Stroke* **2016**, *47*, 2805–2812. [CrossRef]

59. Kong, X.; Huang, X.; Zhao, M.; Xu, B.; Xu, R.; Song, Y.; Yu, Y.; Yang, W.; Zhang, J.; Liu, L.; et al. Platelet Count Affects Efficacy of Folic Acid in Preventing First Stroke. *J. Am. Coll. Cardiol.* **2018**, *71*, 2136–2146. [CrossRef]

60. Hankey, G.J.; Eikelboom, J.W.; Yi, Q.; Lees, K.R.; Chen, C.; Xavier, D.; Navarro, J.C.; Ranawaka, U.K.; Uddin, W.; Ricci, S.; et al. Antiplatelet therapy and the effects of B vitamins in patients with previous stroke or transient ischaemic attack: A post-hoc subanalysis of VITATOPS, a randomised, placebo-controlled trial. *Lancet Neurol.* **2012**, *11*, 512–520. [CrossRef]

61. Assanelli, D.; Bonanome, A.; Pezzini, A.; Albertini, F.; Maccalli, P.; Grassi, M.; Archetti, S.; Negrini, R.; Visioli, F. Folic acid and Vitamin E supplementation effects on homocysteinemia, endothelial function and plasma antioxidant capacity in young myocardial-infarction patients. *Pharmacol. Res.* **2004**, *49*, 79–84. [CrossRef]

62. Aghamohammadi, V.; Gargari, B.P.; Aliasgharzadeh, A. Effect of Folic Acid Supplementation on Homocysteine, Serum Total Antioxidant Capacity, and Malondialdehyde in Patients with Type 2 Diabetes Mellitus. *J. Am. Coll. Nutr.* **2011**, *30*, 210–215. [CrossRef] [PubMed]

63. Lorente, L.; Martín, M.M.; Pérez-Cejas, A.; Abreu-González, P.; Ramos, L.; Argueso, M.; Cáceres, J.J.; Solé-Violán, J.; Jiménez, A. Association between total antioxidant capacity and mortality in ischemic stroke patients. *Ann. Intensive Care* **2016**, *6*, 1–6. [CrossRef] [PubMed]

64. Dam, K.; Füchtemeier, M.; Farr, T.; Boehm-Strum, P.; Foddis, M.; Dirnagal, U.; Jadavji, N.M. Deficiencies in methylenetetrahydrofolate reductase and dietary folic acid alter choline metabolism during chronic hypoperfusion. *Behav. Brain Res.* **2017**, *321*, 201–208. [CrossRef] [PubMed]

65. Arias, N.; Arboleya, S.; Allison, J.; Kaliszewska, A.; Higarza, S.G.; Gueimonde, M.; Arias, J.L. The relationship between choline bioavailability from diet, intestinal microbiota composition, and its modulation of human diseases. *Nutrients* **2020**, *12*, 2340. [CrossRef] [PubMed]

66. Mödinger, Y.; Schön, C.; Wilhelm, M.; Hals, P.A. Plasma kinetics of choline and choline metabolites after a single dose of SuperbaBoost™ krill oil or choline bitartrate in healthy volunteers. *Nutrients* **2019**, *11*, 2548. [CrossRef]

67. Borges, A.A.; Ei-Batah, P.N.; Yamashita, L.F.; dos Santos Santana, A.; Lopes, A.C.; Freymuller-Haapalainen, E.; Coimbra, C.G.; Sinigaglia-Coimbra, R. Neuroprotective effect of oral choline administration after global brain ischemia in rats. *Nutr. Neurosci.* **2015**, *18*, 265–274. [CrossRef]

68. Guseva, M.V.; Hopkins, D.M.; Scheff, S.W.; Pauly, J.R. Dietary Choline Supplementation Improves Behavioral, Histological, and Neurochemical Outcomes in a Rat Model of Traumatic Brain Injury. *J. Neurotrauma* **2008**, *25*, 975–983. [CrossRef]

69. Adibhatla, R.M.; Hatcher, J.F.; Dempsey, R.J. Effects of Citicoline on Phospholipid and Glutathione Levels in Transient Cerebral Ischemia. *Stroke.* **2001**, *32*, 2376–2381. [CrossRef]

70. Hurtado, O.; Cardenas, A.; Pradillo, J.M.; Morales, J.R.; Ortego, F.; Sobrino, T.; Castillo, J.; Moro, M.A.; Lizasoain, I.; Cardenas, A.; et al. A chronic treatment with CDP-choline improves functional recovery and increases neuronal plasticity after experimental stroke. *Neurobiol. Dis.* **2007**, *26*, 105–111. [CrossRef]

71. Ducker, G.S.; Rabinowitz, J.D. One-Carbon Metabolism in Health and Disease. *Cell Metab.* **2017**, *25*, 27–42. [CrossRef]

72. Pérez-Jiménez, A.; Peres, H.; Rubio, V.C.; Oliva-Teles, A. The effect of hypoxia on intermediary metabolism and oxidative status in gilthead sea bream (Sparus aurata) fed on diets supplemented with methionine and white tea. *Comp. Biochem. Physiol. C Toxicol. Pharmacol.* **2012**, *155*, 506–516. [CrossRef] [PubMed]

73. Elango, R. Methionine Nutrition and Metabolism: Insights from Animal Studies to Inform Human Nutrition—PubMed. *J. Nutr.* **2020**, *150*, 2518S–2523S. [CrossRef] [PubMed]

74. Gu, S.X.; Blokhin, I.O.; Wilson, K.M.; Dhanesha, N.; Doddapattar, P.; Grumbach, I.M.; Chauhan, A.K.; Lentz, S.R. Protein methionine oxidation augments reperfusion injury in acute ischemic stroke. *JCI Insight* **2016**, *1*, 1–18. [CrossRef]

75. Swanson, R.A.; Shiraishi, K.; Morton, M.T.; Sharp, F.R. Methionine sulfoximine reduces cortical infarct size in rats after middle cerebral artery occlusion. *Stroke* **1990**, *21*, 322–327. [CrossRef] [PubMed]

76. Yermolaieva, O.; Xu, R.; Schinstock, C.; Brot, N.; Weissbach, H.; Heinemann, S.H.; Hoshi, T. Methionine sulfoxide reductase A protects neuronal cells against brief hypoxia/reoxygenation. *Proc. Natl. Acad. Sci. USA* **2004**, *101*, 1159–1164. [CrossRef]

77. Sbodio, J.I.; Snyder, S.H.; Paul, B.D. Regulators of the transsulfuration pathway. *Br. J. Pharmacol.* **2019**, *176*, 583–593. [CrossRef]

78. Takano, N.; Peng, Y.J.; Kumar, G.K.; Luo, W.; Hu, H.; Shimoda, L.A.; Suematsu, M.; Prabhakar, N.R.; Semenza, G.L. Hypoxia-inducible factors regulate human and rat cystathionine â-synthase gene expression. *Biochem. J.* **2014**, *458*, 203–211. [CrossRef]

79. Wang, C.; Xu, G.; Wen, Q.; Peng, X.; Chen, H.; Zhang, J.; Xu, S.; Zhang, C.; Zhang, M.; Ma, J.; et al. CBS promoter hypermethylation increases the risk of hypertension and stroke. *Clinics* **2019**, *74*, e630. [CrossRef] [PubMed]

80. Sikora, M.; Lewandowska, I.; Kupc, M.; Kubalska, J.; Graban, A.; Marczak, Ł.; Kaźmierski, R.; Jakubowski, H. Serum proteome alterations in human cystathionine β-synthase deficiency and ischemic stroke subtypes. *Int. J. Mol. Sci.* **2019**, *20*, 3096. [CrossRef]

81. Boers Heterozygosity for homocystinuria in premature peripheral and cerebral occlusive arterial disease. *N. Engl. J. Med.* **1974**, *306*, 802–805.

82. Dhar, I.; Svingen, G.F.T.; Ueland, P.M.; Lysne, V.; Svenningsson, M.M.; Tell, G.S.; Nygård, O.K. Plasma cystathionine and risk of incident stroke in patients with suspected stable angina pectoris. *J. Am. Heart Assoc.* **2018**, *7*, 1–12. [CrossRef] [PubMed]

83. Wong, P.T.H.; Qu, K.; Chimon, G.N.; Seah, A.B.H.; Hui, M.C.; Meng, C.W.; Yee, K.N.; Rumpel, H.; Halliwell, B.; Chen, C.P.L.H. High plasma cyst(e)ine level may indicate poor clinical outcome in patients with acute stroke: Possible involvement of hydrogen sulfide. *J. Neuropathol. Exp. Neurol.* **2006**, *65*, 109–115. [CrossRef] [PubMed]

84. Hagen, T.M.; Wierzbicka, G.T.; Sillau, A.H.; Bowman, B.B.; Jones, D.P. Bioavailability of dietary glutathione: Effect on plasma concentration. *Am. J. Physiol. Gastrointest. Liver Physiol.* **1990**, *259*, G524–G529. [CrossRef] [PubMed]

85. Richie, J.P.; Nichenametla, S.; Neidig, W.; Calcagnotto, A.; Haley, J.S.; Schell, T.D.; Muscat, J.E. Randomized controlled trial of oral glutathione supplementation on body stores of glutathione. *Eur. J. Nutr.* **2015**, *54*, 251–263. [CrossRef]

86. Coimbra-Costa, D.; Alva, N.; Duran, M.; Carbonell, T.; Rama, R. Oxidative stress and apoptosis after acute respiratory hypoxia and reoxygenation in rat brain. *Redox Biol.* **2017**, *12*, 216–225. [CrossRef]

87. Dayal, S.; Brown, K.L.; Weydert, C.J.; Oberley, L.W.; Arning, E.; Bottiglieri, T.; Faraci, F.M.; Lentz, S.R. Deficiency of glutathione peroxidase-1 sensitizes hyperhomocysteinemic mice to endothelial dysfunction. *Arterioscler. Thromb. Vasc. Biol.* **2002**, *22*, 1996–2002. [CrossRef]

88. Song, J.; Park, J.; Oh, Y.; Lee, J.E. Glutathione suppresses cerebral infarct volume and cell death after ischemic injury: Involvement of FOXO3 inactivation and Bcl2 expression. *Oxid. Med. Cell. Longev.* **2015**, *2015*, 1–11. [CrossRef]

89. Garcia, M.; Mulvagh, S.L.; Merz, C.N.B.; Buring, J.E.; Manson, J.A.E. Cardiovascular disease in women: Clinical perspectives. *Circ. Res.* **2016**, *118*, 1273–1293. [CrossRef]

90. Wang, Y.; Li, Q.; Wang, J.; Zhuang, Q.K.; Zhang, Y.Y. Combination of thrombolytic therapy and neuroprotective therapy in acute ischemic stroke: Is it important? *Eur. Rev. Med. Pharmacol. Sci.* **2015**, *19*, 416–422.

3

The Role of Genetic Polymorphisms as Related to One-Carbon Metabolism, Vitamin B6 and Gene–Nutrient Interactions in Maintaining Genomic Stability and Cell Viability in Chinese Breast Cancer Patients

Xiayu Wu [1], Weijiang Xu [1], Tao Zhou [1], Neng Cao [1], Juan Ni [1], Tianning Zou [2], Ziqing Liang [1], Xu Wang [1,*] and Michael Fenech [3,*]

[1] School of Life Sciences, The Engineering Research Center of Sustainable Development and Utilization of Biomass Energy, Ministry of Education, Yunnan Normal University, Kunming 650500, Yunnan, China; xiayu.wu@csiro.au or xiayu98wu@163.com (X.W.); sn-xwj@163.com (W.X.); kmzl@163.com (T.Z.); wy2057729@163.com (N.C.); gt_gg30@163.com (J.N.); liang_zq229@hotmail.com (Z.L.)

[2] Third Affiliated Hospital of Kunming Medical College, Kunming 650101, Yunnan, China; zoutn@aliyun.com

[3] Genome Health and Personalized Nutrition, CSIRO Food and Nutrition, P.O. Box 10041, Adelaide SA 5000, Australia

* Correspondence: wangxu@fudan.edu.cn (X.W.); michael.fenech@csiro.au (M.F.)

Academic Editor: Li Yang

Abstract: Folate-mediated one-carbon metabolism (FMOCM) is linked to DNA synthesis, methylation, and cell proliferation. Vitamin B6 (B6) is a cofactor, and genetic polymorphisms of related key enzymes, such as serine hydroxymethyltransferase (SHMT), methionine synthase reductase (MTRR), and methionine synthase (MS), in FMOCM may govern the bioavailability of metabolites and play important roles in the maintenance of genomic stability and cell viability (GSACV). To evaluate the influences of B6, genetic polymorphisms of these enzymes, and gene–nutrient interactions on GSACV, we utilized the cytokinesis-block micronucleus assay (CBMN) and PCR-restriction fragment length polymorphism (PCR-RFLP) techniques in the lymphocytes from female breast cancer cases and controls. GSACV showed a significantly positive correlation with B6 concentration, and 48 nmol/L of B6 was the most suitable concentration for maintaining GSACV in vitro. The GSACV indexes showed significantly different sensitivity to B6 deficiency between cases and controls; the B6 effect on the GSACV variance contribution of each index was significantly higher than that of genetic polymorphisms and the sample state (tumor state). *SHMT C1420T* mutations may reduce breast cancer susceptibility, whereas *MTRR A66G* and *MS A2756G* mutations may increase breast cancer susceptibility. The role of *SHMT, MS*, and *MTRR* genotype polymorphisms in GSACV is reduced compared with that of B6. The results appear to suggest that the long-term lack of B6 under these conditions may increase genetic damage and cell injury and that individuals with various genotypes have different sensitivities to B6 deficiency. FMOCM metabolic enzyme gene polymorphism may be related to breast cancer susceptibility to a certain extent due to the effect of other factors such as stress, hormones, cancer therapies, psychological conditions, and diet. Adequate B6 intake may be good for maintaining genome health and preventing breast cancer.

Keywords: FMOCM; vitamin B6; genetic polymorphisms; gene-nutrient interaction; GSACV; breast cancer

1. Introduction

Folate, vitamin B6 (B6), and vitamin B12 (B12) have been proven to play important roles in the one-carbon metabolism pathway and the prevention of carcinogenesis: (a) in the transformation of homocysteine (Hcy) to methionine for methylation of DNA to ensure gene expression and genomic stability; and (b) in the synthesis of purine precursors and thymidylate of nucleic acid (DNA and RNA) [1–4]. B6 is not only a crucial coenzyme for serine hydroxymethyltransferase (SHMT) in the reversible transformation of serine and tetrahydrofolate (THF) to 5,10-methylene THF and glycine [5,6], a reaction that offers one-carbon units for S-adenosylmethionine (SAM), and for the synthesis of purine and pyrimidine, but it is also a cofactor for cystathionine β-synthase (CBS), which is involved in the transsulfuration pathway where Hcy is converted into cystathionine. Thus, inadequate dietary intake of B6 or deficiency of B6 in plasma might result in a state of missing DNA precursors, aberrations in DNA metabolism and histone methylation, interruption in DNA repair, and imbalance in the synthesis and degradation of Hcy, any of which are likely to be associated with promoting the development of several adverse health effects including carcinogenesis. In addition to its functions in DNA synthesis, methylation, and repair, B6 is also essential for the synthesis of glutathione (GSH) from Hcy via cysteine and cystathionine. GSH plays a key role of detoxification and protection as a cofactor of GSH peroxidases and GSH S-transferases. Additionally, it can protect cells from the oxidative damage of nucleic acids, proteins and lipids [7–9]. Rodent studies have shown that azoxymethane-induced colon tumorigenesis in mice is suppressed by moderate doses of dietary B6, and B6 can suppress endothelial cell angiogenesis and proliferation in part by restraining DNA topoisomerases and DNA polymerase [10,11].

Not only the above-mentioned B6 and SHMT are important in the folate-mediated one-carbon metabolism (FMOCM), which also involves various other enzymes. Among them, 5,10-methylenetetrahydrofolate reductase (MTHFR) irreversibly converts 5,10-methylene THF to 5-methyl THF [12,13]. Methionine synthase (MS) maintains methionine dynamic equilibrium by converting Hcy to methionine (the precursor of SAM) in a cobalamin-dependent reaction, which uses 5-methyl THF as the methyl donor [14]. Methionine synthase reductase (MTRR) is responsible for activating MS by keeping adequate levels of activated B12 [15–18]. The folate metabolism has attracted major attention in relation to breast carcinogenesis. In spite of its significance in the one-carbon metabolism and the elimination of oxidative stress, there is limited basic experimental proof of an association of B6 and the above-mentioned enzymes with susceptibility to cancer, especially breast cancer [19–21]. We previously reported associations among two polymorphisms in the MTHFR gene (677 and 1298 loci), folate (or folic acid), B12 deficiency, genome instability, and increased cell death with breast cancer risk in the Chinese Yunnan population [14,22–24]. Based on previous work, we utilized the cytokinesis-block micronucleus assay (CBMN) and PCR-restriction fragment length polymorphism (PCR-RFLP) techniques to determine the relationships between B6 deficiency, the other above-mentioned genetic polymorphisms in the folate pathway, gene-nutrient interactions and genomic stability and cell viability (GSACV) in vitro.

2. Results

2.1. Dose-Response Relationship between the Concentration of B6 and the Number of Viable Cells (NVC) in Cell Lines

Our goal was to ascertain the dose-response relationship between the concentration of B6 and the NVC. In preliminary experiments, we selected the lowest B6 concentrations to be 0 nmol/L with an experimental concentration gradient of 6, 12, 24, 48, 96, 200, and 4800 nmol/L to culture a breast cancer cell line and a normal cell line (GM13705 and GM12593, respectively) according to the physiological concentrations of B6 in plasma (20–40 nmol/L) [25]. Although vitamin B6 concentration in vivo is unlikely to be zero, we wanted to make sure of the growth status of the cell line in culture without B6, so we selected the lowest concentration to be 0 nmol/L. The results showed a clear dose-response growth relationship in both cell lines at various B6 concentrations, with 24 nmol/L being the lowest concentration of B6 that can lead to an increase in NVC. Because there was no significant difference of growth between 200 and 4800 nmol/L and both cell lines were dead at 0 nmol/L, we selected 6, 12, 24, 48, 96, and 200 nmol/L B6 to culture both lymphocytes from the breast cancer cases and controls in follow-up experiments (Supplementary Figure S1).

2.2. Comparison of GSACV with Different B6 Concentrations in the Breast Cancer Cases or Controls

The levels of GSACV biomarkers in media with different concentrations of B6 are reported in Table 1. A one-way analysis of variance (ANOVA) showed that there were no significant differences among the nuclear division index (NDI) values at different concentrations of B6 in both groups (breast cancer and controls). However, the other GSACV indexes (frequency of micronucleated binucleated cells, MNBN; micronucleated mononucleated cells, MONO; nucleoplasmic bridge cells, NPB; nuclear bud cells, NBUD) showed a decreasing trends with increasing B6 concentrations from 6–24 to 48–200 nmol/L. There were no significant differences in GSACV indexes including MNBN, NPB, NBUD, and MONO frequencies from 48 to 200 nmol/L in the same groups (breast cancer cases or controls). The frequencies of apoptosis (APO) and necrosis (NEC) significantly decreased when the concentration of B6 was raised from 6–12 to 24–200 nmol/L, and there was no significant difference in APO or NEC from 24 to 200 nmol/L B6.

Table 1. The indexes of GSACV in breast cancer cases and controls under various B6 concentrations.

Endpoint	Group	B6 in Medium (nmol/L) ($\bar{x} \pm$ SD) [1,2,3]					
		6	12	24	48	96	200
NDI	Cases	1.30 ± 0.026 [a]	1.28 ± 0.028 [a]	1.29 ± 0.021 [a]	1.36 ± 0.041 [a]	1.30 ± 0.034 [a]	1.30 ± 0.027 [a]
	Controls	1.26 ± 0.027 [a]	1.27 ± 0.031 [a]	1.25 ± 0.015 [a]	1.26 ± 0.030 [a]	1.23 ± 0.027 [a]	1.28 ± 0.025 [a]
‰ MNBN	Cases	27.8 ± 2.05 [a]	25.9 ± 1.60 [b]	22.2 ± 3.24 [b]	18.7 ± 2.44 [c]	17.2 ± 1.62 [c]	17.0 ± 2.63 [c]
	Controls	20.4 ± 2.12 [a]	17.4 ± 1.45 [b]	15.7 ± 3.30 [c]	13.6 ± 2.23 [c,d]	12.07 ± 1.61 [d]	13.44 ± 1.17 [d]
‰ MONO	Cases	2.78 ± 0.45 [a]	1.74 ± 0.40 [b]	1.62 ± 0.65 [b]	1.55 ± 0.53 [b]	1.44 ± 0.23 [b]	1.40 ± 0.42 [b]
	Controls	2.05 ± 0.45 [a]	1.59 ± 0.59 [a]	1.49 ± 0.28 [a,b]	1.30 ± 0.30 [b]	1.29 ± 0.35 [b]	1.33 ± 0.40 [b]
‰ NBUD	Cases	9.30 ± 1.82 [a]	7.98 ± 2.26 [b]	6.13 ± 1.11 [b,c]	5.96 ± 0.74 [c]	5.43 ± 1.33 [c]	6.02 ± 0.95 [c]
	Controls	7.12 ± 1.07 [a]	6.03 ± 1.52 [b]	4.64 ± 1.42 [b]	4.08 ± 1.44 [b,c]	4.21 ± 1.07 [b,c]	4.00 ± 0.68 [c]
‰ NPB	Cases	5.36 ± 0.76 [a]	4.93 ± 1.22 [a]	3.76 ± 0.42 [a,b]	3.41 ± 0.55 [b]	3.08 ± 1.05 [b]	3.11 ± 0.80 [b]
	Controls	4.01 ± 0.27 [a]	3.41 ± 0.56 [a]	2.91 ± 0.67 [b]	2.46 ± 0.60 [b]	2.46 ± 1.02 [b]	2.02 ± 0.12 [b]
% APO	Cases	4.59 ± 0.80 [a]	4.10 ± 0.67 [a,b]	3.58 ± 1.10 [b,c]	3.37 ± 1.11 [b,c]	3.02 ± 0.95 [b,c]	2.86 ± 0.97 [c]
	Controls	5.22 ± 0.55 [a]	5.09 ± 0.80 [a,b]	5.71 ± 0.95 [b]	5.25 ± 0.62 [b,c]	4.24 ± 0.67 [b,c]	3.97 ± 0.67 [c]
% NEC	Cases	7.83 ± 0.53 [a]	5.93 ± 0.40 [b]	5.89 ± 0.60 [b,c]	5.02 ± 0.78 [c]	5.65 ± 0.63 [c]	4.73 ± 0.73 [c]
	Controls	6.37 ± 0.76 [a]	5.79 ± 1.38 [b]	4.65 ± 0.98 [c]	4.05 ± 0.40 [c]	3.85 ± 1.07 [c]	3.69 ± 0.75 [c]

[1] Values are means ± standard deviation (SD); [2] Different letters differ from each other in the same type in different medium; [3] Repeated measures; one-way analysis of variance (ANOVA) of data.

A correlation analysis among the biomarkers showed that the GSACV indexes were obviously positively related to each other ($p < 0.001$–0.05, respectively) and that the GSACV indexes were significantly negatively correlated with the B6 concentration: r = −0.764, −0.615, −0.563, −0.448, −0.761, and −0.601 for MNBN, NPB, NBUD, MONO, APO and NEC ($p < 0.001$–0.05), respectively, in the breast cancer cases, and r = −0.582, −0.609, −0.574, −0.411, −0.663, and −0.510 for MNBN, NPB, NBUD, MONO, APO and NEC ($p < 0.001$–0.05), respectively, in the controls. These results are shown in Tables 2 and 3.

Table 2. Cross-correlation matrix of variables measured in breast cancer cases under various culture media [1,2].

	B6	MNBN	NBUD	NPB	MONO	APO
MNBN	−0.764 ***	-				
NBUD	−0.563 ***	0.712 ***	-			
NPB	−0.615 ***	0.538 ***	0.426 **	-		
MONO	−0.448 ***	0.577 ***	0.440 **	0.234	-	
APO	−0.761 ***	0.739 ***	0.502 ***	0.356 *	0.216 *	-
NEC	−0.601 **	0.621 **	0.605 **	0.362 *	0.516 **	0.523 **

[1] Values are estimated spearman correlation coefficients; [2] *** $p < 0.001$; ** $p < 0.01$; * $p < 0.05$.

Table 3. Cross-correlation matrix of variables measured in controls under various culture media [1,2].

	B6	MNBN	NBUD	NPB	MONO	APO
MNBN	−0.582 ***	-				
NBUD	−0.574 ***	0.701 ***	-			
NPB	−0.609 ***	0.620 ***	0.419 **	-		
MONO	−0.411 ***	0.472 ***	0.504 **	0.381 *	-	
APO	−0.663 ***	0.505 ***	0.528 ***	0.325 *	0.372 *	-
NEC	−0.510 ***	0.610 ***	0.592 ***	0.430 **	0.654 **	0.550 **

[1] Values are estimated spearman correlation coefficients; [2] *** $p < 0.001$; ** $p < 0.01$; * $p < 0.05$.

2.3. Comparison of GSACV at the Same B6 Concentration between the Breast Cancer Cases and Controls

Comparing GSACV between the breast cancer cases and controls, the MNBN, NPB, NBUD, MONO, and NEC frequencies in the controls were notably than those in the breast cancer cases at the same B6 concentrations ($p < 0.001$–0.05) (Figure 1).

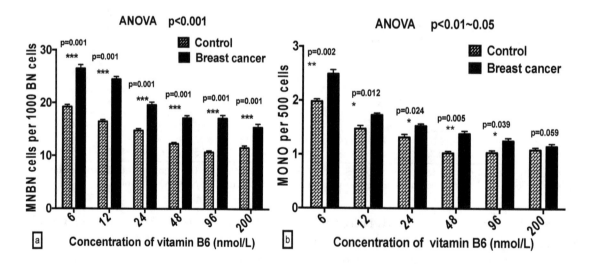

Figure 1. *Cont.*

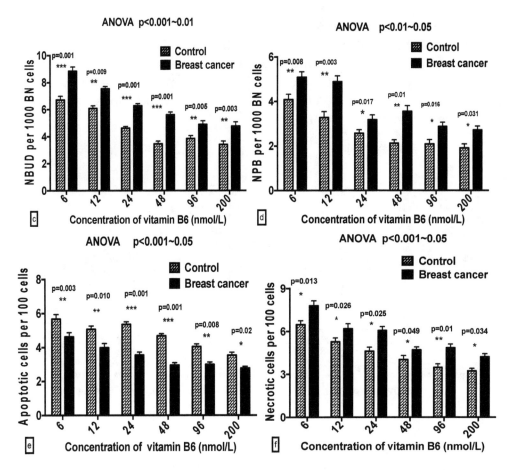

Figure 1. A comparison of: MNBN (**a**); MONO (**b**); NBUD (**c**); NPB (**d**); APO (**e**); and NEC (**f**) frequency between breast cancer cases and controls under various concentrations of B6.

2.4. Effect of B6 and Breast Cancer Status on GSACV

A two-way ANOVA revealed that B6 concentrations accounted for 46.15%, 30.13%, 29.66%, 3.14%, 31.65%, and 41.15% ($p < 0.001$–0.01) of the variance of the MNBN, NPB, NBUD, MONO, APO, and NEC frequencies, respectively, beside the breast cancer status, which accounted for 5.12%, 4.14%, and 5.45% of the variance of the MNBN, NPB, and NEC frequencies, respectively ($p < 0.05$). The investigation suggested that the breast cancer status affected GSACV but that the effect was less significant than that of the B6 concentration (Table 4).

Table 4. Effect of B6 and breast cancer status on GSACV [1,2,3].

Source of Variation	B6	Status	Interaction
	V%	V%	V%
MNBN	46.15 ***	5.12 *	0.88
NPB	30.13 **	4.14 *	0.30
NBUD	29.66 ***	0.48	0.30
MONO	3.14	0.04	1.56
APO	31.65 ***	0.61	1.87
NEC	40.15 ***	5.45 *	2.44

[1] Values determined by two-way ANOVA; [2] *** $p < 0.0001$, ** $p < 0.001$, * $p < 0.05$; [3] Effect size is expressed as the ratio of the differences between the mean values for the two categories of each independent variable.

The breast cancer cases and controls had distinct genomic baselines, which are derived from their different genetic backgrounds. Thus, we performed a Difference in Difference Analysis (DDA) [26] by subtracting the pooled values of the biomarker for 6 to 96 nmol/L from the scores for 200 nmol/L B6. Interestingly, we observed that the MNBN values in the breast cancer cases were significantly higher than those in the respective controls at 6 and 12 nmol/L B6 ($p < 0.05$). Meanwhile, the MONO and NBUD levels were notably higher than those in the controls at only 6 nmol/L ($p < 0.05$). There were no significant differences in the NPB, APO, and NEC occurrences between the breast cancer cases and controls. The analyses showed that there were significant differences in sensitivity to the genotoxic and cytotoxic effects of B6 deficiency between the breast cancer cases and controls with respect to MNBN, MONO, and NBUD frequencies (Figure 2).

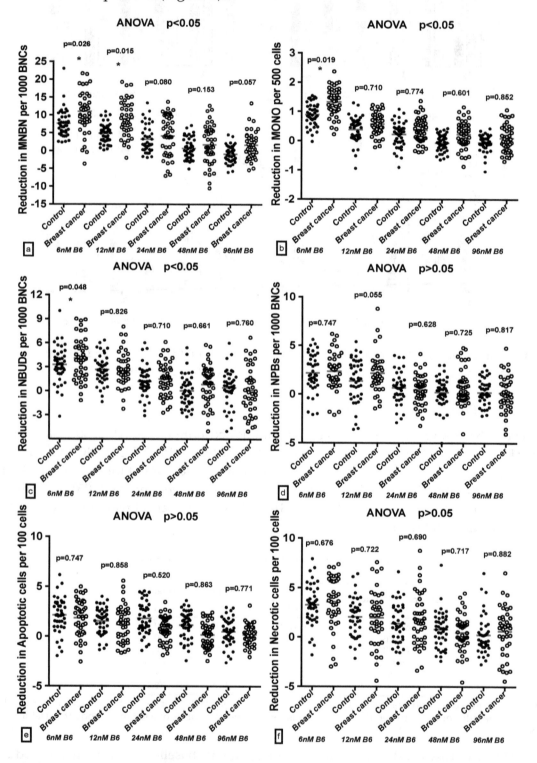

Figure 2. A comparison of reduction of: MNBN (**a**); MONO (**b**); NBUD (**c**); NPB (**d**); APO (**e**); and NEC (**f**) frequency between breast cancer cases and controls using DDA. The results represent the reduction in markers measured relative to 200 nmol/L mean $\pm$ SE.

2.5. The GSACV Indexes in Different SHMT C1420T, MS A2756G, and MTRR A66G Genotypes in Breast Cancer Cases and Controls at Various B6 Concentrations

There were significant differences in the GSACV indexes (MNBN, NPB, NBUD, APO and NEC) that were observed with the different *SHMT C1420T* genotypes at the same B6 concentration in the breast cancer cases. In contrast, no significant differences in the GSACV indexes (NPB, NBUD, MONO, APO and NEC) with the exception of MNBN, were observed with the different *SHMT C1420T* genotypes at the same B6 concentration in the control groups. There was a significant increase in the MNBN frequency for the *SHMT 1420CC* vs *SHMT 1420TT* genotypes at the same concentration of B6 (*p* < 0.001) in both the breast cancer cases and controls. The NBUD, APO, and NEC frequencies of *SHMT 1420CC* were higher than those of *SHMT 1420TT* at 6 and 12 nmol/L B6, while the NPB frequency of *SHMT 1420CC* was higher than that of *SHMT 1420TT* only at 6 nmol/L B6 in the breast cancer cases (Figures 3 and 4).

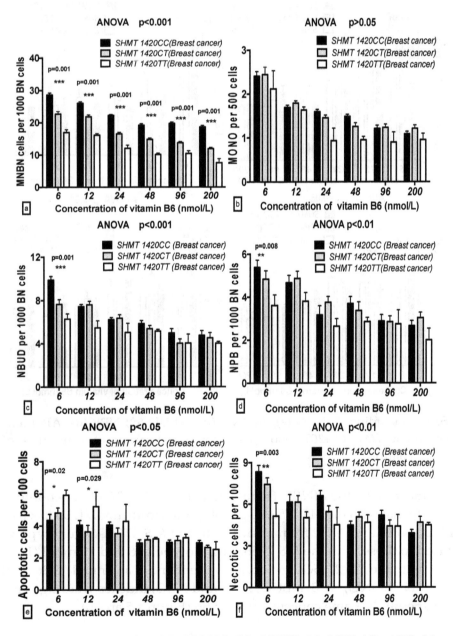

Figure 3. GSACV including: MNBN (**a**); MONO (**b**); NBUD (**c**); NPB (**d**); APO (**e**); and NEC (**f**) frequency in different *SHMT C1420T* genotypes of breast cancer cases at various concentrations of B6 (CC = 24, CT = 16, TT = 2 in breast cancer cases).

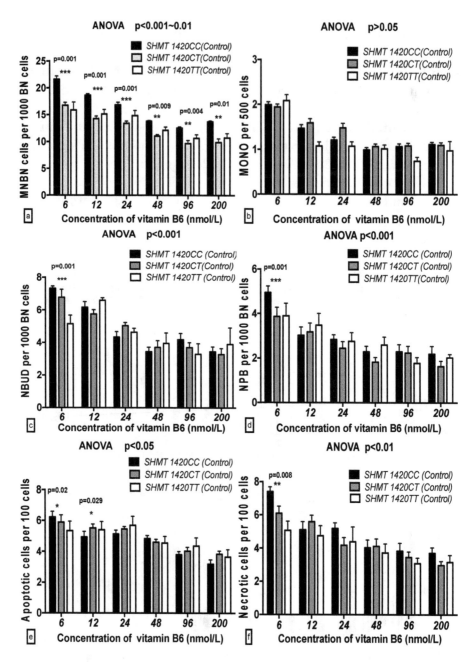

Figure 4. GSACV including: MNBN (**a**); MONO (**b**); NBUD (**c**); NPB (**d**); APO (**e**); and NEC (**f**) frequency in different *SHMT C1420T* genotypes of controls at various concentrations of B6 (*CC* = 17, *CT* = 19, *TT* = 6 in controls).

In the breast cancer cases, the MNBN frequency with the *MS 2756GG* genotype was significantly increased compared to that with the *MS 2756AA* genotype at 6 to 48 nmol/L B6 ($p < 0.001$–0.05), whereas the MONO, NBUD, NPB, and NEC frequencies with the *MS 2756GG* genotype were significantly enhanced compared to those with the *MS 2756AA* genotype at 6 and 12 nmol/L B6 ($p < 0.001$–0.05). The APO frequency with the *MS 2756GG* genotype was enhanced at 6 nmol/L B6. In the controls, none of the GSACV (MNBN, MONO, NPB, NBUD, APO and NEC) indexes were significantly different for the different genotypes at the same concentration of B6 (Figures 5 and 6).

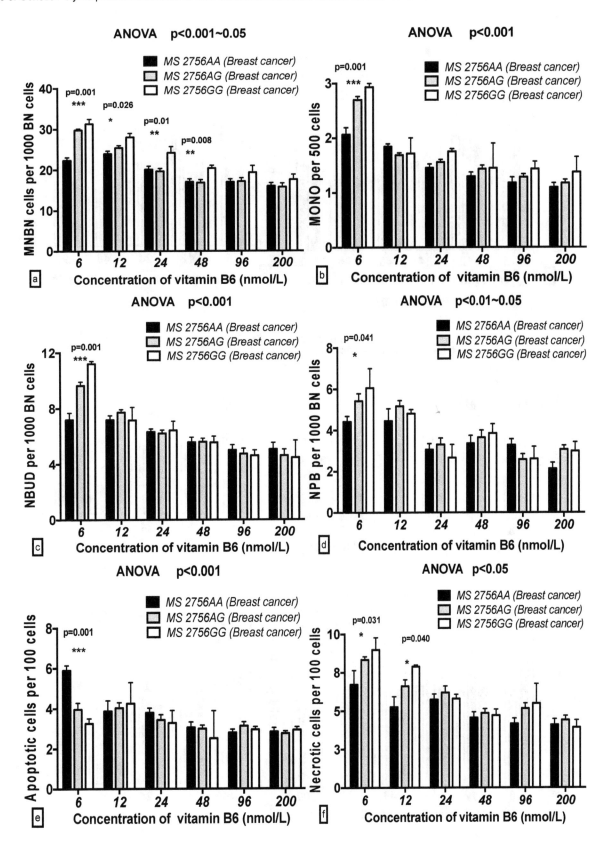

Figure 5. GSACV including: MNBN (**a**); MONO (**b**); NBUD (**c**); NPB (**d**); APO (**e**); and NEC (**f**) frequency in different *MS A2756G* genotypes of breast cancer cases at various B6 concentrations (*AA* = 15, *AG* = 25, *GG* = 2 in breast cancer cases).

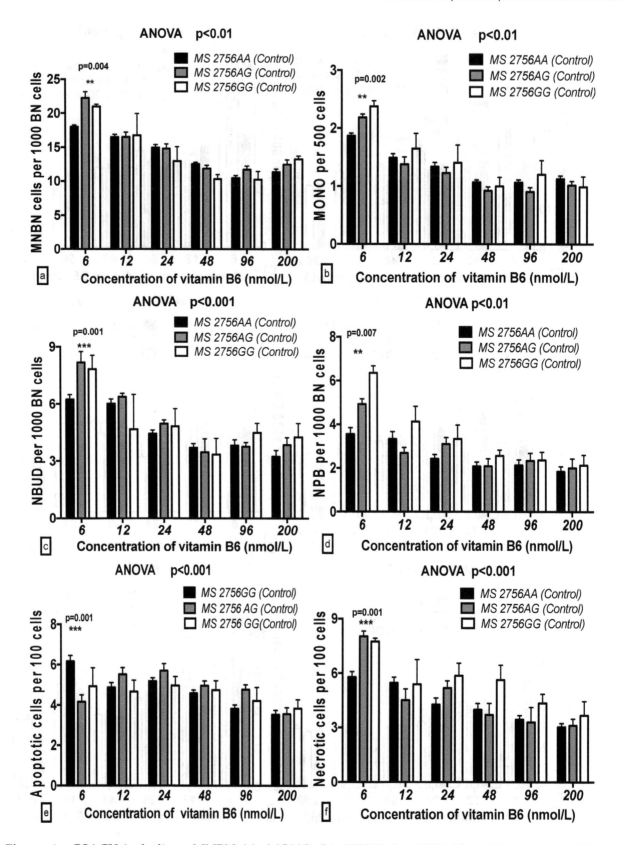

Figure 6. GSACV including: MNBN (**a**); MONO (**b**); NBUD (**c**); NPB (**d**); APO (**e**); and NEC (**f**) frequency in different *MS A2756G* genotypes of controls at various B6 concentrations (*AA* = 29, *AG* = 10, *GG* = 3 in controls).

The MNBN, MONO, and APO frequencies with the *MTRR 66GG* genotype were significantly increased compared to those with the *MTRR 66AA* genotype at 6 nmol/L B6 in both the breast cancer cases and controls. The NBUD frequency with the *MTRR 66AA* genotype was markedly decreased compared to that of *MTRR 66GG* at 6 nmol/L B6 only in the breast cancer cases and not in the controls (Figures 7 and 8).

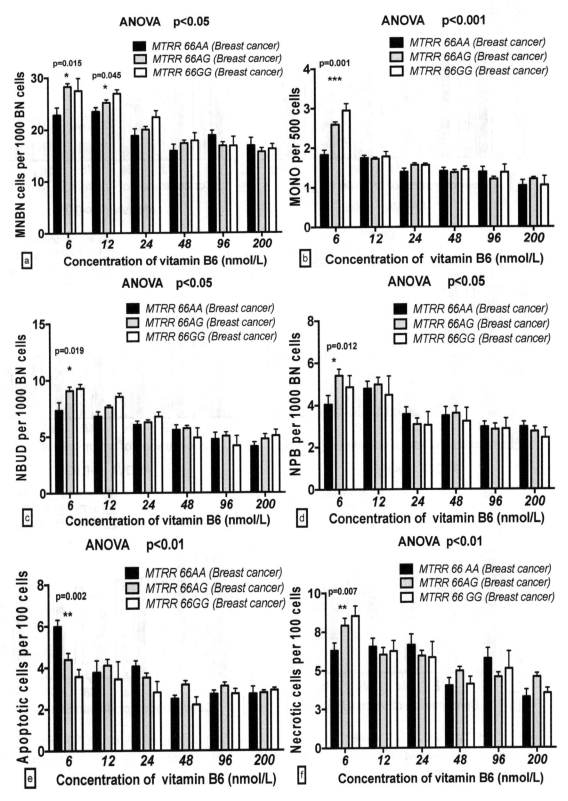

Figure 7. GSACV including: MNBN (**a**); MONO (**b**); NBUD (**c**); NPB (**d**); APO (**e**); and NEC (**f**) frequency in different *MTRR A66G* genotypes of breast cancer cases at various B6 concentrations (*AA* = 8, *AG* = 30, *GG* = 4 in breast cancer cases).

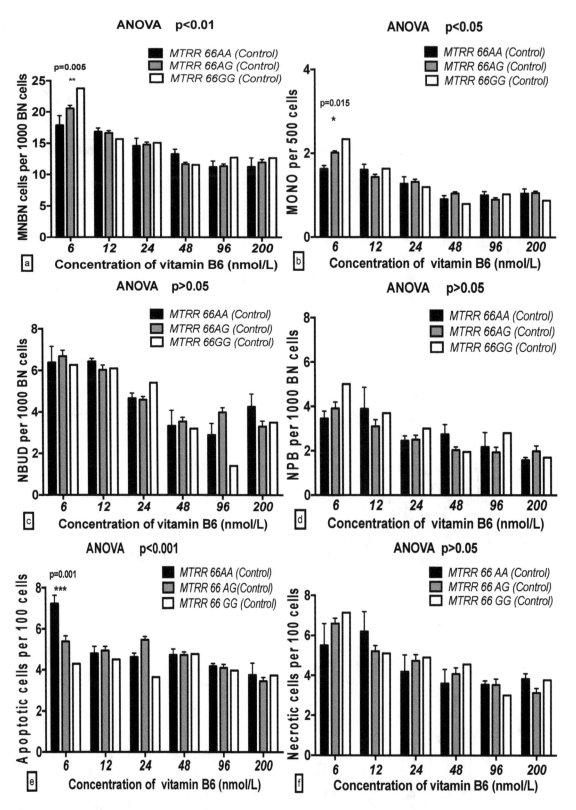

Figure 8. GSACV including: MNBN (**a**); MONO (**b**); NBUD (**c**); NPB (**d**); APO (**e**); and NEC (**f**) frequency in different *MTRR A66G* genotypes of controls at various B6 concentrations (*AA* = 5, *AG* = 36, *GG* = 1 in controls).

2.6. The Effects of the Strength and Variation Analysis of B6 and SHMT C1420T, MS A2756G, and MTRR A66G Polymorphisms on GSACV by Two-Way ANOVA

A two-way ANOVA indicated that the B6 concentration accounted for 36.07%, 20.81%, 30.42%, 41.87%, 19.88%, and 22.73% of the variance of the MNBN, NPB, NBUD, MONO, NEC, and APO frequencies, respectively ($p < 0.001$). However, the *SHMT C1420T* polymorphisms only explained 21.10%, 2.18%, and 2.31%, of the MNBN, MONO, and NEC frequencies ($p < 0.001$–0.01), respectively, in the controls. The B6 concentration accounted for 16.58%, 7.19%, 11.94%, 21.60%, 5.68%, and 13.09% of the variance of the MNBN, NPB, NBUD, MONO, NEC, and APO frequencies, respectively ($p < 0.001$). However, the *SHMT C1420T* polymorphisms only explained 30.36%, 1.56%, and 3.21% of the MNBN, MONO, and NBUD frequencies ($p < 0.001$–0.01), respectively, in the breast cancer cases. There was only an interaction between the B6 concentration and the *SHMT C1420T* polymorphisms for the NBUD biomarker in the breast cancer cases (Table 5).

The B6 concentration accounted for 28.45%, 20.23%, 17.77%, 35.30%, 18.19%, and 7.98% of the variance of the MNBN, NPB, NBUD, MONO, NEC, and APO frequencies, respectively ($p < 0.001$). However, the *MS A2756G* polymorphisms only explained 1.31%, 1.45%, and 2.76% of the MNBN, NBUD, and NPB frequencies ($p < 0.001$–0.01), respectively, in the controls. The B6 concentration accounted for 20.68%, 11.68%, 19.86%, 23.69%, 12.71%, and 6.98% of the variance of the MNBN, NPB, NBUD, MONO, NEC, and APO frequencies, respectively ($p < 0.001$). However, the *MS A2756G* polymorphisms only explained 2.89%, 2.23%, and 3.57% of the MNBN, MONO, and NEC frequencies ($p < 0.001$–0.01), respectively, in the breast cancer cases. There was an interaction between the B6 concentration and the *MS A2756G* polymorphisms for the MNBN, MONO, APO, and NEC biomarkers in the breast cancer cases and for the MNBN, MONO, NBUD, and APO biomarkers in the controls (Table 6).

The B6 concentration accounted for 13.79%, 17.03%, 10.03%, 11.74%, 5.09%, and 3.73% of the variance of the MNBN, NPB, NBUD, MONO, NEC, and APO frequencies, respectively ($p < 0.001$). However, there were no effects on the biomarkers for the *MTRR A66G* polymorphisms in the controls. The B6 concentration explained 26.69%, 11.95%, 25.31%, 32.47%, 17.72%, and 13.95% of the variance of the MNBN, NPB, NBUD, MONO, NEC, and APO frequencies, respectively ($p < 0.001$). However, the *MTRR A66G* polymorphisms only explained 1.40% and 1.44% of the MONO and NBUD frequencies ($p < 0.01$–0.05), respectively, in the breast cancer cases. There was only an interaction between the B6 concentration and the *MTRR A66G* polymorphisms for the NBUD biomarker in the breast cancer cases (Table 7).

Table 5. Effect contribution to the strength and variation analysis of B6 and *SHMT C1420T* polymorphisms on GSACV by two-way ANOVA analysis.

GSACV	MNBN			MONO			NBUD			NPB			APO			NEC		
	F	p	% of Variation	F	p	% of Variation	F	p	% of Variation	F	p	% of Variation	F	p	% of Variation	F	p	% of Variation
Controls																		
Genotype (*SHMT*)	97.87	0.001 ***	21.10	6.36	0.002 **	2.18	0.383	0.682	0.17	2.54	0.081	1.47	0.764	0.467	0.43	4.161	0.017 *	2.31
B6	66.92	0.001 ***	36.07	48.82	0.001 ***	41.87	26.88	0.001 ***	30.42	14.41	0.001 ***	20.81	16.32	0.001 ***	22.73	14.30	0.001 ***	19.88
B6-genotype interaction	1.677	0.087	1.81	1.83	0.056	3.14	1.755	0.07	3.97	0.78	0.647	2.25	0.82	0.609	2.29	1.009	0.436	2.81
Cases																		
Genotype (*SHMT*)	25.31	0.001 ***	30.36	4.788	0.009 **	1.56	8.286	0.001 ***	3.21	1.690	0.187	1.03	1.322	0.266	0.83	2.10	0.125	1.17
B6	49.97	0.001 ***	16.58	26.51	0.001 ***	21.6	12.33	0.001 ***	11.94	4.720	0.001 ***	7.19	8.377	0.001 ***	13.09	4.071	0.002 **	5.68
B6-genotype interaction	1.116	0.35	0.74	1.012	0.434	1.65	2.014	0.033*	3.90	0.478	0.904	1.46	0.839	0.591	2.62	1.30	0.232	3.63

*** $p < 0.001$; ** $p < 0.01$; * $p < 0.05$.

Table 6. Effect contribution to the strength and variation analysis of B6 and *MS A2756G* polymorphisms on GSACV by two-way ANOVA.

GSACV	MNBN			MONO			NBUD			NPB			APO			NEC		
	F	p	% of Variation	F	p	% of Variation	F	p	% of Variation	F	p	% of Variation	F	p	% of Variation	F	p	% of Variation
Controls																		
Genotype (MS)	5.134	0.007 **	1.31	2.147	0.119	0.76	3.334	0.037 *	1.45	4.775	0.009 **	2.76	0.289	0.749	0.16	4.174	0.017 *	2.18
B6	44.52	0.001 ***	28.45	39.95	0.001 ***	35.3	16.31	0.001 ***	17.77	14.01	0.001 ***	20.23	5.942	0.001 ***	7.98	13.93	0.001 ***	18.19
B6-genotype interaction	3.465	0.001 ***	4.43	1.89	0.046 *	3.35	1.615	0.103	3.52	1.621	0.101	4.68	3.653	0.001 ***	9.81	1.957	0.039 *	5.11
Cases																		
Genotype (MS)	10.33	0.001 ***	2.89	8.801	0.001 ***	2.23	1.766	0.173	0.72	2.256	0.107	1.28	2.637	0.078	1.54	6.208	0.002 **	3.57
B6	29.62	0.001 ***	20.68	37.41	0.001 ***	23.69	19.57	0.001 ***	19.86	8.249	0.001 ***	11.68	4.779	0.001 ***	6.98	8.837	0.001 ***	12.71
B6-genotype interaction	4.164	0.001 ***	5.81	3.507	0.001 ***	4.44	2.275	0.003 **	5.58	1.011	0.435	2.86	2.565	0.006 **	7.49	0.648	0.772	1.86

*** $p < 0.001$; ** $p < 0.01$; * $p < 0.05$.

Table 7. Effect contribution to the strength and variation analysis of B6 and *MTRR A66G* polymorphisms on GSACV by two-way ANOVA analysis.

GSACV	MNBN			MONO			NBUD			NPB			APO			NEC		
	F	p	% of Variation	F	p	% of Variation	F	p	% of Variation	F	p	% of Variation	F	p	% of Variation	F	p	% of Variation
Controls																		
Genotype (MTRR)	0.626	0.536	0.19	0.383	0.682	0.13	0.221	0.801	0.10	2.229	0.11	1.33	1.117	0.329	0.64	0.265	0.877	0.04
B6	18.01	0.001 ***	13.79	13.75	0.001 ***	11.74	9.152	0.001 ***	10.03	11.38	0.001 ***	17.03	2.618	0.025 *	3.37	3.534	0.004 **	5.09
B6-genotype interaction	1.105	0.360	1.69	1.193	0.296	2.04	0.866	0.566	1.90	0.924	0.512	2.76	1.595	0.109	4.55	0.517	0.937	1.49
Cases																		
Genotype (MTRR)	2.625	0.075	0.84	5.499	0.005 **	1.40	3.36	0.036 *	1.44	0.501	0.606	0.29	2.879	0.058	1.72	0.335	0.716	0.19
B6	33.38	0.001 ***	26.69	51.12	0.001 ***	32.47	23.67	0.001 ***	25.31	8.116	0.001 ***	11.95	9.355	0.001 ***	13.95	12.31	0.001 ***	17.72
B6-genotype interaction	1.949	0.040 *	3.12	4.457	0.001 ***	5.66	0.610	0.516	1.97	0.919	0.805	1.80	1.845	0.054	5.50	1.502	0.139	4.32

$*** \, p < 0.001; \, ** \, p < 0.01; \, * \, p < 0.05.$

3. Discussion

In the present study, we evaluated the response of the lymphocytes from women with breast cancer to B6 deficiency and gene-nutrient interactions by analyzing the induction of genomic damage and the effect of B6 on cell proliferation and viability. A deficiency of B6 increased genomic instability in binucleated cells. This was an expected result because folate and B6 have been shown to be connected to breast carcinogenesis [27,28]. B6, as a critical coenzyme, acts in two different steps of the folate metabolism pathway: one is the synthesis of 5,10-methylenetetrahydrofolate, which is crucial for DNA synthesis, DNA repair, and DNA methylation [29,30], and the other is the Hcy to glutathione catabolism, which plays vital roles in the detoxification as well as in the defense of cells from oxidative DNA damage [31]. Secondly, the results showed that cell viability increased at 24 nmol/L B6, indicating that proper B6 nutrition is a key determinant of cell growth and proliferation. The CBMN analysis is a thorough system for evaluating genomic damage, cytotoxicity, and cytostasis. Genomic damage events are marked especially in once-divided binucleated (BN) cells, which include three indexes: (a) the chromosome breakage and/or whole chromosome loss biomarker of micronuclei (MNi); (b) the DNA misrepair and/or telomere end-fusions biomarker of NPBs; and (c) the elimination of amplified DNA and/or DNA repair complexes biomarker of NBUDs. The cytostatic events are scored, including frequencies of mononucleated cells, binucleated cells, and multinucleated cells, and cytotoxic events are counted via necrotic and apoptotic cell proportions.

3.1. Influences of B6 on GSACV

We hypothesized that decline in the MNBN frequencies with increasing B6 concentration may be due to a slowdown of the cell proliferation speed or to the wear of strongly damaged cells [22–24]. Anyhow, the cells will not arrive at the mitotic telophase when MNBNs are marked in BN cells. The responses to DNA damage are serious and can decrease cell viability, and they can further induce the activation of surveillance systems, which either postpones cell cycle progression until the damaged DNA is repaired or eliminated, or induces apoptosis in case the damage is irreparable [32]. Additionally, we inspected whether the B6 deficiency-induced MNBNs from 9 day would be accompanied by a reduction in NVC and the NDI of the breast cancer cases and controls. Interestingly, our results showed that there was no difference in NDI among the different concentrations of B6. B6 deficiency cultures showed a regular progression through the cell cycle, which maintained the cells' proliferation ability without suffering either cell loss or the prospective mitotic delay regardless of the persistent DNA lesions [33,34].

We separately analyzed the pooled data from this study and verified that the B6 concentration correlated significantly negative with all of these markers of DNA damage and cell death. DNA damage was minimized at 48 to 200 nmol/L B6 in the breast cancer cases and controls; these concentrations are greater than those normally observed in plasma (20–40 nmol/L) [25]. Cell death was minimized at 24 to 200 nmol/L B6, which suggested that the B6 concentration in plasma may only maintain cell viability, but is not sufficient for maintaining genomic stability. We conclude that 48 nmol/L B6 is the optimal concentration for cell viability and genome stabilization in vitro. More interestingly, we observed that the MNBN, NPB, NBUD, and NEC frequencies correlated significantly and positively, suggesting that whole chromosomes or fragments that lag behind at anaphase may be related to increased chromosome rearrangement and gene amplification [35].

The notion that genetic susceptibility to carcinogenesis is connected to genomic instability was originally observed in rare disorders such as xeroderma pigmentosum and ataxia telangiectasia, which are associated with in vitro and in vivo chromosomal instability and defective DNA repair capacity [36]. The matched-pair Student's t-test revealed that the breast cancer status in the cases contributed to the variations in the measured biomarkers. The MNBN, NPB, NBUD, MONO, APO, and NEC frequencies in the cancer cases were markedly modified by the B6 concentrations as compared to the controls. This result suggests that breast cancer cases are more sensitive to B6 deficiency than matched controls, considering genomic instability and cell death, which stresses the possibility that

B6 may be more important to genome maintenance in cancer groups than in healthy groups. As there have been no studies to date on the relationship between B6 and genomic stability in breast cells, we cannot exclude the possibility that the sensitivities of lymphocyte cells and breast epithelium to B6 deficiency may be different and that the estrogen level in different individuals may have influenced our results. Therefore, future research on the effects of micronutrient deficiency on GSACV should be considered in breast cells, lymphocytes, and tumor patients by including different cancer cells, types of cells, and hormone expression levels.

3.2. Influences of Genetic Polymorphisms on GSACV

We examined the association between GSACV and three enzyme polymorphisms, *SHMT C1420T*, *MS A2756G*, and *MTRR A66G*, under B6 deficiency, which was based on functional polymorphisms and previous reports of associations with breast cancer risk. Functional polymorphisms in these genes may alter the availability of folate in the synthesis and methylation of DNA, and may consequently influence the susceptibility to cancer. To our knowledge, this is also the first report examining the association between *MTHFR C677T* polymorphisms and GSACV in a Chinese population, though the data are limited for most other populations [37].

In our study, we found an association between the individual *SHMT C1420T* polymorphism studied and genomic stability. *SHMT 1420TT* genotypes were found to have reduced DNA damage in the breast cancer cases and controls as compared to *CC* genotype. One key reason is that the variant SHMT enzyme may lead to accumulation of THF and reduced production of 5,10-methylene THF, although the exact biological effect of this phenomenon or the complete mechanism leading to DNA damage is not certain. Our previous study underlines the capacity of the *SHMT C1420T* polymorphism being able to directly reduce breast cancer risk. [14,38]. The study found risk reduction for the *SHMT 1420TT* genotype in malignant lymphomas [39], adult acute lymphocytic leukemia [40], and also in a wide spectrum of diseases including Parkinson's disease (PD), coronary artery disease (CAD) and systemic lupus erythematosus (SLE) [38]. These suggested that the reduction of DNA damage in the *SHMT 1420TT* genotype might be the main reason for the risk reduction of different cancers and a wide spectrum of diseases. The variant SHMT enzyme may result in decreased production of 5,10-methylene THF and decreased accumulation of THF, even though the accurate and complete biology mechanism leading to DNA damage is not recognized.

For the *MS 2756AG* polymorphism, increased GSCAV was found for the *AA* genotype as compared to the *GG* genotype. For *MTRR A66G*, the results indicated elevated GSACV for carriers of the homozygote wild-type genotype (*AA*) as compared to the other genotypes. The main reason for increased GSCAV is that the *A2756G* mutation in the *MS* gene leads to the Asp919Gly substitution in the MS enzyme, which further results in more valid production of methionine and remethylation and the elevation of Hcy, as well as DNA hypomethylation [41]. For *MTRR A66G*, it was revealed that the *66GG* genotype was inversely related to Hcy levels in plasma. Additionally, the mutation of *MTRR 66AG* easily showed the irregular methylation of DNA and abnormal nucleotide synthesis and altered repair. Our previous study showed that *MS 2756GG* and *MTRR 66GG* genotypes had significantly increased risk among Chinese women, which might be due to higher GSCAV.

3.3. Influences of Gene-Nutrient Interactions on GSACV

The interaction between *SHMT C1420T*, *MS A2756G*, and *MTRR A66G* polymorphisms and B6 deficiency was addressed in vitro with human lymphocytes cultured at different concentrations of B6. The different modifying effect of the *SHMT C1420T*, *MS A2756G*, and *MTRR A66G* polymorphisms on various cytogenetic markers may indicate that under B6 deprivation, MNi and NPBs arise through different mechanisms. The results suggest that B6, *SHMT C1420T*, and *MS A2756G* are three of the basic determining factors of lymphocyte growth in culture medium, while *MTRR A66G* has less effect on it. In addition, it is evident that the *SHMT 1420TT* and *MS 2756AA* genotypes provided a notable growth advantage over the *SHMT 1420CC* and *MS 2756GG* genotypes. The growth advantage of the

SHMT 1420TT, MS 2756AA, and *MTRR 66AA* genotypes may be concerned with decreased cell cycle delay, which may result from the NBUDs formation process which happens during S-phase [42–44]. The cells bearing *SHMT 1420TT, MS 2756AA,* and *MTRR 66AA* express significantly fewer NBUDs than *SHMT 1420CC, MS 2756GG,* and *MTRR 66GG* cells. An alternative interpretation is the slight reduction in the APO frequency in *SHMT 1420TT, MS 2756AA,* and *MTRR 66AA* cells compared with *SHMT 1420CC, MS 2756GG,* and *MTRR 66GG* cells. Lee et al. examined the relationship between polymorphisms of *MTHFR A1298C,* and *C677T, MTRR A66G* and *MTR A2756G* and non-obstructive male infertility in a Korean population. They found that *MTHFR C677T, MTRR A66G,* and *MS A2756G* genotypes were independently related to male infertility [45]. Ethnic differences, gender, geographic variation, the distribution of folate-related enzyme gene polymorphisms, as well as gene-nutrient, gene-environmental, and gene-ethnic interactions have been shown to influence the impact of GSACV.

There were limitations in the present study: (a) the sample number in this study is relatively small, especially the *MTRR 66GG* genotype of the controls which has only one subject, which could decrease the statistical credibility of finding divergence between breast cancer cases and controls; and (b) all samples were selected from one hospital and all samples were limited to females, which could not explain populations in other places and males. Therefore, a larger number of samples and geographic variation studies are greatly needed for studies in the future.

4. Materials and Methods

4.1. Cell Lines

The GM12593 and GM13705 cell lines are both human B lymphoblastoid cell lines. Both cell lines are from NIGMS Human Genetic Mutant Cell Bank (NIGMS Human Genetic Mutant Cell Repository), and were supplied by Prof. Michael Fenech, Adelaide, Australia. GM12593 came from the spleen of a 34-year-old Caucasian female, while GM13705 was derived from a 38-year-old Caucasian female carrying a positive family history of breast cancer and with a germline *BRCA1* mutation at exon 11, codon 1252. The mutation results in the production of a truncated protein [46].

4.2. Characteristics of the Study Population

Consent for our study was acquired from the Yunnan Scientific and Technological Committee and the National Natural Sciences Foundation of China (NSFC). All breast cancer cases and controls agreed to participate and provided written informed consent. Pathology tests were fulfilled, and a number of active manifestations were recruited from each patient. The breast cancer cases were randomly picked from January 2010 to April 2011 in the Third Affiliated Hospital of Kunming Medical College, Kunming, Yunnan, China. In view of the hospital chart number, the breast cancer cases included 42 females consecutively selected from subjects with a first confirmed histopathologic breast carcinoma diagnosis in the age range of 49.83 ± 13.6 years, and 42 female controls comprising individuals without a history of cancer with ages in the range of 43.15 ± 12.6 years were simultaneously recruited from the health examination clinics in the same hospital during the same study period. These samples are the same as in our previous study [14].

4.3. Genotyping Analysis

Peripheral blood lymphocytes were collected from each subject for CBMN assay. Genomic DNA was extracted from fresh or frozen whole blood using a commercially available FlexiGen DNA isolation kit (Qiagen, Valencia, CA, USA). Characteristics of the studied polymorphisms of *SHMT C1420T, MS A2756G,* and *MTRR A66G* are reported in our previous study [14]. All genotypes were determined by PCR-based assays followed by RFLP analysis according to published methods [14,47–49]. In addition, for internal quality control, 90% of samples were repeated. The genotypes of *SHMT 1420CC/MTRR 66AA/MS 2756AA* were defined as wild homozygous, *SHMT 1420CT/MTRR 66AG/MS 2756AG* as mutant heterozygous, and *SHMT 1420TT/MTRR 66GG/MS 2756GG* as mutant homozygous.

4.4. Cell Lines and Lymphocytes Culture

Before culturing, GM13705 and GM12593 cell lines were washed with fresh Hank's balanced salt solution (HBSS, Biochrom AG, Berlin, Germany) three times. Cells were prepared at a concentration of 0.25×10^6 viable cells/mL for 2 mL volumes in Roswell Park Memorial Institute Medium (RPMI) 1640 culture medium containing doses of B6 (0, 6, 12, 24, 48, 96, and 200 nmol/L). B6 in regular RPMI 1640 medium (4800 nmol/L) was used as a control. The lymphocytes were cultured at 0.5×10^6 viable cells/mL in 2 mL volume in RPMI 1640 culture medium containing different doses of B6 (6, 12, 24, 48, 96, and 200 nmol/L). Mitogenesis was stimulated by the addition of phytohaemagglutinin (45 g/mL) (PHA; Murex Biotech, Kent, UK) and cultures were incubated at 37 °C and 5% CO_2 in a humidified incubator. After 3 days, cell number and viability were determined using a Coulter counter and Trypan blue exclusion, respectively. The cultures were continued in 4.7 mL fresh medium and 0.3 mL "conditioned" medium from the previous 3-day culture with 0.5×10^6 viable cells/mL. The components of fresh medium were the same as above but without PHA. Medium change was repeated at 6 days post-PHA treatment and a final viable cell count was measured on day 9. On the eighth day post-PHA treatment, two 750 µL aliquots of each culture were transferred to 6 mL culture tubes for the CBMN. Cytochalasin B (4.5 g/mL; Sigma Chemical Co., Darmstadt, Germany) was added to each tube and approximately 28 h later cells were harvested onto microscope slides using a cyto-centrifuge (Shandon Southern Products, Cheshire, UK). All other constituents of the medium were standard for RPMI 1640 and CBMN assay was performed as previously described [14,50,51]. All experiments in this study were conducted in the dark to avoid light influences.

4.5. Statistical Analysis

The results for comparison of GSACV with different B6 concentrations in the breast cancer cases or controls were compared using a one-way ANOVA. The GSACV of two groups were compared using the matched-pair Student's t-test. The significant differences between B6 and genotype were determined by a repeated-measure two-way ANOVA. The differences in sensitivity to B6 deficiency between the breast cancer and control groups were determined using a DDA [26]. The mean values of the GSACS indexes for the breast cancer cases and controls with different genotypes under various concentrations of B6 were determined using the Newman-Keuls ANOVA post-test (two-tailed). The graphical analysis and statistical analyses were conducted using the Prism 6.0 software (GraphPad, San Diego, CA, USA) and SPSS Statistical Package,Version 12.0 (IBM SPSS Inc., Chicago, IL, USA).

5. Conclusions

In conclusion, this research indicates that B6 deficiency induces the formation of MNBNs, NPBs, and NBUDs, decreases APO and increases NEC frequencies in vitro, which shows that it may be a risk factor for cancer by inducing genomic instability/hypermutability/gene amplification in cells via chromosome breakage/rearrangement and breakage-fusion-bridge cycles. Human genome instability can be induced by vitamin B6 deficiency, and 48 nmol/L B6 was the most suitable concentration to maintain genomic stability in lymphocytes in vitro. Although in vitro conditions might not precisely estimate internal B6 requirements, these conditions offer a valuable guideline for the optimal concentration range to maintain genome health. Breast cancer patients are more sensitive to B6 deficiency than controls with respect to genomic stability, suggesting that a low intake of B6 in the long term could increase DNA damage and further exacerbate genomic instability. Adequate B6 intake was believed to be beneficial for breast cancer prevention. In addition, this research showed that the *SHMT C1420T* mutation may reduce breast cancer susceptibility. In contrast, the *MS A2756G* and *MTRR A66G* mutations may increase breast cancer susceptibility, but the role of polymorphisms in *SHMT*, *MS*, and *MTRR* in genome stability is reduced compared to that of B6, which is consistent with our previous results [17]. These results suggest that individuals with various genotypes have different sensitivities to B6 deficiency. FMOCM metabolic enzyme gene polymorphisms may be associated with breast cancer.

Acknowledgments: This research was supported by the National Natural Science Foundation of China (Project No. 31260268 and 31560307), the cooperative project with the United Gene High-Tech Group, the Yunnan Normal University Ph.D. Startup Project and China Scholarship Council (CSC).

Author Contributions: Xiayu Wu was responsible for the majority of this work, including the execution of experiments, data analysis, and writing and publication of this report; Weijiang Xu performed CBMN and genotype analysis; Tao Zhou contributed to cell culture; Neng Cao provided some of the data analysis and spell revision; Juan Ni provided instructions and data proofreading; Tianning Zou was responsible for providing samples; Ziqing Liang performed proofreading; and Xu Wang and Michael Fenech were the corresponding authors and were responsible for the overall work, including the experiments and publication. All authors have read and approved the final manuscript.

References

1. Cheng, T.Y.; Makar, K.W.; Neuhouser, M.L.; Miller, J.W.; Song, X.; Brown, E.C.; Beresford, S.A.; Zheng, Y.; Poole, E.M.; Galbraith, R.L.; et al. Folate-mediated one-carbon metabolism genes and interactions with nutritional factors on colorectal cancer risk: Women's Health Initiative Observational Study. *Cancer* **2015**, *121*, 3684–3691. [CrossRef] [PubMed]

2. Zeng, F.F.; Liu, Y.T.; Lin, X.L.; Fan, Y.Y.; Zhang, X.L.; Xu, C.H.; Chen, Y.M. Folate, vitamin B6, vitamin B12 and methionine intakes and risk for nasopharyngeal carcinoma in Chinese adults: A matched case-control study. *Br. J. Nutr.* **2016**, *115*, 121–128. [CrossRef] [PubMed]

3. Rajdl, D.; Racek, J.; Trefil, L.; Stehlik, P.; Dobra, J.; Babuska, V. Effect of Folic Acid, Betaine, Vitamin B6, and Vitamin B12 on Homocysteine and Dimethylglycine Levels in Middle-Aged Men Drinking White Wine. *Nutrients* **2016**, *8*, E34. [CrossRef] [PubMed]

4. Gong, Z.; Yao, S.; Zirpoli, G.; David Cheng, T.Y.; Roberts, M.; Khoury, T.; Ciupak, G.; Davis, W.; Pawlish, K.; Jandorf, L.; et al. Genetic variants in one-carbon metabolism genes and breast cancer risk in European American and African American women. *Int. J. Cancer* **2015**, *137*, 666–677. [CrossRef] [PubMed]

5. Assies, J.; Mocking, R.J.; Lok, A.; Koeter, M.W.; Bockting, C.L.; Visser, I.; Pouwer, F.; Ruhé, H.G.; Schene, A.H. Erythrocyte fatty acid profiles and plasma homocysteine, folate and vitamin B6 and B12 in recurrent depression: Implications for co-morbidity with cardiovascular disease. *Psychiatry Res.* **2015**, *229*, 992–998. [CrossRef] [PubMed]

6. Bourquin, F.; Capitani, G.; Grütter, M.G. PLP-dependent enzymes as entry and exit gates of sphingolipid metabolism. *Protein Sci.* **2011**, *20*, 1492–1508. [CrossRef] [PubMed]

7. Bessler, H.; Djaldetti, M. Vitamin B6 Modifies the Immune Cross-Talk between Mononuclear and Colon Carcinoma Cells. *Folia Biol. (Praha)* **2016**, *62*, 47–52. [PubMed]

8. Zuo, H.; Ueland, P.M.; Eussen, S.J.; Tell, G.S.; Vollset, S.E.; Nygård, O.; Midttun, Ø.; Meyer, K.; Ulvik, A. Markers of vitamin B6 status and metabolism as predictors of incident cancer: The Hordaland Health Study. *Int. J. Cancer* **2015**, *136*, 2932–2939. [CrossRef] [PubMed]

9. Ferrari, A.; de Carvalho, A.M.; Steluti, J.; Teixeira, J.; Marchioni, D.M.; Aguiar, S., Jr. Folate and nutrients involved in the 1-carbon cycle in the pretreatment of patients for colorectal cancer. *Nutrients* **2015**, *7*, 4318–4335. [CrossRef] [PubMed]

10. Matsubara, K.; Komatsu, S.; Oka, T.; Kato, N. Vitamin B6-mediated suppression of colon tumorigenesis, cell proliferation, and angiogenesis (review). *J. Nutr. Biochem.* **2003**, *14*, 246–250. [CrossRef]

11. Matsubara, K.; Matsumoto, H.; Mizushina, Y.; Lee, J.S.; Kato, N. Inhibitory effect of pyridoxal 5′-phosphate on endothelial cell proliferation, replicative DNA polymerase and DNA topoisomerase. *Int. J. Mol. Med.* **2003**, *12*, 51–55. [CrossRef] [PubMed]

12. Fenech, M.; Kirsch-Volders, M.; Natarajan, A.T. Molecular mechanisms of micronucleus, nucleoplasmic bridge and nuclear bud formation in mammalian and human cells. *Mutagenesis* **2010**, *26*, 125–132. [CrossRef] [PubMed]

13. Jiang, S.; Li, J.; Zhang, Y.; Venners, S.A.; Tang, G.; Wang, Y.; Li, Z.; Xu, X.; Wang, B.; Huo, Y. Methylenetetrahydrofolate Reductase C677T Polymorphism, Hypertension, and Risk of Stroke: A Prospective, Nested Case-Control Study. *Int. J. Neurosci.* **2016**, *29*, 1–22. [CrossRef] [PubMed]

14. Wu, X.; Zou, T.; Cao, N.; Ni, J.; Xu, W.; Zhou, T.; Wang, X. Plasma homocysteine levels and genetic polymorphisms in folate metabolism are associated with breast cancer risk in Chinese women. *Hered. Cancer Clin. Pract.* **2014**, *12*, 1198–1206. [CrossRef] [PubMed]

15. Li, X.Y.; Ye, J.Z.; Ding, X.P.; Zhang, X.H.; Ma, T.J.; Zhong, R.; Ren, H.Y. Association between methionine synthase reductase A66G polymorphism and primary infertility in Chinese males. *Genet. Mol. Res.* **2015**, *14*, 3491–3500. [CrossRef] [PubMed]

16. Hou, N.; Chen, S.; Chen, F.; Jiang, M.; Zhang, J.; Yang, Y.; Zhu, B.; Bai, X.; Hu, Y.; Huang, H.; et al. Association between premature ovarian failure, polymorphisms in MTHFR and MTRR genes and serum homocysteine concentration. *Reprod. Biomed.* **2016**, *32*, 407–413. [CrossRef] [PubMed]

17. Zwart, S.R.; Gregory, J.F.; Zeisel, S.H.; Gibson, C.R.; Mader, T.H.; Kinchen, J.M.; Ueland, P.M.; Ploutz-Snyder, R.; Heer, M.A.; Smith, S.M. Genotype, B-vitamin status, and androgens affect spaceflight-induced ophthalmic changes. *FASEB J.* **2016**, *30*, 141–148. [CrossRef] [PubMed]

18. Liu, K.; Zhao, R.; Shen, M.; Ye, J.; Li, X.; Huang, Y.; Hua, L.; Wang, Z.; Li, J. Role of genetic mutations in folate-related enzyme genes on Male Infertility. *Sci. Rep.* **2015**, *5*, 15548. [CrossRef] [PubMed]

19. Agnoli, C.; Grioni, S.; Krogh, V.; Pala, V.; Allione, A.; Matullo, G.; di Gaetano, C.; Tagliabue, G.; Pedraglio, S.; Garrone, G.; et al. Plasma Riboflavin and Vitamin B-6, but Not Homocysteine, Folate, or Vitamin B-12, Are Inversely Associated with Breast Cancer Risk in the European Prospective Investigation into Cancer and Nutrition-Varese Cohort. *J. Nutr.* **2016**. [CrossRef] [PubMed]

20. Galluzzi, L.; Vacchelli, E.; Michels, J.; Garcia, P.; Kepp, O.; Senovilla, L.; Vitale, I.; Kroemer, G. Effects of vitamin B6 metabolism on oncogenesis, tumor progression and therapeutic responses. *Oncogene* **2013**, *32*, 4995–5004. [CrossRef] [PubMed]

21. Cancarini, I.; Krogh, V.; Agnoli, C.; Grioni, S.; Matullo, G.; Pala, V.; Pedraglio, S.; Contiero, P.; Riva, C.; Muti, P.; et al. Micronutrients Involved in One-Carbon Metabolism and Risk of Breast Cancer Subtypes. *PLoS ONE* **2015**, *10*, e0138318. [CrossRef] [PubMed]

22. Wu, X.Y.; Ni, J.; Xu, W.J.; Zhou, T.; Wang, X. Interactions between MTHFR C677T-A1298C variants and folic acid deficiency affect breast cancer risk in a Chinese population. *Asian Pac. J. Cancer Prev.* **2012**, *13*, 2199–2206. [CrossRef] [PubMed]

23. Wu, X.Y.; Cheng, J.; Lu, L. Vitamin B12 and methionine deficiencies induce genome damage measured using the cytokinesis-block micronucleus cytome assay in human B lymphoblastoid cell lines. *Nutr. Cancer* **2013**, *65*, 866–873. [CrossRef] [PubMed]

24. Wu, X.Y.; Liang, Z.; Zou, T.; Wang, X. Effects of folic acid deficiency and MTHFRC677T polymorphisms on cytotoxicity in human peripheral blood lymphocytes. *Biochem. Biophys. Res. Commun.* **2009**, *379*, 732–737. [CrossRef] [PubMed]

25. Herrmann, M. *Vitamins in the Prevention of Human Diseases*; Walter de Gruyter GmbH & Co. KG.: Berlin, Germany; New York, NY, USA, 2011; pp. 305–307.

26. Andrew, J.V.; Douglas, G.A. Analysing controlled trials with baseline and follow up measurements. *Br. Med. J.* **2001**, *323*, 1123–1124.

27. Gong, Z.; Ambrosone, C.B.; McCann, S.E.; Zirpoli, G.; Chandran, U.; Hong, C.C.; Bovbjerg, D.H.; Jandorf, L.; Ciupak, G.; Pawlish, K.; et al. Associations of dietary folate, Vitamins B6 and B12 and methionine intake with risk of breast cancer among African American and European American women. *Int. J. Cancer* **2014**, *134*, 1422–1435. [CrossRef] [PubMed]

28. Pirouzpanah, S.; Taleban, F.A.; Mehdipour, P.; Atri, M. Association of folate and other one-carbon related nutrients with hypermethylation status and expression of RARB, BRCA1, and RASSF1A genes in breast cancer patients. *J. Mol. Med.* **2015**, *93*, 917–934. [CrossRef] [PubMed]

29. Jung, A.Y.; van Duijnhoven, F.J.; Nagengast, F.M.; Botma, A.; Heine-Bröring, R.C.; Kleibeuker, J.H.; Vasen, H.F.; Harryvan, J.L.; Winkels, R.M.; Kampman, E. Dietary B vitamin and methionine intake and MTHFR C677T genotype on risk of colorectal tumors in Lynch syndrome: the GEOLynch cohort study. *Cancer Causes Control* **2014**, *25*, 1119–1129. [CrossRef] [PubMed]

30. Kune, G.; Watson, L. Colorectal cancer protective effects and the dietary micronutrients folate, methionine, vitamins B6, B12, C, E, selenium, and lycopene. *Nutr. Cancer* **2006**, *56*, 11–21. [CrossRef] [PubMed]

31. Shen, J.; Lai, C.Q.; Mattei, J. Association of vitamin B-6 status with inflammation, oxidative stress, and chronic inflammatory conditions: The Boston Puerto Rican Health Study. *Am. J. Clin. Nutr.* **2010**, *91*, 337–342. [CrossRef] [PubMed]

32. Bodakuntla, S.; Libi, A.V.; Sural, S.; Trivedi, P.; Lahiri, M. N-nitroso-N-ethylurea activates DNA damage surveillance pathways and induces transformation in mammalian cells. *BMC Cancer* **2014**, *14*, 287. [CrossRef] [PubMed]

33. Takeuchi, P.L.; Antunes, L.M.; Takahashi, C.S. Evaluation of the clastogenicity and anticlastogenicity of vitamin B6 in human lymphocyte cultures. *Toxicol. Vitr.* **2007**, *21*, 665–670. [CrossRef] [PubMed]

34. Sharp, A.A.; Fedorovich, Y. Teratogenic effects of pyridoxine on the spinal cord and dorsal root ganglia of embryonic chickens. *Neuroscience* **2015**, *289*, 233–241. [CrossRef] [PubMed]

35. Fenech, M.; Crott, J.W. Micronuclei, nucleoplasmic bridges and nuclear buds induced in folic acid deficient human lymphocytes-evidence for breakage-fusion-bridge cycles in the cytokinesis-block micronucleus assay. *Mutat. Res.* **2002**, *504*, 131–136. [CrossRef]

36. El-Zein, R.; Vral, A.; Etzel, C.J. Cytokinesis-blocked micronucleus assay and cancer risk assessment. *Mutagenesis* **2011**, *26*, 101–106. [CrossRef] [PubMed]

37. Yilmaz, M.; Kacan, T.; Sari, I.; Kilickap, S. Lack of association between the MTHFRC677T polymorphism and lung cancer in a Turkish population. *Asian Pac. J. Cancer Prev.* **2014**, *15*, 6333–6337. [CrossRef] [PubMed]

38. Naushad, S.M.; Vijayalakshmi, S.V.; Rupasree, Y.; Kumudini, N.; Sowganthika, S.; Naidu, J.V.; Ramaiah, M.J.; Rao, D.N.; Kutala, V.K. Multifactor dimensionality reduction analysis to elucidate the cross-talk between one-carbon and xenobiotic metabolic pathways in multi-disease models. *Mol. Biol. Rep.* **2015**, *42*, 1211–1224. [CrossRef] [PubMed]

39. Hishida, A.; Matsuo, K.; Hamajima, N.; Ito, H.; Ogura, M.; Kagami, Y.; Taji, H.; Morishima, Y.; Emi, N.; Tajima, K. Associations between polymorphisms in the thymidylate synthase and serine hydroxymethyltransferase genes and susceptibility to malignant lymphoma. *Haematologica* **2003**, *88*, 159–166. [PubMed]

40. Skibola, C.F.; Smith, M.T.; Hubbard, A.; Shane, B.; Roberts, A.C.; Law, G.R.; Rollinson, S.; Roman, E.; Cartwright, R.A.; Morgan, G.J. Polymorphisms in the thymidylate synthase and serine hydroxymethyltransferase genes and risk of adult acute lymphocytic leukemia. *Blood* **2002**, *99*, 3786–3791. [CrossRef] [PubMed]

41. Matsuo, K.; Suzuki, R.; Hamajima, N.; Ogura, M.; Kagami, Y.; Taji, H.; Kondoh, E.; Maeda, S.; Asakura, S.; Kaba, S.; et al. Association between polymorphisms of folate- and methionine-metabolizing enzymes and susceptibility to malignant lymphoma. *Blood* **2001**, *97*, 3205–3209. [CrossRef] [PubMed]

42. Tsuchiya, D.; Lacefield, S. Cdk1 modulation ensures the coordination of cell-cycle events during the switch from meiotic prophase to mitosis. *Curr. Biol.* **2013**, *23*, 1505–1513. [CrossRef] [PubMed]

43. Thomas, P.; Fenech, M. Buccal Cytome Biomarkers and Their Association with Plasma Folate, Vitamin B12 and Homocysteine in Alzheimer's Disease. *J. Nutrigenet. Nutrigenom.* **2015**, *8*, 57–69. [CrossRef] [PubMed]

44. Fenech, M.; Holland, N.; Zeiger, E.; Chang, W.P.; Burgaz, S.; Thomas, P.; Bolognesi, C.; Knasmueller, S.; Kirsch-Volders, M.; Bonassi, S. The HUMN and HUMNxL international collaboration projects on human micronucleus assays in lymphocytes and buccal cells—Past, present and future. *Mutagenesis* **2011**, *26*, 239–245. [CrossRef] [PubMed]

45. Lee, H.C.; Jeong, Y.M.; Lee, S.H.; Cha, K.Y.; Song, S.H.; Kim, N.K.; Lee, K.W.; Lee, S. Association study of four polymorphisms in three folate-related enzyme genes with non-obstructive male infertility. *Hum. Reprod.* **2006**, *21*, 3162–3170. [CrossRef] [PubMed]

46. Aressy, B.; Greenberg, R.A. DNA Damage: Placing BRCA1 in the Proper Context. *Curr. Biol.* **2012**, *22*, R806–R808. [CrossRef] [PubMed]

47. Vaughn, J.D.; Bailey, L.B.; Shelnutt, K.P.; Dunwoody, K.M.; Maneval, D.R.; Davis, S.R.; Quinlivan, E.P.; Gregory, J.F., 3rd; Theriaque, D.W.; Kauwell, G.P. Methionine synthase reductase 66A→G polymorphism is associated with increased plasma homocysteine concentration when combined with the homozygous methylenetetrahydrofolate reductase 677C→T variant. *J. Nutr.* **2004**, *134*, 2985–2990. [PubMed]

48. Scazzone, C., Acuto, S.; Guglielmini, E.; Campisi, G.; Bono, A. Methionine synthase reductase (MTRR) A66G polymorphism is not related to plasma homocysteine concentration and the risk for vascular disease. *Exp. Mol. Pathol.* **2009**, *86*, 131–133. [CrossRef] [PubMed]

49. Lightfoot, T.J.; Johnston, W.T.; Painter, D.; Simpson, J.; Roman, E.; Skibola, C.F.; Smith, M.T.; Allan, J.M.; Taylor, G.M.; United Kingdom Childhood Cancer Study. Genetic variation in the folate metabolic pathway and risk of childhood leukemia. *Blood* **2010**, *115*, 3923–3929. [CrossRef] [PubMed]

50. Moore, G.E.; Woods, L.K. Culture media for human cells—RPMI 1603, RPMI 1634, RPMI 1640 and GEM 1717. *Methods Cell Sci.* **1977**, *3*, 503–509. [CrossRef]

51. Fenech, M. Cytokinesis-block micronucleus assay evolves into a "cytome" assay of chromosomal instability, mitotic dysfunction and cell death. *Mutat. Res.* **2006**, *600*, 58–66. [CrossRef] [PubMed]

4

Potential Links between Impaired One-Carbon Metabolism Due to Polymorphisms, Inadequate B-Vitamin Status, and the Development of Alzheimer's Disease

Barbara Troesch *, Peter Weber and M. Hasan Mohajeri

DSM Nutritional Products Ltd., Wurmisweg 576, Kaiseraugst 4303, Switzerland;
peter.weber@dsm.com (P.W.); hasan.mohajeri@dsm.com (M.H.M.)
* Correspondence: barbara.troesch@dsm.com

Abstract: Alzheimer's disease (AD) is the major cause of dementia and no preventive or effective treatment has been established to date. The etiology of AD is poorly understood, but genetic and environmental factors seem to play a role in its onset and progression. In particular, factors affecting the one-carbon metabolism (OCM) are thought to be important and elevated homocysteine (Hcy) levels, indicating impaired OCM, have been associated with AD. We aimed at evaluating the role of polymorphisms of key OCM enzymes in the etiology of AD, particularly when intakes of relevant B-vitamins are inadequate. Our review indicates that a range of compensatory mechanisms exist to maintain a metabolic balance. However, these become overwhelmed if the activity of more than one enzyme is reduced due to genetic factors or insufficient folate, riboflavin, vitamin B6 and/or vitamin B12 levels. Consequences include increased Hcy levels and reduced capacity to synthetize, methylate and repair DNA, and/or modulated neurotransmission. This seems to favor the development of hallmarks of AD particularly when combined with increased oxidative stress e.g., in apolipoprotein E (ApoE) ε4 carriers. However, as these effects can be compensated at least partially by adequate intakes of B-vitamins, achieving optimal B-vitamin status for the general population should be a public health priority.

Keywords: homocysteine; dementia; Alzheimer's disease; nutrition; one-carbon metabolism; B-vitamins; polymorphism; prevention; therapy

1. Introduction

Alzheimer's disease (AD) is the most frequent type of dementia, causing around two-thirds of cases [1]. The condition becomes more common with increasing age, affecting between 5% and 8%, 15% and 20%, and 25% and 50% of those in the age groups $\geq$65 years, $\geq$75 years and $\geq$85 years, respectively [1]. The number of people aged $\geq$65 years is estimated to increase from ~500 million in 2008 to ~1.3 billion in 2040 [2]. A significant increase in absolute numbers, but also in the proportion of the population affected by the disease, is expected for the coming decades. In Europe, the predicted increase in numbers of individuals with dementia from ~36 million in 2010 to ~115 million in 2050 will result in an around €250 billion health care cost with respect to the condition by 2030 [1]. In the U.S., the cost is projected to exceed $1 trillion by 2050 if the disease continues to progress at its current pace [3]. Even more importantly, despite intensive research, there is currently no treatment available to cure or reverse AD [4]. This is reflected in the alarming mortality rates: for diseases such as human immunodeficiency virus, cardiovascular disease (CVD) and some cancers, important decreases in the death rate were achieved between 2000 and 2010, while for AD, the death rate increased by nearly 70% during the same period [5].

While many questions remain concerning its etiology, treatment is further complicated by the early onset of neuro-pathological changes: postmortem studies have revealed specific hallmarks of AD such as amyloid plaque formations in cognitively normal elderly [6]. It has been postulated that they develop decades before even mild symptoms of dementia manifest [7]. By the time the disease is diagnosed, cellular damage and amyloid plaque deposition might therefore already be too advanced for treatment to be successful [8,9]. Consequently, preventing the development o AD seems to be a promising avenue for improving health and quality of life for the elderly and to reduce the burden for society.

For a preventive approach to be successful, a better understanding of risk factors for AD is crucial. Some rare genetic mutations have been identified as the cause of early onset of the disease [10], but only a relatively small fraction of cases falls into this category. We will therefore concentrate on the significantly more common late-onset type, which is thought to be triggered by a combination of genetic, epigenetic and environmental factors [11]. It has been well established that apolipoprotein E (ApoE) is a very important genetic risk factor for age-dependent chronic diseases, including CVD and AD [12]. Due to two major polymorphisms on the encoding exon 4 of this gene, three major protein isoforms, ApoE ε2, ApoE ε3 and ApoE ε4 exist [13]. It has been shown that homozygous carriers of the ApoE ε4 allele have a more than 10-fold increased risk of developing AD, possibly due to increased cholesterol levels, altered brain development early in life [12] or increased oxidative brain damage [14].

Environmental factors such as nutrition seem to play a role in the development of the disease [11 In particular, some B-vitamins are thought to be implicated, even though the mechanism linking low status of B-vitamins and the development of AD is poorly understood. However, it seems that elevated levels of homocysteine (Hcy), a non-protein sulfur-containing amino acid implicated in the etiology of a range of medical conditions such as CVD [15], play an important role. Insufficiency of B-vitamins may also affect the development of the diseases via their role in DNA methylation [16], synthesis and/or repair [17] or in modulating neurotransmission [18]. Polymorphisms in genes encoding for specific enzymes can significantly affect their activity [19]. Therefore, studying mutations at critical steps in the metabolism of B-vitamins might help resolve some of the inconsistencies reported for their protective effect on the development of AD. Our aim is to evaluate the role of common polymorphisms of key enzymes in one-carbon metabolism (OCM; See Table 1) in the etiology of AD, particularly when intakes of the relevant B-vitamins are inadequate.

Table 1. Polymorphisms relating to key enzymes in the one-carbon metabolism that are potentially relevant to the development of Alzheimer's disease (AD).

Enzyme	Polymorphism	Reference
MTHFR	C677T A1298C T1317C	Schwahn and Rozen 2001 [20], Yamada et al., 2001 [21], Guenther et al., 1999 [22] Weisberg et al., 2001 [23] Weisberg et al., 1998 [24]
MS	A2756G	Leclerc et al., 1996 [25], Chen et al., 1997 [26]
MSR	A66G C524T	Olteanu et al., 2002 [27] Olteanu et al., 2002 [27]
CBS	68 bp insertion at exon 8 G9276A 31 bp variable number of tandem repeats	Sebastio et al., 1995 [28] Nienaber-Rousseau et al., 2013 [29] Lievers et al., 2001 [30]
SHMT	C1420T	Heil et al., 2001 [31]

bp: base pairs; CBS: Cystathionine β-synthase; MSR: Methionine synthase reductase; MS: Methionine synthase; MTHFR: Methylenetetrahydrofolate reductase; SHMT: Serine hydroxymethyltransferase.

2. Evidence Linking B-Vitamins, Hcy and the Pathogenesis of AD

2.1. Observational Trials

Epidemiological studies provide evidence that AD patients tend to have higher Hcy plasma levels than controls, while there are trends for lower levels of B-vitamins [9,32]. Follow-up of a cohort with initially dementia-free elderly for a median of eight years found that plasma Hcy level >14 µmol/L at baseline doubled the risk of developing AD [33]. In addition, the inverse association between Hcy levels and cognitive decline seemed to exist even when the former was in what is generally accepted as the normal range (≤15 µmol/L) [34]. A meta-analysis in 2011 concluded that Hcy levels were clearly higher in AD patients compared to controls [32]. However, based on the available evidence, they could not establish that hyperhomocysteinemia preceded AD [32]. McCaddon and Miller [35] concluded that the available evidence showed a strong and coherent relationship, biological plausibility, dose-response relationship and temporality, and therefore, most of the criteria necessary to establish causality between elevated Hcy and dementia were fulfilled. In the studies they reviewed, elevated Hcy predated hallmarks of AD such as dementia, brain atrophy or neurofibrillary tangles by 5–35 years [35]. They felt what was needed were well-designed intervention trials showing a clear effect of Hcy lowering on cognitive decline [35] (see below). A more recent meta-analysis concluded that the relative risk of developing AD due to elevated Hcy levels or low folate levels were ~1.8 (95% confidence interval 1.37–2.16) and ~2.1 (95% confidence interval 1.51–2.71), respectively, while the data for vitamin B12 and AD was inconclusive, even though AD patients had lower serum levels than controls [36].

2.2. Evidence from Supplementation with B-Vitamins

While somewhat inconsistent, some of the studies supplementing B vitamins show promising results: In a randomized placebo-controlled trial in elderly men, supplementation with 2 mg folic acid, 25 mg vitamin B6 and 400 µg vitamin B12 daily for 2 years decreased Hcy levels and reduced the rate of increase in circulating levels of amyloid-β1-40, an indicator for AD [37]. Supplementation with 800 µg folic acid daily for 3 years also led to a reduced progression of cognitive decline in parallel with a decrease in Hcy plasma levels compared to a control group receiving a placebo [38]. Moreover, an intervention with B-vitamins (800 µg folic acid, 500 µg vitamin B12 and 20 mg vitamin B6 per day for 2 years) in elderly with mild cognitive impairment was shown to slow down the progression of brain atrophy and reduce Hcy levels, both of which were associated with improved cognitive performance [39]. More specifically, this intervention decelerated shrinkage of the grey matter regions of the brain that are particularly affected by AD and the protective effect of the B-vitamins was limited to those with elevated Hcy levels [40]. Doses of these vitamins well above the recommended daily intakes in elderly men (aged ≥75 years) who were not specifically selected for elevated Hcy levels led to an improvement in vitamin status and Hcy levels [37]. In addition, these doses slowed the increase in circulating levels of amyloid beta, a proposed indicator for amyloid plaque formation, even though it did not reach statistical significance [37]. An intervention with supplements in a similar range improved memory and reduced the rate of atrophy in regions particularly affected by AD in elderly with mild cognitive impairment, particularly if they had elevated Hcy levels [39,40].

However, despite some encouraging results, a study on the benefits of Hcy lowering on heart health concluded that the evidence did not support the recommendation of routine supplementation with B-vitamins [41]. Similarly, despite lowering Hcy by around 25%, B-vitamin supplementation only had a marginal effect on cognitive aging [42]. McCaddon and Miller [35] pointed out that most individuals included did not actually experience such a decline and they highlighted the need for further studies specifically designed to assess such an effect.

3. Role of Key Polymorphisms in the OCM

3.1. Overview of the Enzymes of the OCM

The OCM is a complex metabolic pathway in which reduced tetrahydrofolate (THF), the active form of folate, acts as co-enzyme in the transfer of methyl groups [43]. It consists of three interrelated cycles, which are the methionine, thymidylate and purine cycles [44] (Figure 1A). Hcy can either be fed into the methionine or the thymidylate cycle (Figure 1A–C): When methionine levels are low, Hcy is remethylated into methionine (Figure 1B,D). For this, a methyl group is transferred from methylenetetrahydrofolate (MTHF) to Hcy by the methionine synthase (MS), resulting in THF and methionine. The latter can be further metabolized into *S*-adenosylmethionine (SAM), which plays a crucial role as a methyl-donor in other metabolic pathways such as DNA methylation or synthesis of neurotransmitters, phospholipids and myelin [44].

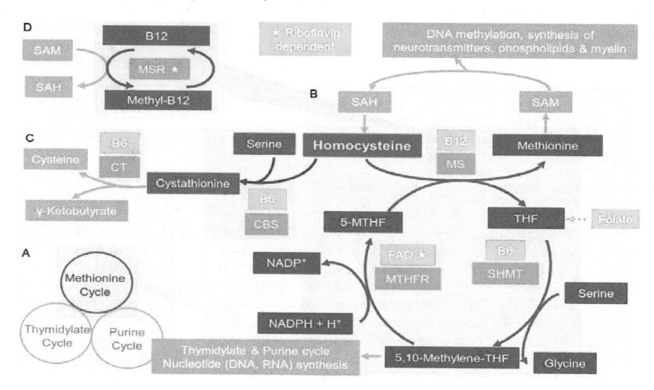

Figure 1. Metabolic pathways of the one-carbon metabolism: (**A**) Overview of the three cycles; (**B**) Methionine cycle: remethylation of homocysteine to methionine; (**C**) Transsulfuartion pathway: Irreversible conversion of homocysteine into cysteine; (**D**) Remethylation of vitamin B12 to its active form; CBS: cystathionine β-synthase; CT: γ-cystathionase; FAD: flavin adenine dinucleotide; MTHF: methylenetetrahydrofolate; MTHFR: methylenetetrahydrofolate reductase; MS: methionine synthase; MSR: methionine synthase reductase; NADP(H): (Hydroxy) Nicotinamide adenine dinucleotide phosphate; SAH: *S*-adenosylhomocysteine; SAM: *S*-adenosylmethionine; SHMT: serine hydroxymethyltransferase THF: tetrahydrofolate.

S-adenosylhomocysteine (SAH), remaining after the one-carbon transfer from SAM, is then hydrolyzed back to Hcy [45]. Serine and THF are turned into glycine and 5,10-methylene-THF in a reaction catalyzed by the serine hydroxymethyltransferase (SHMT) [46]. Then, 5,10-methylene-THF is reduced to 5-methylenetetrahydrofolate (MTHF) by the action of the methylenetetrahydrofolate reductase (MTHFR) [47], closing the cycle. If sufficient methionine is available or Hcy is accumulating, Hcy condenses with serine to form cystathionine and subsequently cysteine [45]. This reaction is called the transsulfuration pathway and is mediated by two vitamin B6-dependent enzymes (cystathionine β-synthase (CBS) and γ-cystathionase) [45].

MS depends on methyl-cobalamin, the active form of vitamin B12 [44], as an intermediate methyl carrier, and consequently, adequate amounts of the nutrient are essential to keep the cycle going [48]. Vitamin B12 is regenerated into its active form by the methionine synthase reductase (MSR) through remethylation with one-carbon units from SAM [49,50]. MSR is a flavoprotein [51] and therefore riboflavin dependent. SHMT consists of four subunits and each of those uses pyridoxal-5'-phosphate, the active form of vitamin B6, as a cofactor [52]. MTHFR also uses flavin adenine dinucleotide (FAD), derived from riboflavin, as a cofactor [51]. This highlights the important role B-vitamins play in the OCM and how deficiencies of each of them are likely to disturb its balance in specific ways.

3.2. Polymorphisms in Key Enzymes of the OCM

The relationship between B-vitamins, relevant polymorphisms and AD has not been studied in great detail and the potential mechanisms are poorly understood. The association between MTHFR C677T and AD has been studied in most detail, while for the other polymorphism the available evidence is very limited. In addition, a great shortcoming of the majority of studies is that no information on nutritional status in general and on B-vitamins more specifically is provided. We will also review how reduced enzymatic activity due to polymorphisms combined with lack of cofactors caused by inadequate dietary intake might unbalance these metabolic processes, thereby potentially favoring the development of AD.

3.2.1. Methylenetetrahydrofolate Reductase (MTHFR) Polymorphisms

MTHFR is by far the most widely studied enzyme in regard to polymorphisms affecting the OCM and their effect on Hcy levels. While deficiency is relatively rare in humans [53], three common mutations of the MTHFR gene, namely C677T, A1298C, and T1317C, have been proposed for an association with various pathological conditions. However, the T1317C mutation appears to be a silent polymorphism [24]; very limited evidence is available and none of it shows any association with Hcy levels or B-vitamin intakes [54,55], let alone AD and this will therefore not be discussed further in this review.

Globally, the frequency of population homozygote for the MTHFR 677TT mutation is thought to range from close to 0% in Sub-Saharan Africans to 32% in Mexicans [56,57]. Homozygotes for the polymorphism were reported to be more likely to have elevated Hcy levels compared to the population average [58–68] and the mutation constitutes the most frequent cause of moderate hyperhomocysteinemia due to genetic factors [20]. There is some evidence for gender-specific differences: one study found men who were homozygous carriers of the mutation had a much higher risk for significantly elevated Hcy levels than women [61]. In addition, a French study corroborated the above results by showing that genotype affected Hcy levels in men, but not in women [69]. Interestingly, one study found the age-dependent increase in Hcy masked the effect of the mutation and only showed a significant association in the older participants [70].

The enzyme activity seems to be reduced by up to 50% [20] due to reduced stability of the association with its cofactor FAD [21,22]. The addition of folate derivatives was shown to stabilize the FAD-MTHFR-folate complex in *Escherichia coli* with the 677TT mutation [22]. In line with this, the effect of the mutation on Hcy levels was more pronounced if folate levels were low [48,54,60,61,63,70–72] and it was not apparent in persons with high intakes from supplements ($\geq$400 µg/day) [66]. It was shown that the odds ratio for elevated Hcy levels in this genotype increased from 15 to 175 if plasma folate was $\leq$3.7 nmol/L [73]. Moreover, hyperhomocysteinemia in persons homozygous for the 677T mutation could be reversed or reduced with folic acid supplementation [47,73], while this had no effect in persons carrying the wild type allele [47]. A folate depletion–repletion study in elderly women showed a more pronounced decrease in serum folate levels accompanied by a steeper increase of Hcy levels in homozygous carriers of the mutation compared to the wild type [74]. After repletion, both serum folate and Hcy levels normalized to levels comparable with those of the participants with the wild type [74]. All this indicates that individuals with the MTHFR 677TT genotype may have higher folate requirements and might benefit even more from supplementation [71] as increasing folate intakes could compensate for the reduced activity of the MTHFR. Multivitamin supplements showed a positive impact on levels of other B-vitamins such as vitamin B12 and pyridoxal 5'-phosphate [47] and might therefore also beneficially affect Hcy levels. Riboflavin status was also negatively associated with Hcy levels in carriers of at least one copy of this polymorphism [75]. In particular, Hcy levels were increased in persons homozygous for 677TT with marginal or low riboflavin status compared to heterozygous and wild types, which was not the case if the vitamin status was adequate [72]. In line with this, daily supplementation with 1.6 mg improved riboflavin status in all subjects with low levels at baseline, but Hcy levels only decreased significantly (by 40%) in subjects who were homozygous carriers of the mutation [76]. Moreover, the impact of riboflavin status on Hcy levels was more important in homozygous carriers of the 677TT mutation with low folate status [77]. Consequently, these data indicate that both riboflavin and folate can independently compensate the decreased MTHFR enzymatic activity due to the mutation.

While the effect of vitamin B6 on Hcy was found to be inconsistent, Hustad and colleagues [78] suggest that the effect is particularly evident in persons homozygous for the MTHFR 677T mutation and that interactions with other B vitamins might further complicate the relationship. Hcy levels were found to be inversely associated with vitamin B6 status if riboflavin levels were adequate, but plasma folate levels were low [72]. If re-methylation of Hcy via the methionine cycle (Figure 1B) is not possible due to lack of folate, the alternative pathway for Hcy is condensation with serine to cystathionine and this is catalyzed by the vitamin B6-dependent CBS (Figure 1C). However, if this pathway is also disturbed due to insufficient levels of vitamin B6, Hcy seems to accumulate. The role of vitamin B12 in persons with 677TT genotype is not completely clear: Vitamin B12 levels did not seem to have any effect on the risk of hyperhomocysteinemia in the 677TT genotype in some studies [60,71], while others reported a negative association between Hcy and serum vitamin B12 levels, particularly in person homozygous for 677T [54,79]. Moreover, Hcy levels were found to be higher in homozygous carriers of the mutation with low vitamin B12 levels, particularly if they did not take folate supplements [66]. The mechanism for such an effect is unknown, but it has been suggested it might be due to a coexisting mutation within the OCM [48].

The A1298C mutation in MTHFR gene was reported in approximately 10% of Canadians [24]. The prevalence seems to differ between ethnic groups: while non-Hispanic whites in the U.S. showed a similar prevalence of homozygous carriers (~12%) as that reported for Canadians, in Mexican Americans, the prevalence was ~20% and in non-Hispanic blacks it was just over 1% [66]. In itself, the A1298C mutation was not associated with elevated Hcy levels in either heterozygotes or homozygotes in most studies [54,61–63,66,70,80,81] and the reduction in MTHFR activity is lower than for the 677TTTT mutation (~70% of wild type) [23]. However, in vitro studies indicate a synergistic effect for the two mutations [23], Hcy levels were found to be highest [61,82] and the corresponding red cell folate level lowest in individuals with both mutations [61]. No significant effects were found for the combinations of genotypes and serum folate or vitamin B12, but this might be due to the low prevalence of the recombinant genotype [61,82]. In other studies, the activity of MTHFR was further reduced than what would have been expected from C677T alone in individuals heterozygous for C677T and A1298C (none of the subjects was homozygous for both mutations), which was accompanied by increased Hcy and decreased plasma folate [23,24,83]. Carriers of the wild type for both polymorphisms on the other hand were found to have the lowest Hcy levels compared with other combinations of the genotypes [84]. Again, the effect seems to be more pronounced in individuals with low folate levels [23].

In addition, plasma vitamin B6 levels were lower in individuals heterozygous for C677T carrying at least one copy of the mutation for A1298C compared to those who were homozygous for A1298C, but this might have been due to differences in supplement use between the groups [23]. Moreover, in doubly heterozygous subjects, plasma vitamin B12 was a significant predictor of Hcy levels, which was not the case for those who were wild type for at least one of the polymorphisms [48]. The authors conclude that these people would benefit from an increase in vitamin B12 status, as this would help reducing or normalizing Hcy levels [48].

3.2.2. Methionine Synthase (MS) Polymorphism

Several polymorphisms in MS have been identified, which might potentially be relevant for the Hcy metabolism [25,26]. The most prevalent is the A2756G polymorphism with an allele frequency of around 20% [25,26,85–87]. A number of studies in both healthy and sick individuals of different age and gender groups assessed its effect on Hcy or B-vitamin levels and found no or only marginal effects that failed to reach statistical significance [61,86–91]. Given the relatively low prevalence of homozygous mutation in the gene encoding for MS, larger studies might be able to shed more light on the relationship between the different genotypes, levels of B-vitamins and Hcy concentrations. One study in more than 1200 healthy men between the ages of 50 and 61 years found that carriers homozygous for the more common AA genotype had higher Hcy levels than those with at least one copy of the G mutation, independent of folate or vitamin B12 status [60]. Similarly, fasting and post-methionine load Hcy levels were lower in individuals with at least one copy of the 2756G allele [59]. Moreover, an additive effect on Hcy levels was reported in carriers who have at least one copy of the MTHFR 677T allele and who are homozygous for MS 2756A [60].

In addition, Ma and colleagues report a trend towards a protective effect of the GG genotype for colorectal cancer despite the lack of association with Hcy, indicating an effect via a different mechanism, possibly via DNA methylation [91]. In line with this, the AG genotype was associated with increased erythrocyte folate and lower risk for myocardial infarction, but not Hcy or vitamin B12 levels, compared to the wild type (only one patient was homozygous for the mutation and was therefore not included in the analysis) [92]. Reduced activity of MS and the resulting decrease in SAM could affect DNA methylation and/or synthesis of neurotransmitters, phospholipids and myelin (Figure 1B), which in turn could contribute to the development of the AD. Hcy levels could still be kept in the normal range by condensing it with serine to cystathionine (Figure 1C). This is in line with the finding that the mutation correlated with cystathionine levels [70], indicating a preference for transsulfuration rather than re-methylation in the 2756AG/GG genotype. In line with this, one study found moderately increased Hcy levels in persons with the AA genotype, which increased with decreasing levels of vitamin B6, but seemed independent of folate and vitamin B12 status [93].

Moreover, a study in American men aged ~40 to 80 years found that Hcy levels decreased with increasing number of copies of the 2756G allele in healthy controls, but not in cases with a history of myocardial infarction [94]. It has been proposed that in conditions of elevated oxidative stress, functional vitamin B12 deficiency arises as the recycling into its active form cannot keep up with the rate of its oxidation [95]. Consequently, it can be speculated that the effect of the polymorphism on enzyme activity in the above-mentioned patients is masked by the stronger effect of vitamin B12 oxidation. Whether this underlying mechanism is relevant for the etiology of AD needs to be established. However, it is conceivable to assume such a link given the elevated levels of oxidative stress found in AD patients' brains.

3.2.3. Methionine Synthase Reductase (MSR) Polymorphism

Another relatively common mutation affecting an enzyme of the OCM is the A66G mutation in the gene encoding for the MSR. In a range of studies, it was reported that ~25% to 30% of Caucasians were homozygous carriers of the mutation [61,72,96]. Data from case-control studies indicate a great range between countries (for a review see [97]), but also between ethnic groups within one country: In the U.S. ~30% non-Hispanic whites were found to be homozygous for the mutation compared to ~20% Ashkenazi Jews, ~8% to 10% non-Hispanic blacks and ~7% Mexican Americans [66,98], while in Muslims in India, ~50% were carriers of two copies of the mutation [97].

It was reported that the mutation lead to a less efficient regeneration of vitamin B12 [27] and it has been proposed as a risk factor for elevated Hcy levels [51] as it reduces its conversion into methionine. Another consequence of this impairment of the OCM is the reduced availability of SAM for DNA methylation [97]. However, the majority of studies does not confirm an effect on Hcy levels [66,70,82,88,96,99–101] and only two studies found significantly [49,102] and borderline significantly higher Hcy [61] levels in homozygous carriers of the mutation.

Given the role of MSR in recycling vitamin B12 and thereby contributing to the remethylation of Hcy, the decreased activity caused by the mutation can be assumed to be particularly critical if vitamin B12 levels are low. This was confirmed by a study showing that in persons with low plasma cobalamin levels ($\leq$273 pmol/L), Hcy levels were higher in carriers of the mutant allele, if their riboflavin status was adequate [72]. In other words, adequate vitamin B12 levels seem to be able to compensate the reduced enzymatic activity, and the impairment due to inadequate riboflavin levels masks that due to genetic variation. If Hcy cannot be turned into methionine, the transsulfuration pathway involving the vitamin B6-dependent CBS will be activated to regulate its levels (Figure 1C). It is therefore not surprising that vitamin B6 status has an impact on the effect of the A66G polymorphism on Hcy levels [72].

There might also be an interaction between the different genotypes: in non-Hispanic whites homozygous for MTHFR 677T, there was a significant trend towards lower Hcy levels with increasing numbers of copies of 66G, which was not the case for the 677CC or CT genotypes [66]. While the MSR genotype in itself had no effect on Hcy in a study in healthy women, there seems to be an effect in combination with the MTHFR 677TT genotype [82]. However, the authors conclude that due to the small sample size in the MTHFR 677TT/MSR 66AA and GG groups, they failed to detect potential differences in plasma Hcy between these groups.

Further research is needed to assess the effect of this mutation, particularly in combination with other polymorphisms affecting the OCM and/or in individuals with inadequate status of one or more of the relevant B-vitamins. Brown and colleagues [100] showed an effect of the mutation on the risk for coronary artery disease, but not on Hcy levels, indicating that a mechanism other than elevated Hcy levels might be relevant. Given that vascular diseases seem to increase the risk of developing AD [103], this link should be further investigated.

Less is known about the C524T mutation in the gene encoding for MSR, for which ~14% homozygous carriers were found in a group of healthy Spaniards, while nearly 60% had at least one copy of the mutation [72]. It seems to affect the enzyme structure in the region between the binding domains for flavin mononucleotide and FAD/(Hydroxy) Nicotinamide adenine dinucleotide phosphate (NADPH), respectively [27]. As for the A66G variant, this mutation reduced the efficacy of B12 regeneration by MSR [27]. In carriers of the C524T mutation, Hcy was significantly higher than in controls if vitamin B12 levels were low, while riboflavin status had no clear effect [72]. For both mutations of the MSR, vitamin B6 levels were inversely associated with Hcy levels in persons with optimal riboflavin and vitamin B12 levels [72], highlighting again the importance of the transsulfuration pathway for keeping Hcy in the normal range when re-methylation is impaired.

3.2.4. Cystathionine β-Synthase (CBS) Polymorphism

Relatively rare mutations of the gene encoding for CBS are frequently found in patients with homocystinuria, but they do not seem to be more common in persons with moderately elevated plasma Hcy levels and were consequently considered to be of minor importance as risk factors for the general population [90,104–107]. In addition, some rare mutations in the gene encoding for CBS have been reported to have beneficial, albeit statistically not significant effects on Hcy levels. These mutations, however, were not regarded as significant due to their low prevalence [108]. However, a more common 68 base pair (bp) insertion in exon 8 in the gene encoding for CBS [28] might be relevant. The prevalence of this insertion in healthy men and women from Northern Ireland was around 18% [61] and around 12% in healthy US controls [109]. In the US, allele frequency has been reported to be significantly higher in non-Hispanic blacks (~26%) compared to non-Hispanic whites (~8%) or Mexican American individuals (~6%) [66]. It had been proposed that insertion had no effect on the enzyme activity [109] and assessed on its own, its effect on Hcy is inconsistent: while some found no effect on Hcy [61,70], others showed a trend towards lower levels at least in specific subpopulations [59,60,66,89,110].

A few studies that assessed the effect of combined polymorphisms found that the insertion is capable of compensating the negative effect of MTHFR 677TT and MS 2756 AA [59,60,108]. However, in another study, a combination of homozygous 677T and 68 bd led to a further increase in Hcy levels, albeit in a very small sample ($n = 4$) [70]. While in black South Africans, the insertion itself had no effect on Hcy, in combination with MTHFR 677TT, those without the insertion had the highest Hcy levels [29]. Similarly, a different mutation of CBS (9276 GA genotype compared to 9276 GG, no 9276 AA in the study) led to an increase in Hcy levels in individuals homozygous for the MTHFR 677T mutation compared to other genotypes [29]. Moreover, increasing numbers of repeat units of the 31-bp *variable number of tandem repeats* polymorphism in the non-coding sequence of CBS at the boundary of exon 13 to intron 13 were found to decrease CBS activity and increase Hcy levels [30]. Frequency and position of these seem to vary between different ethnic groups [111]. Albeit inconsistent, these results highlight the importance of the transsulfuration pathway as an alternative to catabolize Hcy if remethylation is impaired. In line with this, the protective effect of the insertion on Hcy appears to be independent of folate and vitamin B12 status [60].

3.2.5. Serine Hydroxymethyltransferase (SHMT) Polymorphism

For SHMT, a polymorphism has been described at the position C1420T. While it has not been studied extensively, one study reports that women with the 1420CC genotype had significantly increased Hcy and decreased red cell and plasma folate levels [31]. In another study in patients with coronary artery disease, the mutation was also associated with lower levels of Hcy, higher plasma folate concentrations and decreased markers of oxidative stress [112].

4. Proposed Mechanisms Linking Polymorphisms, Hcy, B-Vitamins and AD

The data presented on polymorphisms in the genes encoding for key enzymes in the OCM and their interaction with various B-vitamins highlights the complex relationship between the various steps of these metabolic pathways. Genetic factors affecting the OCM alone are likely to play a relatively minor role in the overall risk of developing AD: 9% of variation in Hcy levels could be explained by differences in the polymorphisms for MTHFR, MS, MTR and CBS, while folate and vitamin B12 status are thought to be responsible for 35% of the variance [61]. Combining these genetic and nutritional factors increased the effect to 42%in relatively young subjects (20–25 years of age) [61]. The authors chose this age group as they expected the genetic effects to be less masked by a range of environmental influences that accumulate over a lifetime [61]. They suggest that more subtle genetic effects might only manifest in combination with longer-term exposure to other factors such as smoking [61]. In any case, polymorphisms help to understand the complexity of the metabolic system and explain some of the inconsistencies encountered in studies trying to link nutritional factors with risks for diseases.

The evidence presented above shows that lack of substrate or reduced enzymatic activity in one step in the OCM can be compensated at least partially or results in a shift to a different pathway. Consequently, it seems that health is only affected if these copying mechanisms fail due to a combination of more than one polymorphisms and/or inadequate supply of relevant vitamins (Figure 2). It is therefore not surprising that studies concentrating on a single polymorphism and its association with AD failed to show a consistent picture: A number of studies did not detect a difference in the frequency of the MTHFR C677T genotype in AD patients and controls [113–126], which is probably only partially due to the small sample sizes. Other studies and meta-analyses found an effect of the C677T polymorphism on AD [127–129], but there seemed to be some differences between the ethnicities [127,130]. Unfortunately, no study actually took into account the different polymorphisms of key enzymes in the OCM in combination with B-vitamin status. Importantly, one study showed that despite a lack of difference in C677T genotypes or Hcy levels between patients and controls, plasma Hcy concentrations were significantly higher in patients with dementia who were either TT or CT and had low folate levels (<5.7 nmol/L) compared to those with adequate folate levels or CC genotype [131].

AD is a multifactorial disease, which is poorly understood and a range of hypothesis have been proposed for its etiology, which are reviewed in detail elsewhere [9,132]. According to the authors of a recent review, low folate and vitamin B12 status contribute to the development of cognitive impairment directly and via elevated Hcy levels [16]. These mechanisms will be discussed in the following sections.

4.1. Proposed Mechanism Linking Hcy & AD

A range of mechanisms have been proposed for the link between elevated Hcy and AD and preclinical studies show that hyperhomocysteinemia, induced by genetic manipulation or by B-vitamin deficiency, causes known hallmarks of AD such as accumulation of amyloid-β peptide [133–136] and intensified tau protein hyperphosphorylation in the brain [137]. An autopsy study showed a clear association between Hcy levels and neurofibrillary tangles, a known hallmark of AD, with an odds ratio of having such deposits of 2.60 (95% confidence interval 1.28–5.28) when comparing the top with the bottom Hcy quartile [138]. A prospective study showed greater brain atrophy in AD patients with higher Hcy levels [116] and this association between Hcy and grey matter atrophy has been confirmed by a range of studies (See review by Smith and Refsum [16]).

Amyloid plaque formation is thought to be an important event in the etiology of AD [139,140] and there is evidence that elevated levels of Hcy can impact the plaque formation by reducing the clearing rate of amyloid-β in the brain of mice [141]. Moreover, amyloid-β levels increased in rats after injection of Hcy into their brain and this was accompanied by loss in spatial memory [142]. Folate and vitamin B12 supplementation was able to lessen these effects [142]. A further piece of the puzzle is the finding that Hcy can bind to amyloid-β in vivo and in vitro, thereby triggering the formation of interconnections and subsequently aggregates [143]. Moreover, these deposits can induce oxidative stress, another important element in the etiology of AD [144,145].

The effect of elevated Hcy on brain capillaries is a further mechanism through which an impaired OCM might facilitate the development of AD [146] (Figure 2C). It has been postulated that elevated Hcy levels due to genetics or dietary inadequacies may compromise vascular health, thereby contributing to dementia and AD [131]. Hcy is thought to affect endothelial integrity by promoting the generation of peroxides, but also by reducing the availability of nitric oxide through a reduction of intracellular glutathione peroxide levels [147]. Moreover, while these vascular effects might be more prominent in individuals who are not otherwise genetically predisposed to AD, it has been speculated that there might be a more direct effect on brain cells in those with the ApoE ε4 genotype [146].

Increased levels of Hcy were shown to be a risk factor for shrinkage of specific brain regions including the bilateral hippocampus and parahippocampal gyrus, retrosplenial precuneus, lingual and fusiform gyrus, which is a key component of the AD process and is associated with cognitive decline [40]. In rats, it has been shown that exposure to Hcy leads to apoptosis in hippocampal neurons by inducing a cascade that results in DNA damage, decline of mitochondrial membrane potential and eventually nuclear disintegration, possibly triggered by nicotinamide adenine dinucleotide and adenosine triphosphate depletion [148]. Hcy was shown to accumulate in neurons as it is rapidly taken up via specific membrane transporters [149]. These changes might then increase the vulnerability of neuronal cells to oxidative stress and further contribute to the development of AD [148].

Evidence from animal studies also indicates that Hcy is likely to contribute to cognitive decline, but also that its levels further increase as a result of neurodegeneration [150]. The authors conclude that dietary intake or supplementation with B-vitamins might be able to break this vicious cycle. Moreover, in many conditions that are related to oxidative stress, including neurodegenerative diseases, a simultaneous elevation of Hcy and reduced level of B-vitamins, particularly folate, has been reported [151]. It has consequently been proposed that folate requirements might be increased due to irreversible oxidation and that hyperhomocysteinemia might be a consequence of the pro-oxidative environment and not just a result of inadequate intakes [151,152].

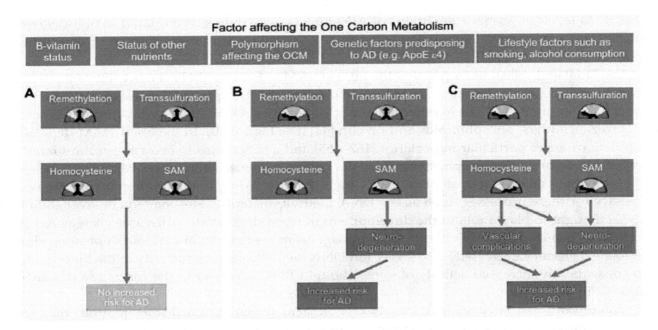

Figure 2. Proposed framework for the effect on genetic, nutritional and lifestyle factors on the development of Alzheimer's disease: (**A**) Balance between remethylation and transsulfuration results in adequate levels of homocysteine, DNA synthesis, repair and methylation as well as synthesis of neurotransmitter, phospholipids and myelin and consequently no increase in the risk of Alzheimer's disease; (**B**) Remethylation is decreased, while homocysteine is still kept in the normal range via transsulfuration, resulting in reduced DNA synthesis, repair and methylation as well as synthesis of neurotransmitter, phospholipids and myelin and consequently, an increase in the risk of Alzheimer's, but not vascular disease; (**C**) Remethylation and transsulfuration are decreased, resulting in reduced DNA synthesis, repair and methylation as well as synthesis of neurotransmitter, phospholipids and myelin and consequently, an increase in the risk of Alzheimer's, also due to compromised vascular health; AD: Alzheimer's disease; ApoE: Apolipoprotein E; OCM: One-carbon metabolism; SAM: *S*-adenosylmethionine.

4.2. Further Mechanisms Linking an Impaired OCM to the Development of AD

As the framework in Figure 2 shows, Hcy levels in the normal range do not necessarily mean that there is no disturbance of the OCM. Mechanisms such as DNA repair can be reduced due to specific polymorphisms alone or in combination with low levels of folate, riboflavin and/or vitamin B12, while Hcy is catabolized via transsulfuration. This pathway has been known to be upregulated if methionine recycling is reduced in order to keep Hcy levels low [153]. However, as the switch affects the substrates or methyl donors for essential pathways, such imbalances not only compromise DNA synthesis, repair and methylation, but also the availability of neurotransmitters, phospholipids and myelin (See below). Hcy can further be re-methylated to methionine via the betaine pathway in the liver or kidney [154], but not in the brain [155]. The balance between these pathways depends on an elaborate feedback loop, but also on the availability of nutrients such as folate, vitamin B6, B12 and methionine as well as the methyl-donors choline and betaine [154]. Interestingly, one study found that choline was a strong positive predictor of Hcy levels in Mexican American men with the MTHFR 677TT, but not the 677CC, genotype who had low folate levels [156].

It has also been shown that decreased activity in one enzyme of the OCM can trigger downregulation in the gene expression for key enzymes in alternative pathways, thereby affecting the balance, e.g., between DNA methylation and synthesis [157]. In addition, there is evidence that during folate deficiency, mechanisms are in place to preserve thymidylate and consequently DNA synthesis at the expense of Hcy remethylation [158]. Even though one has to be careful to draw causative conclusions from associations, it is conceivable that such imbalances contribute to the development of

AD as SAM levels in postmortem brains of AD patients were reduced compared to non-demented controls [159] and changed methylation patterns were found in postmortem analysis of specific brain regions of AD patients [160].

Van Driel and colleagues argue that the ratio of SAM to SAH might be a more relevant predictor of health outcomes due to impaired OCM [161] and this might also apply in the case of AD. SAM plays a crucial role as methyl-donor in other metabolic pathways such as DNA methylation or synthesis of neurotransmitters, phospholipids and myelin [44] (See Figure 1B). In the brain, SAM-dependent methylations are of particular importance [162–165] and a lack seems to favor the accumulation of amyloid precursor protein and phosphorylated tau protein, validated hallmarks of AD [133,137,166–168]. SAM is the major methyl-group donor for DNA methylation; it is involved in the regulation of enzymes necessary for these processes, such as the DNA methyltransferase, and inadequate availability of SAM is thought to play a role in the development of neurodegenerative diseases such as AD (For review see Fuso 2013 [169]). Evidence from transgenic mouse model of amyloid deposition shows that folate deficiency decreased SAM levels and DNA methyltransferase activity in the hippocampus and consequently increased activity of genes thought to be involved in the formation of amyloid plaque [170].

Polyunsaturated fatty acids, docosahexaenoic acid (DHA) in particular, play an important role in cognitive health as they are implicated in synaptic functions and signaling pathways, but also for the structure of membranes in the brain and imbalances are thought to be implicated in a range of neuropsychiatric diseases including AD (See review by Liu and colleagues [171]). A crucial step to ensure adequate supply with essential fatty acids to tissues such as the brain includes the methylation of phosphatidylethanolamine to phosphatidylcholine, which requires the phosphatidylethanolamine methyltransferase (PEMT) [172]. PEMT is thought to be regulated by SAM and SAH concentrations [173] and an impaired OCM can therefore be expected to limit the availability of essential fatty acids such as DHA to the brain. This is in line with the findings of a study that found significantly decreased DHA mobilization from the liver likely due to elevated levels of Hcy and SAH AD patients compared to healthy controls [18]. Moreover, DHA levels in the brains of AD patients were lower than in those of controls and at least in some regions of the brain (temporal and mix-frontal cortex, but not cerebellum) they were negatively correlated with the degree of cognitive decline [174].

It has been postulated that early on in the disease, oxidative stress levels increase due to mechanisms most likely unrelated to the OCM [95]. As a consequence, functional vitamin B12 deficiency can develop if the rate of oxidation surpasses its recycling [95]. This effect is likely more pronounced if the activity of MSR is reduced due to a polymorphism. Elevated Hcy levels would therefore be a consequence of changes occurring due to the AD pathophysiology, but they might then also contribute to its progression [95]. The MSR A66G was found to be correlated not only with Hcy levels, but also with markers of oxidative stress [112]. It has been suggested that the reduction in MS activity due to lack of vitamin B12 might mask the more subtle decrease in activity due to an MS polymorphism, thereby further complicating the association between the genotype and AD [175].

Dorszewska and colleagues [176] report an increase of markers for oxidative stress as well as Hcy levels in AD patients, while in elderly controls, there was an age-related, but less pronounced increase in the latter, but not the former. Moreover, even though ApoE ε4 itself does not seem to be linked to elevated Hcy levels [115], the increased level of oxidative damage thought to be linked to the ApoE ε4 genotype might be aggravated if the OCM is disturbed. Studies in mice demonstrate that folate might play an important role in countering the effect of elevated oxidative stress prevalent in brains of ApoE ε4carriers [177,178]. Markers of oxidative stress in the central nervous system of ApoE knockout mice only increased following an iron challenge if folate was deficient [178]. Folate deficiency was associated with increased Hcy and a reduced ability to counter oxidative stress as it was shown to decrease the activity of key antioxidant enzymes, namely the Cu-Zn superoxide dismutase and the glutathione peroxidase [179]. While it was long assumed that the oxidative pentose phosphate pathway was the main source of NADPH, it was recently shown that the OCM is equally important in providing this important reducing agent [180]. An impaired OCM can therefore be expected to increase the vulnerability to oxidative stress by decreasing the cell's oxidative defense mechanisms. Wakutani and colleagues therefore propose that an impaired folate metabolism due to the MTHFR polymorphism or inadequate dietary supply might enhance the adverse effect of ApoE ε4 on the etiology of AD [181].

In addition, studies in mice that are not genetically predisposed to AD show that inadequate supply with B vitamins in itself can cause cognitive decline [146]. One potential mechanism is that impaired DNA repair due to deficiency of folate seems to increase oxidative neuronal damage induced by amyloid beta-peptide [182]. It is postulated that damage to mitochondrial DNA accumulating with age leads to increased oxidative stress, which—in the absence of efficient repair mechanisms—causes neurodegeneration (for a review see Swerdlow et al. 2014 [17]). The activity of CBS is thought to increase in response to oxidative stress [183], which might result in a further imbalance of the OCM that could potentially contribute to the development of the disease.

Age itself might further contribute to impaired OCM as there was an age-dependent decrease in THF accompanied by an increase in products of its oxidation, which are biologically inactive [184]. Hcy levels were elevated in both dementia patients and elderly controls when compared to a younger group of neurological patients without dementia [131]. Similarly, an association between age and Hcy levels as well as a negative association between the former and serum folate and vitamin B12 concentrations were found in the combined as well as stratified analysis of AD patients and controls [10]. In addition to the aging process, lifestyle factors such as alcohol consumption and smoking might also influence the interaction between B-vitamins, polymorphisms of the OCM and AD [60,91]. A vicious circle between impaired OCM and oxidative stress seems to develop in the elderly, particularly in certain genotypes prone to impaired cognitive health. It was suggest that carriers of the 677T mutation might still be able to compensate the imbalance in the folate metabolism under normal circumstances, but if vitamin B12 supply is also inadequate, an effective compensation might no longer be possible [185]. This ties in with the findings of another study that reported a weak, but significant association between the MSR 66G mutation and the risk for AD as well as with the severity of the disease, particularly in combination with the ApoEε4 genotype [123].

Many questions remain concerning the proposed mechanisms and given their key roles in a range of processes pertinent to brain health, it is likely that more than one is relevant for the etiology of AD.

5. Dietary Intake of B-Vitamins

Current intake recommendations do not take into account potentially increased needs due to reduced enzymatic activity caused by a polymorphism, as the mechanisms are not understood well enough to adapt them accordingly. Until this is possible, it is advisable to assure intakes of B-vitamins in all age groups are in line with the available recommendations to reduce the risk of the developments that eventually result in AD.

Worryingly, for part of the general population even in affluent countries, this is not the case. A relatively recent analysis of data from the National Health and Nutrition Examination Survey reported elevated Hcy levels in ~6% of the U.S. population aged ≥19 years, with levels ranging from >3% in 19–39 year-olds to ~18% in those ≥60 years old [186]. Despite mandatory folic acid fortification, around 5% and 15% of men and women, respectively, in the age range of ≥19years have folate intakes below the Estimated Average Requirement (EAR) in the United States [187]. Similar figures were given by Agarwal and colleagues [188], who also report intakes of vitamin B6 to be low for ~15%. In different European countries, intakes below EAR range from 0% to 40% for vitamin B12 and from 10% to just over 90% for folate in adults aged 19–64 years [189]. In Ireland, voluntary fortification as well as dietary supplements significantly contributed to achieving adequate folate intakes, but still, nearly 70% of women aged 18–50 years had suboptimal serum folate levels [190]. Vitamin B12 deficiency is typically seen as a problem of the elderly due to malabsorption [191–194].

However, Bailey and colleagues argue that even if the proportions of people with deficiencies in the general population are not very high, the absolute number of affected persons is still significant [186].

As is often the case in nutrition, B-vitamins can only function properly if the supply of other essential nutrients is assured: It has been shown that an intervention with B-vitamins in elderly with mild cognitive impairment only showed beneficial effects if their omega-3 fatty acid status, particularly DHA, was adequate [195]. Worryingly, it has been shown that intakes of DHA are low in many regions of the world [196]. Other nutritional inadequacies likely also play a role in the development of AD, which further highlights the importance of a diet that supplies all essential nutrients in adequate amounts through.

6. Conclusions

The evidence presented shows that persons with specific genotypes are more susceptible to imbalances in the OCM, resulting in increased levels of Hcy, insufficient DNA repair, methylation and/or synthesis as well as reduced availability of neurotransmitters, phospholipids and myelin. This can facilitate the development of AD via a range of—as of yet—poorly understood mechanisms, particularly, but not exclusively, if other risk factors such as the ApoE ε4 polymorphism predispose an individual to the disease. The reduced enzymatic activity can be compensated at least to some degree by adequate intakes of the relevant B-vitamins. Even though supplementation with folate, vitamin B6 and B12 might be able to slow the progression of dementia at an early stage [37,39,40], by the time overt clinical signs appear it might be too late to reverse the decline [197]. This emphasizes the importance of a life-long adequate intake of B-vitamins for prevention of cognitive decline and dementia.

The relationship between polymorphisms of the OCM, intakes of B-vitamins and AD can only be resolved with well-designed long-term cohort studies with detailed neuropsychological and vascular measurements. Given the long latency period between the occurrence of elevated Hcy as well as oxidative stress levels and the first symptoms of cognitive decline, studies should be initiated with healthy, middle-aged subjects. Moreover, these indicators have to be assessed at regular intervals to allow for a more in-depth understanding of the mechanisms eventually leading to AD. Until these issues are resolved, efforts should be made to ensure adequate intakes of all B-vitamins via the diet, fortified foods and possibly dietary supplements.

Acknowledgments: The cost of the publication was covered by DSM Nutritional Products Ltd., Kaiseraugst, Switzerland.

Author Contributions: All authors defined the scope of the publication; Barbara Troesch and M. Hasan Mohajeri wrote the paper; and Barbara Troesch, M. Hasan Mohajeri and Peter Weber had primary responsibility for the final content.

References

1.   Duthey, B. *Priority Medicines for Europe and the World Update Report-Background Paper "Alzheimer's Disease and Other Dementias"*; World Health Organization: Geneva, Switzerland, 2013.

2.   Kinsella, K.; He, W. *An Aging World: 2008 International Population Reports*; U.S. Department of Health and Human Services, National Institute of Health, National Institute of Aging: Washington, DC, USA, 2009.

3.   Alzheimer's Association Website. Available online: Http://www.Alz.Org (accessed on 19 September 2016).

4.   Lindsley, C.W. Alzheimer's disease: Development of disease-modifying treatments is the challenge for our generation. *ACS Chem Neurosci* **2012**, *3*, 804–805. [CrossRef] [PubMed]

5.   Alzheimer's Association Website. Available online: Http://www.Alz.Org (accessed on 21 November 2014).

6.   Serrano-Pozo, A.; Frosch, M.P.; Masliah, E.; Hyman, B.T. Neuropathological alterations in Alzheimer's disease. *Cold Spring Harb. Perspect. Med.* **2011**, *1*, a006189. [CrossRef] [PubMed]

7.   Selkoe, D.J. Resolving controversies on the path to Alzheimer's therapeutics. *Nat. Med.* **2011**, *17*, 1060–1065. [CrossRef] [PubMed]

8.   Moyer, M.W. Alzheimer's researchers call for clinical revamp. *Nat. Med.* **2011**, *17*, 235. [CrossRef] [PubMed]

9.	Mohajeri, M.H.; Troesch, B.; Weber, P. Inadequate supply of vitamins and DHA in the elderly: Implications for brain aging and Alzheimer-type dementia. *Nutrition* **2015**, *31*, 261–275. [CrossRef] [PubMed]

10.	Coppedè, F.; Tannorella, P.; Pezzini, I.; Migheli, F.; Ricci, G.; Caldarazzo Ienco, E.; Piaceri, I.; Polini, A.; Nacmias, B.; Monzani, F.; et al. Folate, homocysteine, vitamin B12, and polymorphisms of genes participating in one-carbon metabolism in late-onset Alzheimer's disease patients and healthy controls. *Antioxid. Redox Signal.* **2011**, *17*, 195–204. [CrossRef] [PubMed]

11.	Migliore, L.; Coppedè, F. Genetics, environmental factors and the emerging role of epigenetics in neurodegenerative diseases. *Mutat. Res. Fundam.Mol. Mech. Mutagen.* **2009**, *667*, 82–97. [CrossRef] [PubMed]

12.	Finch, C.E. Evolution of the human lifespan and diseases of aging: Roles of infection, inflammation, and nutrition. *Proc. Natl. Acad.Sci. USA* **2010**, *107*, 1718–1724. [CrossRef] [PubMed]

13.	Egert, S.; Rimbach, G.; Huebbe, P. Apoe genotype: From geographic distribution to function and responsiveness to dietary factors. *Proc. Nutr. Soc.* **2012**, *71*, 410–424. [CrossRef] [PubMed]

14.	Ramassamy, C.; Averill, D.; Beffert, U.; Bastianetto, S.; Theroux, L.; Lussier-Cacan, S.; Cohn, J.S.; Christen, Y.; Davignon, J.; Quirion, R.; et al. Original contributions: Oxidative damage and protection by antioxidants in the frontal cortex of Alzheimer's disease is related to the apolipoprotein e genotype. *Free Radic. Biol. Med.* **1999**, *27*, 544–553. [CrossRef]

15.	Selhub, J. Public health significance of elevated homocysteine. *Food Nutr. Bull.* **2008**, *29*, S116–S125. [CrossRef] [PubMed]

16.	Smith, A.D.; Refsum, H. Homocysteine, B vitamins, and cognitive impairment. *Annu. Rev. Nutr.* **2016**, *36*, 211–239. [CrossRef] [PubMed]

17.	Swerdlow, R.H.; Burns, J.M.; Khan, S.M. The Alzheimer's disease mitochondrial cascade hypothesis: Progress and perspectives. *Biochim. Biophys. Acta* **2014**, *1842*, 1219–1231. [CrossRef] [PubMed]

18.	Selley, M.L. A metabolic link between *S*-adenosylhomocysteine and polyunsaturated fatty acid metabolism in Alzheimer's disease. *Neurobiol. Aging* **2007**, *28*, 1834–1839. [CrossRef] [PubMed]

19.	Troesch, B.; Hoeft, B.; Weber, P.; Eggersdorfer, M. Understanding the genome: Implications for human nutrition? *Vitam. Miner.* **2014**, *3*. [CrossRef]

20.	Schwahn, B.; Rozen, R. Polymorphisms in the methylenetetrahydrofolate reductase gene: Clinical consequences. *Am. J. Pharmacogenom.* **2001**, *1*, 189–201. [CrossRef]

21.	Yamada, K.; Chen, Z.; Rozen, R.; Matthews, R.G. Effects of common polymorphisms on the properties of recombinant human methylenetetrahydrofolate reductase. *Proc. Natl. Acad.Sci. USA* **2001**, *98*, 14853–14858. [CrossRef] [PubMed]

22.	Guenther, B.D.; Sheppard, C.A.; Tran, P.; Rozen, R.; Matthews, R.G.; Ludwig, M.L. The structure and properties of methylenetetrahydrofolate reductase from *Escherichia coli* suggest how folate ameliorates human hyperhomocysteinemia. *Nat. Struct. Mol. Biol.* **1999**, *6*, 359–365.

23.	Weisberg, I.S.; Jacques, P.F.; Selhub, J.; Bostom, A.G.; Chen, Z.; Curtis Ellison, R.; Eckfeldt, J.H.; Rozen, R. The 1298a→c polymorphism in methylenetetrahydrofolate reductase (MTHFR): In vitro expression and association with homocysteine. *Atherosclerosis* **2001**, *156*, 409–415. [CrossRef]

24.	Weisberg, I.; Tran, P.; Christensen, B.; Sibani, S.; Rozen, R. A second genetic polymorphism in methylenetetrahydrofolate reductase (MTHFR) associated with decreased enzyme activity. *Mol. Genet. Metab.* **1998**, *64*, 169–172. [CrossRef] [PubMed]

25.	Leclerc, D.; Campeau, E.; Goyette, P.; Adjalla, C.E.; Christensen, B.; Ross, M.; Eydoux, P.; Rosenblatt, D.S.; Rozen, R.; Gravel, R.A. Human methionine synthase: cDNA cloning and identification of mutations in patients of the cblg complementation group of folate/cobalamin disorders. *Hum. Mol. Genet.* **1996**, *5*, 1867–1874. [CrossRef] [PubMed]

26.	Chen, L.H.; Liu, M.-L.; Hwang, H.-Y.; Chen, L.-S.; Korenberg, J.; Shane, B. Human methionine synthase: cDNA cloning, gene localization, and expression. *J. Biol. Chem.* **1997**, *272*, 3628–3634. [CrossRef] [PubMed]

27.	Olteanu, H.; Munson, T.; Banerjee, R. Differences in the efficiency of reductive activation of methionine synthase and exogenous electron acceptors between the common polymorphic variants of human methionine synthase reductase. *Biochemistry* **2002**, *41*, 13378–13385. [CrossRef] [PubMed]

28.	Sebastio, G.; Sperandeo, M.P.; Panico, M.; de Franchis, R.; Kraus, J.P.; Andria, G. The molecular basis of homocystinuria due to cystathionine beta synthase deficiency in italian families, and report of four novel mutations. *Am. J. Hum. Genet.* **1995**, *56*, 1324–1333. [PubMed]

29. Nienaber-Rousseau, C.; Ellis, S.M.; Moss, S.J.; Melse-Boonstra, A.; Towers, G.W. Gene-environment and gene-gene interactions of specific MTHFR, MTR and CBS gene variants in relation to homocysteine in black south africans. *Gene* **2013**, *530*, 113–118. [CrossRef] [PubMed]

30. Lievers, K.J.; Kluijtmans, L.A.; Heil, S.G.; Boers, G.H.; Verhoef, P.; van Oppenraay-Emmerzaal, D.; den Heijer, M.; Trijbels, F.J.; Blom, H.J. A 31 bp VNTR in the cystathionine beta-synthase (CBS) gene is associated with reduced cbs activity and elevated post-load homocysteine levels. *Eur. J. Hum. Genet.* **2001**, *9*, 583–589. [CrossRef] [PubMed]

31. Heil, S.G.; Van der Put, N.M.J.; Waas, E.T.; den Heijer, M.; Trijbels, F.J.M.; Blom, H.J. Is mutated serine hydroxymethyltransferase (SHMT) involved in the etiology of neural tube defects? *Mol. Genet. Metabol.* **2001**, *73*, 164–172. [CrossRef] [PubMed]

32. Ho, R.C.M.; Cheung, M.W.L.; Fu, E.; Win, H.H.; Zaw, M.H.; Ng, A.; Mak, A. Is high homocysteine level a risk factor for cognitive decline in elderly? A systematic review, meta-analysis, and meta-regression. *Am. J. Geriatr. Psychiatry* **2011**, *19*, 607–617. [CrossRef] [PubMed]

33. Seshadri, S.; Beiser, A.; Selhub, J.; Jacques, P.F.; Rosenberg, I.H.; D'Agostino, R.B.; Wilson, P.W.F.; Wolf, P.A. Plasma homocysteine as a risk factor for dementia and Alzheimer's disease. *N. Engl. J. Med.* **2002**, *346*, 476–483. [CrossRef] [PubMed]

34. Schafer, J.H.; Glass, T.A.; Bolla, K.I.; Mintz, M.; Jedlicka, A.E.; Schwartz, B.S. Homocysteine and cognitive function in a population-based study of older adults. *J. Am. Geriatr. Soc.* **2005**, *53*, 381–388. [CrossRef] [PubMed]

35. McCaddon, A.; Miller, J.W. Assessing the association between homocysteine and cognition: Reflections on bradford hill, meta-analyses, and causality. *Nutr. Rev.* **2015**, *73*, 723–735. [CrossRef] [PubMed]

36. Shen, L.; Ji, H.F. Associations between homocysteine, folic acid, vitamin B12 and Alzheimer's disease: Insights from meta-analyses. *J. Alzheimers Dis.* **2015**, *46*, 777–790. [CrossRef] [PubMed]

37. Flicker, L.; Martins, R.N.; Thomas, J.; Acres, J.; Taddei, K.; Vasikaran, S.D.; Norman, P.; Jamrozik, K.; Almeida, O.P. B-vitamins reduce plasma levels of beta amyloid. *Neurobiol. Aging* **2008**, *29*, 303–305. [CrossRef] [PubMed]

38. Durga, J.; van Boxtel, M.P.J.; Schouten, E.G.; Kok, F.J.; Jolles, J.; Katan, M.B.; Verhoef, P. Effect of 3-year folic acid supplementation on cognitive function in older adults in the facit trial: A randomised, double blind, controlled trial. *Lancet* **2007**, *369*, 208–216. [CrossRef]

39. Smith, A.D.; Smith, S.M.; de Jager, C.A.; Whitbread, P.; Johnston, C.; Agacinski, G.; Oulhaj, A.; Bradley, K.M.; Jacoby, R.; Refsum, H. Homocysteine-lowering by B vitamins slows the rate of accelerated brain atrophy in mild cognitive impairment: A randomized controlled trial. *PLoS ONE* **2010**, *5*, e12244. [CrossRef] [PubMed]

40. Douaud, G.; Refsum, H.; de Jager, C.A.; Jacoby, R.; Nichols, T.E.; Smith, S.M.; Smith, A.D. Preventing Alzheimer's disease-related gray matter atrophy by B-vitamin treatment. *Proc. Natl. Acad. Sci. USA* **2013**, *110*, 9523–9528. [CrossRef] [PubMed]

41. Clarke, R.; Halsey, J.; Bennett, D.; Lewington, S. Homocysteine and vascular disease: Review of published results of the homocysteine-lowering trials. *J. Inherit. Metab. Dis.* **2011**, *34*, 83–91. [CrossRef] [PubMed]

42. Clarke, R.; Bennett, D.; Parish, S.; Lewington, S.; Skeaff, M.; Eussen, S.J.; Lewerin, C.; Stott, D.J.; Armitage, J.; Hankey, G.J.; et al. Effects of homocysteine lowering with B vitamins on cognitive aging: Meta-analysis of 11 trials with cognitive data on 22,000 individuals. *Am. J. Clin. Nutr.* **2014**, *100*, 657–666. [CrossRef] [PubMed]

43. Fox, J.T.; Stover, P.J. Chapter 1 folate-mediated one-carbon metabolism. In *Vitamins & Hormones*; Gerald, L., Ed.; Academic Press: New York, NY, USA, 2008; Volume 79, pp. 1–44.

44. Shane, B. Folate and vitamin B12 metabolism: Overview and interaction with riboflavin, vitamin B6, and polymorphisms. *Food Nutr. Bull.* **2008**, *29*, S5–S16. [CrossRef] [PubMed]

45. Selhub, J. Homocysteine metabolism. *Annu. Rev. Nutr.* **1999**, *19*, 217–246. [CrossRef] [PubMed]

46. Gregory, J.F., 3rd. Chemical and nutritional aspects of folate research: Analytical procedures, methods of folate synthesis, stability, and bioavailability of dietary folates. *Adv. Food Nutr. Res.* **1989**, *33*, 1–101. [PubMed]

47. Malinow, M.R.; Nieto, F.J.; Kruger, W.D.; Duell, P.B.; Hess, D.L.; Gluckman, R.A.; Block, P.C.; Holzgang, C.R.; Anderson, P.H.; Seltzer, D.; et al. The effects of folic acid supplementation on plasma total homocysteine are modulated by multivitamin use and methylenetetrahydrofolate reductase genotypes. *Arterioscler. Thromb. Vasc. Biol.* **1997**, *17*, 1157–1162. [CrossRef] [PubMed]

48. Bailey, L.B.; Duhaney, R.L.; Maneval, D.R.; Kauwell, G.P.A.; Quinlivan, E.P.; Davis, S.R.; Cuadras, A.; Hutson, A.D.; Gregory, J.F. Vitamin B-12 status is inversely associated with plasma homocysteine in young women with C677T and/or a1298c methylenetetrahydrofolate reductase polymorphisms. *J. Nutr.* **2002**, *132*, 1872–1878. [PubMed]

49. Gaughan, D.J.; Kluijtmans, L.A.J.; Barbaux, S.; McMaster, D.; Young, I.S.; Yarnell, J.W.G.; Evans, A.; Whitehead, A.S. The methionine synthase reductase (MTRR) A66G polymorphism is a novel genetic determinant of plasma homocysteine concentrations. *Atherosclerosis* **2001**, *157*, 451–456. [CrossRef]

50. Ludwig, M.L.; Matthews, R.G. Structure-based perspectives on B12-dependent enzymes. *Annu. Rev. Biochem.* **1997**, *66*, 269–313. [CrossRef] [PubMed]

51. Leclerc, D.; Wilson, A.; Dumas, R.; Gafuik, C.; Song, D.; Watkins, D.; Heng, H.H.Q.; Rommens, J.M.; Scherer, S.W.; Rosenblatt, D.S.; et al. Cloning and mapping of a cDNA for methionine synthase reductase, a flavoprotein defective in patients with homocystinuria. *Proc. Natl. Acad. Sci. USA* **1998**, *95*, 3059–3064. [CrossRef] [PubMed]

52. Renwick, S.B.; Snell, K.; Baumann, U. The crystal structure of human cytosolic serine hydroxymethyltransferase: A target for cancer chemotherapy. *Structure* **1998**, *6*, 1105–1116. [CrossRef]

53. Rosenblatt, D.S. Inherited disorders of folate transport and metabolism. In *The Metabolic Basis of Inherited Disease*; Seriver, A.L., Beaudet, W.S., Sly, W.S., Valle, D., Eds.; McGraw-Hill: New York, NY, USA, 1995; Volume 2, pp. 3111–3128.

54. Pereira, A.C.; Schettert, I.T.; Morandini Filho, A.A.F.; Guerra-Shinohara, E.M.; Krieger, J.E. Methylenetetrahydrofolate reductase (MTHFR) C677T gene variant modulates the homocysteine folate correlation in a mild folate-deficient population. *Clin. Chim. Acta* **2004**, *340*, 99–105. [CrossRef] [PubMed]

55. Meisel, C.; Cascorbi, I.; Gerloff, T.; Stangl, V.; Laule, M.; Müller, J.M.; Wernecke, K.D.; Baumann, G.; Roots, I.; Stangl, K. Identification of six methylenetetrahydrofolate reductase (MTHFR) genotypes resulting from common polymorphisms: Impact on plasma homocysteine levels and development of coronary artery disease. *Atherosclerosis* **2001**, *154*, 651–658. [CrossRef]

56. Botto, L.D.; Yang, Q. 5,10-methylenetetrahydrofolate reductase gene variants and congenital anomalies: A huge review. *Am. J. Epidemiol.* **2000**, *151*, 862–877. [CrossRef] [PubMed]

57. Wilcken, B.; Bamforth, F.; Li, Z.; Zhu, H.; Ritvanen, A.; Redlund, M.; Stoll, C.; Alembik, Y.; Dott, B.; Czeizel, A.; et al. Geographical and ethnic variation of the 677c>t allele of 5,10 methylenetetrahydrofolate reductase (MTHFR): Findings from over 7000 newborns from 16 areas world wide. *J. Med. Genet.* **2003**, *40*, 619–625. [CrossRef] [PubMed]

58. Harmon, D.L.; Woodside, J.V.; Yarnell, J.W.G.; McMaster, D.; Young, I.S.; McCrum, E.E.; Gey, K.F.; Whitehead, A.S.; Evans, A.E. The Common 'Thermolabile' Variant of Methylene Tetrahydrofolate Reductase is a Major Determinant of Mild Hyperhomocysteinaemia. *QJM* **1996**, *89*, 571–578. [CrossRef] [PubMed]

59. Tsai, M.Y.; Bignell, M.; Yang, F.; Welge, B.G.; Graham, K.J.; Hanson, N.Q. Polygenic influence on plasma homocysteine: Association of two prevalent mutations, the 844INS68 of cystathionine β-synthase and A2756G of methionine synthase, with lowered plasma homocysteine levels. *Atherosclerosis* **2000**, *149*, 131–137. [CrossRef]

60. Dekou, V.; Gudnason, V.; Hawe, E.; Miller, G.J.; Stansbie, D.; Humphries, S.E. Gene-environment and gene-gene interaction in the determination of plasma homocysteine levels in healthy middle-aged men. *Thromb. Haemost.* **2001**, *85*, 67–74. [PubMed]

61. Kluijtmans, L.A.J.; Young, I.S.; Boreham, C.A.; Murray, L.; McMaster, D.; McNulty, H.; Strain, J.J.; McPartlin, J.; Scott, J.M.; Whitehead, A.S. Genetic and Nutritional Factors Contributing to Hyperhomocysteinemia in Young Adults. *Blood* **2003**, *101*, 2483–2488. [CrossRef] [PubMed]

62. Narayanan, S.; McConnell, J.; Little, J.; Sharp, L.; Piyathilake, C.J.; Powers, H.; Basten, G.; Duthie, S.J. Associations between two common variants C677T and A1298C in the methylenetetrahydrofolate reductase gene and measures of folate metabolism and DNA stability (strand breaks, misincorporated uracil, and DNA methylation status) in human lymphocytes in vivo. *Cancer Epidemiol. Biomark. Prev.* **2004**, *13*, 1436–1443.

63. Devlin, A.M.; Clarke, R.; Birks, J.; Evans, J.G.; Halsted, C.H. Interactions among polymorphisms in folate-metabolizing genes and serum total homocysteine concentrations in a healthy elderly population. *Am. J. Clin. Nutr.* **2006**, *83*, 708–713. [PubMed]

64. DeVos, L.; Chanson, A.; Liu, Z.; Ciappio, E.D.; Parnell, L.D.; Mason, J.B.; Tucker, K.L.; Crott, J.W. Associations between single nucleotide polymorphisms in folate uptake and metabolizing genes with blood folate, homocysteine, and DNA uracil concentrations. *Am. J. Clin. Nutr.* **2008**, *88*, 1149–1158. [PubMed]

65. Kim, J.-M.; Stewart, R.; Kim, S.-W.; Yang, S.-J.; Shin, I.-S.; Shin, H.-Y.; Yoon, J.-S. Methylenetetrahydrofolate reductase gene and risk of Alzheimer's disease in koreans. *Int. J. Geriatr. Psychiatry* **2008**, *23*, 454–459. [CrossRef] [PubMed]

66. Yang, Q.-H.; Botto, L.D.; Gallagher, M.; Friedman, J.; Sanders, C.L.; Koontz, D.; Nikolova, S.; Erickson, J.D.; Steinberg, K. Prevalence and effects of gene-gene and gene-nutrient interactions on serum folate and serum total homocysteine concentrations in the united states: Findings from the third national health and nutrition examination survey DNA bank. *Am. J. Clin. Nutr.* **2008**, *88*, 232–246. [PubMed]

67. Zappacosta, B.; Graziano, M.; Persichilli, S.; Di Castelnuovo, A.; Mastroiacovo, P.; Iacoviello, L. 5,10-methylenetetrahydrofolate reductase (MTHFR) C677T and A1298C polymorphisms: Genotype frequency and association with homocysteine and folate levels in middle-southern italian adults. *Cell Biochem. Funct.* **2014**, *32*, 1–4. [CrossRef] [PubMed]

68. Zhu, Y.; Zhu, R.-X.; He, Z.-Y.; Liu, X.; Liu, H.-N. Association of MTHFR C677T with total homocysteine plasma levels and susceptibility to parkinson's disease: A meta-analysis. *Neurol. Sci.* **2015**, *36*, 945–951. [CrossRef] [PubMed]

69. Chango, A.; Potier De Courcy, G.; Boisson, F.; Guilland, J.C.; Barbe, F.; Perrin, M.O.; Christides, J.P.; Rabhi, K.; Pfister, M.; Galan, P.; et al. 5,10-methylenetetrahydrofolate reductase common mutations, folate status and plasma homocysteine in healthy french adults of the supplementation en vitamines et mineraux antioxydants (su.Vi.Max) cohort. *Br. J. Nutr.* **2000**, *84*, 891–896. [PubMed]

70. Geisel, J.; Zimbelmann, I.; Schorr, H.; Knapp, J.P.; Bodis, M.; Hübner, U.; Herrmann, W. Genetic defects as important factors for moderate hyperhomocysteinemia. *Clin. Chem. Lab. Med.* **2001**, *39*, 698–704. [CrossRef] [PubMed]

71. Jacques, P.F.; Bostom, A.G.; Williams, R.R.; Ellison, R.C.; Eckfeldt, J.H.; Rosenberg, I.H.; Selhub, J.; Rozen, R. Relation between folate status, a common mutation in methylenetetrahydrofolate reductase, and plasma homocysteine concentrations. *Circulation* **1996**, *93*, 7–9. [CrossRef] [PubMed]

72. García-Minguillán, C.J.; Fernandez-Ballart, J.D.; Ceruelo, S.; Ríos, L.; Bueno, O.; Berrocal-Zaragoza, M.I.; Molloy, A.M.; Ueland, P.M.; Meyer, K.; Murphy, M.M. Riboflavin status modifies the effects of methylenetetrahydrofolate reductase (MTHFR) and methionine synthase reductase (mtrr) polymorphisms on homocysteine. *Genes Nutr.* **2014**, *9*, 435. [CrossRef] [PubMed]

73. Guttormsen, A.B.; Ueland, P.M.; Nesthus, I.; Nyg, E.O.; Schneede, J.; Vollset, S.E.; Refsum, H. Determinants and vitamin responsiveness of intermediate hyperhomocysteinemia (> or = 40 micromol/liter). The hordaland homocysteine study. *J. Clin. Investig.* **1996**, *98*, 2174–2183. [CrossRef] [PubMed]

74. Kauwell, G.P.; Wilsky, C.E.; Cerda, J.J.; Herrlinger-Garcia, K.; Hutson, A.D.; Theriaque, D.W.; Boddie, A.; Rampersaud, G.C.; Bailey, L.B. Methylenetetrahydrofolate reductase mutation (677c->t) negatively influences plasma homocysteine response to marginal folate intake in elderly women. *Metabolism* **2000**, *49*, 1440–1443. [CrossRef] [PubMed]

75. Hustad, S.; Ueland, P.M.; Vollset, S.E.; Zhang, Y.; Bjørke-Monsen, A.L.; Schneede, J. Riboflavin as a determinant of plasma total homocysteine: Effect modification by the methylenetetrahydrofolate reductase C677T polymorphism. *Clin. Chem.* **2000**, *46*, 1065–1071. [PubMed]

76. McNulty, H.; Dowey, L.R.C.; Strain, J.J.; Dunne, A.; Ward, M.; Molloy, A.M.; McAnena, L.B.; Hughes, J.P.; Hannon-Fletcher, M.; Scott, J.M. Riboflavin lowers homocysteine in individuals homozygous for the MTHFR 677c→t polymorphism. *Circulation* **2006**, *113*, 74–80. [CrossRef] [PubMed]

77. Jacques, P.F.; Kalmbach, R.; Bagley, P.J.; Russo, G.T.; Rogers, G.; Wilson, P.W.F.; Rosenberg, I.H.; Selhub, J. The relationship between riboflavin and plasma total homocysteine in the framingham offspring cohort is influenced by folate status and the C677T transition in the methylenetetrahydrofolate reductase gene. *J. Nutr.* **2002**, *132*, 283–288. [PubMed]

78. Hustad, S.; Midttun, Ø.; Schneede, J.; Vollset, S.E.; Grotmol, T.; Ueland, P.M. The methylenetetrahydrofolate reductase 677c→t polymorphism as a modulator of a B vitamin network with major effects on homocysteine metabolism. *Am. J. Hum. Genet.* **2007**, *80*, 846–855. [CrossRef] [PubMed]

79. D'Angelo, A.; Coppola, A.; Madonna, P.; Fermo, I.; Pagano, A.; Mazzola, G.; Galli, L.; Cerbone, A.M. The role of vitamin B12 in fasting hyperhomocysteinemia and its interaction with the homozygous C677T mutation of the methylenetetrahydrofolate reductase (MTHFR) gene a case-control study of patients with early-onset thrombotic events. *Thromb. Haemost.* **2000**, *83*, 563–570. [PubMed]

80. Trimmer, E.E. Methylenetetrahydrofolate reductase: Biochemical characterization and medical significance. *Curr. Pharm. Design* **2013**, *19*, 2574–2593. [CrossRef]

81. Friedman, G.; Goldschmidt, N.; Friedlander, Y.; Ben-Yehuda, A.; Selhub, J.; Babaey, S.; Mendel, M.; Kidron, M.; Bar-On, H. A common mutation A1298C in human methylenetetrahydrofolate reductase gene: Association with plasma total homocysteine and folate concentrations. *J. Nutr.* **1999**, *129*, 1656–1661. [PubMed]

82. Vaughn, J.D.; Bailey, L.B.; Shelnutt, K.P.; Dunwoody, K.M.V.-C.; Maneval, D.R.; Davis, S.R.; Quinlivan, E.P.; Gregory, J.F.; Theriaque, D.W.; Kauwell, G.P.A. Methionine synthase reductase 66a→g polymorphism is associated with increased plasma homocysteine concentration when combined with the homozygous methylenetetrahydrofolate reductase 677c→t variant. *J. Nutr.* **2004**, *134*, 2985–2990. [PubMed]

83. van der Put, N.M.; Gabreëls, F.; Stevens, E.M.; Smeitink, J.A.; Trijbels, F.J.; Eskes, T.K.; van den Heuvel, L.P.; Blom, H.J. A second common mutation in the methylenetetrahydrofolate reductase gene: An additional risk factor for neural-tube defects? *Am. J. Hum. Genet.* **1998**, *62*, 1044–1051. [CrossRef] [PubMed]

84. Cabo, R.; Hernes, S.; Slettan, A.; Haugen, M.; Ye, S.; Blomhoff, R.; Mansoor, M.A. Effect of genetic polymorphisms involved in folate metabolism on the concentration of serum folate and plasma total homocysteine (p-thcy) in healthy subjects after short-term folic acid supplementation: A randomized, double blind, crossover study. *Genes Nutr.* **2015**, *10*, 7. [CrossRef] [PubMed]

85. Morrison, K.; Edwards, Y.H.; Lynch, S.A.; Burn, J.; Hol, F.; Mariman, E. Methionine synthase and neural tube defects. *J. Med. Genet.* **1997**, *34*, 958. [CrossRef] [PubMed]

86. van der Put, N.M.; van der Molen, E.F.; Kluijtmans, L.A.; Heil, S.G.; Trijbels, J.M.; Eskes, T.K.; Van Oppenraaij-Emmerzaal, D.; Banerjee, R.; Blom, H.J. Sequence analysis of the coding region of human methionine synthase: Relevance to hyperhomocysteinaemia in neural-tube defects and vascular disease. *QJM* **1997**, *90*, 511–517. [CrossRef] [PubMed]

87. Morita, H.; Kurihara, H.; Sugiyama, T.; Hamada, C.; Kurihara, Y.; Shindo, T.; Oh-hashi, Y.; Yazaki, Y. Polymorphism of the methionine synthase gene: Association with homocysteine metabolism and late-onset vascular diseases in the japanese population. *Arterioscler. Thromb. Vasc. Biol.* **1999**, *19*, 298–302. [CrossRef] [PubMed]

88. Jacques, P.F.; Bostom, A.G.; Selhub, J.; Rich, S.; Curtis Ellison, R.; Eckfeldt, J.H.; Gravel, R.A.; Rozen, R. Effects of polymorphisms of methionine synthase and methionine synthase reductase on total plasma homocysteine in the NHLBI family heart study. *Atherosclerosis* **2003**, *166*, 49–55. [CrossRef]

89. Wang, X.L.; Duarte, N.; Cai, H.; Adachi, T.; Sim, A.S.; Cranney, G.; Wilcken, D.E.L. Relationship between total plasma homocysteine, polymorphisms of homocysteine metabolism related enzymes, risk factors and coronary artery disease in the australian hospital-based population. *Atherosclerosis* **1999**, *146*, 133–140. [CrossRef]

90. Tsai, M.Y.; Welge, B.G.; Hanson, N.Q.; Bignell, M.K.; Vessey, J.; Schwichtenberg, K.; Yang, F.; Bullemer, F.E.; Rasmussen, R.; Graham, K.J. Genetic causes of mild hyperhomocysteinemia in patients with premature occlusive coronary artery diseases. *Atherosclerosis* **1999**, *143*, 163–170. [CrossRef]

91. Ma, J.; Stampfer, M.J.; Christensen, B.; Giovannucci, E.; Hunter, D.J.; Chen, J.; Willett, W.C.; Selhub, J.; Hennekens, C.H.; Gravel, R.; et al. A polymorphism of the methionine synthase gene: Association with plasma folate, vitamin B12, homocyst(e)ine, and colorectal cancer risk. *Cancer Epidemiol. Biomark. Prev.* **1999**, *8*, 825–829.

92. Hyndman, M.E.; Bridge, P.J.; Warnica, J.W.; Fick, G.; Parsons, H.G. Effect of heterozygosity for the methionine synthase 2756 a→g mutation on the risk for recurrent cardiovascular events. *Am. J. Cardiol.* **2000**, *86*, 1144–1146. [CrossRef]

93. Harmon, D.L.; Shields, D.C.; Woodside, J.V.; McMaster, D.; Yarnell, J.W.G.; Young, I.S.; Peng, K.; Shane, B.; Evans, A.E.; Whitehead, A.S. Methionine synthase D919G polymorphism is a significant but modest determinant of circulating homocysteine concentrations. *Genet. Epidemiol.* **1999**, *17*, 298–309. [CrossRef]

94   Chen, J.; Stampfer, M.J.; Ma, J.; Selhub, J.; Malinow, M.R.; Hennekens, C.H.; Hunter, D.J. Influence of a methionine synthase (D919G) polymorphism on plasma homocysteine and folate levels and relation to risk of myocardial infarction. *Atherosclerosis* **2001**, *154*, 667–672. [CrossRef]

95. McCaddon, A.; Regland, B.; Hudson, P.; Davies, G. Functional vitamin B(12) deficiency and Alzheimer's disease. *Neurology* **2002**, *58*, 1395–1399. [CrossRef] [PubMed]

96. Wilson, A.; Platt, R.; Wu, Q.; Leclerc, D.; Christensen, B.; Yang, H.; Gravel, R.A.; Rozen, R. A common variant in methionine synthase reductase combined with low cobalamin (vitamin B12) increases risk for spina bifida. *Mol. Genet. Metab.* **1999**, *67*, 317–323. [CrossRef] [PubMed]

97. Rai, V.; Yadav, U.; Kumar, P.; Yadav, S.K. Analysis of methionine synthase reductase polymorphism (A66G) in indian muslim population. *Indian J. Hum. Genet.* **2013**, *19*, 183–187. [CrossRef] [PubMed]

98. Rady, P.L.; Szucs, S.; Grady, J.; Hudnall, S.D.; Kellner, L.H.; Nitowsky, H.; Tyring, S.K.; Matalon, R.K. Genetic polymorphisms of methylenetetrahydrofolate reductase (MTHFR) and methionine synthase reductase (MTRR) in ethnic populations in texas; a report of a novel MTHFR polymorphic site, G1793A. *Am. J. Med. Genet.* **2002**, *107*, 162–168. [CrossRef] [PubMed]

99. Brilakis, E.S.; Berger, P.B.; Ballman, K.V.; Rozen, R. Methylenetetrahydrofolate reductase (MTHFR) 677C>T and methionine synthase reductase (MTRR) 66A>G polymorphisms: Association with serum homocysteine and angiographic coronary artery disease in the era of flour products fortified with folic acid. *Atherosclerosis* **2003**, *168*, 315–322. [PubMed]

100. Brown, C.A.; McKinney, K.Q.; Kaufman, J.S.; Gravel, R.A.; Rozen, R. A common polymorphism in methionine synthase reductase increases risk of premature coronary artery disease. *J. Cardiovasc. Risk* **2000**, *7*, 197–200. [CrossRef] [PubMed]

101. O'Leary, V.B.; Parle-McDermott, A.; Molloy, A.M.; Kirke, P.N.; Johnson, Z.; Conley, M.; Scott, J.M.; Mills, J.L. MTRR and MTHFR polymorphism: Link to down syndrome? *Am. J. Med. Genet.* **2002**, *107*, 151–155. [CrossRef] [PubMed]

102. Gaughan, D.J.; Kluijtmans, L.A.J.; Barbaux, S.; McMaster, D.; Young, I.S.; Yarnell, J.W.G.; Evans, A.; Whitehead, A.S. Corrigendum to "the methionine synthase reductase (MTRR) A66G polymorphism is a novel genetic determinant of plasma homocysteine concentrations" [ath 157 (2001) 451–456]. *Atherosclerosis* **2003**, *167*, 373. [CrossRef]

103. De Bruijn, R.F.A.G.; Ikram, M.A. Cardiovascular risk factors and future risk of Alzheimer's disease. *BMC Med.* **2014**, *12*, 130. [CrossRef] [PubMed]

104. Kluijtmans, L.A.; van den Heuvel, L.P.; Boers, G.H.; Frosst, P.; Stevens, E.M.; van Oost, B.A.; den Heijer, M.; Trijbels, F.J.; Rozen, R.; Blom, H.J. Molecular genetic analysis in mild hyperhomocysteinemia: A common mutation in the methylenetetrahydrofolate reductase gene is a genetic risk factor for cardiovascular disease. *Am. J. Hum. Genet.* **1996**, *58*, 35–41. [PubMed]

105. Gallagher, P.M.; Meleady, R.; Shields, D.C.; Tan, K.S.; McMaster, D.; Rozen, R.; Evans, A.; Graham, I.M.; Whitehead, A.S. Homocysteine and risk of premature coronary heart disease: Evidence for a common gene mutation. *Circulation* **1996**, *94*, 2154–2158. [CrossRef] [PubMed]

106. Hu, F.L.; Gu, Z.; Kozich, V.; Kraus, J.P.; Ramesh, V.; Shih, V.E. Molecular basis of cystathionine beta-synthase deficiency in pyridoxine responsive and nonresponsive homocystinuria. *Hum. Mol. Genet.* **1993**, *2*, 1857–1860. [CrossRef] [PubMed]

107. Kraus, J.P. Komrower lecture. Molecular basis of phenotype expression in homocystinuria. *J. Inherit. Metab. Dis.* **1994**, *17*, 383–390. [CrossRef] [PubMed]

108. De Stefano, V.; Dekou, V.; Nicaud, V.; Chasse, J.F.; London, J.; Stansbie, D.; Humphries, S.E.; Gudnason, V. Linkage disequilibrium at the cystathionine beta synthase (CBS) locus and the association between genetic variation at the CBS locus and plasma levels of homocysteine. The ears II group. European atherosclerosis research study. *Ann. Hum. Genet.* **1998**, *62*, 481–490. [CrossRef] [PubMed]

109. Tsai, M.Y.; Bignell, M.; Schwichtenberg, K.; Hanson, N.Q. High prevalence of a mutation in the cystathionine beta-synthase gene. *Am. J. Hum. Genet.* **1996**, *59*, 1262–1267. [PubMed]

110. Kluijtmans, L.A.; Boers, G.H.; Trijbels, F.J.; van Lith-Zanders, H.M.; van den Heuvel, L.P.; Blom, H.J. A common 844INS68 insertion variant in the cystathionine beta-synthase gene. *Biochem. Mol. Med.* **1997**, *62*, 23–25. [CrossRef] [PubMed]

111. Gan, Y.Y.; Chen, C.F. Novel alleles of 31-bp VNTR polymorphism in the human cystathionine beta-synthase (CBS) gene were detected in healthy asians. *J. Genet.* **2010**, *89*, 449–455. [CrossRef] [PubMed]

112. Vijaya Lakshmi, S.V.; Naushad, S.; Seshagiri Rao, D.; Kutala, V. Oxidative stress is associated with genetic polymorphisms in one-carbon metabolism in coronary artery disease. *Cell Biochem. Biophys.* **2013**, *67*, 353–361. [CrossRef] [PubMed]

113. Prince, J.A.; Feuk, L.; Sawyer, S.L.; Gottfries, J.; Ricksten, A.; Nagga, K.; Bogdanovic, N.; Blennow, K.; Brookes, A.J. Lack of replication of association findings in complex disease: An analysis of 15 polymorphisms in prior candidate genes for sporadic Alzheimer's disease. *Eur. J. Hum. Genet.* **2001**, *9*, 437–444. [CrossRef] [PubMed]

114. Linnebank, M.; Linnebank, A.; Jeub, M.; Klockgether, T.; Wüllner, U.; Kölsch, H.; Heun, R.; Koch, H.G.; Suormala, T.; Fowler, B. Lack of genetic dispositions to hyperhomocysteinemia in Alzheimer's disease. *Am. J. Med. Genet.* **2004**, *131 A*, 101–102. [CrossRef] [PubMed]

115. Religa, D.; Styczynska, M.; Peplonska, B.; Gabryelewicz, T.; Pfeffer, A.; Chodakowska, M.; Luczywek, E.; Wasiak, B.; Stepien, K.; Golebiowski, M.; et al. Homocysteine, apolipoproteine E and methylenetetrahydrofolate reductase in Alzheimer's disease and mild cognitive impairment. *Dement. Geriatr. Cogn. Disord.* **2003**, *16*, 64–70. [CrossRef] [PubMed]

116. Clarke, R.; Smith, A.D.; Jobst, K.A.; Refsum, H.; Sutton, L.; Ueland, P.M. Folate, vitamin B12, and serum total homocysteine levels in confirmed Alzheimer's disease. *Arch. Neurol.* **1998**, *55*, 1449–1455. [CrossRef] [PubMed]

117. Chapman, J.; Wang, N.; Treves, T.A.; Korczyn, A.D.; Bornstein, N.M. Ace, MTHFR, factor v leiden, and apoe polymorphisms in patients with vascular and Alzheimer's dementia. *Stroke* **1998**, *29*, 1401–1404. [CrossRef] [PubMed]

118. Kida, T.; Kamino, K.; Yamamoto, M.; Kanayama, D.; Tanaka, T.; Kudo, T.; Takeda, M. C677T polymorphism of methylenetetrahydrofolate reductase gene affects plasma homocysteine level and is a genetic factor of late-onset Alzheimer's disease. *Psychogeriatrics* **2004**, *4*, 4–10. [CrossRef]

119. Brunelli, T.; Bagnoli, S.; Giusti, B.; Nacmias, B.; Pepe, G.; Sorbi, S.; Abbate, R. The C677T methylenetetrahydrofolate reductase mutation is not associated with Alzheimer's disease. *Neurosci. Lett.* **2001**, *315*, 103–105. [CrossRef]

120. Postiglione, A.; Milan, G.; Ruocco, A.; Gallotta, G.; Guiotto, G.; Di Minno, G. Plasma folate, vitamin B12, and total homocysteine and homozygosity for the C677T mutation of the 5,10-methylene tetrahydrofolate reductase gene in patients with Alzheimer's dementia: A case-control study. *Gerontology* **2001**, *47*, 324–329. [CrossRef] [PubMed]

121. Zuliani, G.; Ble, A.; Zanca, R.; Munari, M.R.; Zurlo, A.; Vavalle, C.; Atti, A.R.; Fellin, R. Genetic polymorphisms in older subjects with vascular or Alzheimer's dementia. *Acta Neurol. Scand.* **2001**, *103*, 304–308. [CrossRef] [PubMed]

122. Seripa, D.; Dal Forno, G.; Matera, M.G.; Gravina, C.; Margaglione, M.; Palermo, M.T.; Wekstein, D.R.; Antuono, P.; Davis, D.G.; Daniele, A.; et al. Methylenetetrahydrofolate reductase and angiotensin converting enzyme gene polymorphisms in two genetically and diagnostically distinct cohort of Alzheimer patients. *Neurobiol. Aging* **2003**, *24*, 933–939. [CrossRef]

123. Bosco, P.; Gueant-Rodriguez, R.; Anello, G.; Romano, A.; Namour, B.; Spada, R.; Caraci, F.; Tringali, G.; Ferri, R.; Gueant, J. Association of IL-1 RN*2 allele and methionine synthase 2756 AA genotype with dementia severity of sporadic Alzheimer's disease. *J. Neurol. Neurosurg. Psychiatry* **2004**, *75*, 1036–1038. [CrossRef] [PubMed]

124. Wehr, H.; Bednarska-Makaruk, M.; Łojkowska, W.; Graban, A.; Hoffman-Zacharska, D.; Kuczyńska-Zardzewiały, A.; Mrugała, J.; Rodo, M.; Bochyńska, A.; Sułek, A.; et al. Differences in risk factors for dementia with neurodegenerative traits and for vascular dementia. *Dement. Geriatr. Cogn. Disord.* **2006**, *22*, 1–7. [CrossRef] [PubMed]

125. Styczynska, M.; Strosznajder, J.B.; Religa, D.; Chodakowska-Zebrowska, M.; Pfeffer, A.; Gabryelewicz, T.; Czapski, G.A.; Kobrys, M.; Karciauskas, G.; Barcikowska, M. Association between genetic and environmental factors and the risk of Alzheimer's disease. *Folia Neuropathol. Assoc. Pol. Neuropathol. Med. Res. Centre Pol. Acad. Sci.* **2008**, *46*, 249–254.

126. Fernandez, L.L.; Scheibe, R.M. Is MTHFR polymorphism a risk factor for Alzheimer's disease like apoe? *Arquivos de Neuro-Psiquiatria* **2005**, *63*, 1–6. [CrossRef] [PubMed]

127. Zhang, M.-Y.; Miao, L.; Li, Y.-S.; Hu, G.-Y. Meta-analysis of the methylenetetrahydrofolate reductase C677T polymorphism and susceptibility to Alzheimer's disease. *Neurosci. Res.* **2010**, *68*, 142–150. [CrossRef] [PubMed]

128. Rai, V. Folate pathway gene methylenetetrahydrofolate reductase C677T polymorphism and Alzheimer's disease risk in asian population. *Indian J. Clin. Biochem.* **2016**, *31*, 245–252. [CrossRef] [PubMed]

129. Keikhaee, M.; Hashemi, S.; Najmabadi, H.; Noroozian, M. C677T methylentetrahydrofulate reductase and angiotensin converting enzyme gene polymorphisms in patients with Alzheimer's disease in iranian population. *Neurochem. Res.* **2006**, *31*, 1079–1083. [CrossRef] [PubMed]

130. Da Silva, V.C.; Ramos, F.J.D.C.; Freitas, E.M.; De Brito-Marques, P.R.; Cavalcanti, M.N.D.H.; D'Almeida, V.; Cabral-Filho, J.E.; Muniz, M.T.C. Alzheimer's disease in brazilian elderly has a relation with homocysteine but not with MTHFR polymorphisms. *Arquivos de Neuro-Psiquiatria* **2006**, *64*, 941–945. [CrossRef] [PubMed]

131. Bottiglieri, T.; Parnetti, L.; Arning, E.; Ortiz, T.; Amici, S.; Lanari, A.; Gallai, V. Plasma total homocysteine levels and the C677T mutation in the methylenetetrahydrofolate reductase (MTHFR) gene: A study in an italian population with dementia. *Mech. Ageing Dev.* **2001**, *122*, 2013–2023. [CrossRef]

132. McGarel, C.; Pentieva, K.; Strain, J.J.; McNulty, H. Emerging roles for folate and related b-vitamins in brain health across the lifecycle. *Proc. Nutr. Soc.* **2015**, *74*, 46–55. [CrossRef] [PubMed]

133. Fuso, A.; Nicolia, V.; Cavallaro, R.A.; Ricceri, L.; D'Anselmi, F.; Coluccia, P.; Calamandrei, G.; Scarpa, S. B-vitamin deprivation induces hyperhomocysteinemia and brain *S*-adenosylhomocysteine, depletes brain *S*-adenosylmethionine, and enhances ps1 and bace expression and amyloid-β deposition in mice. *Mol. Cell. Neurosci.* **2008**, *37*, 731–746. [CrossRef] [PubMed]

134. Sai, X.; Kawamura, Y.; Kokame, K.; Yamaguchi, H.; Shiraishi, H.; Suzuki, R.; Suzuki, T.; Kawaichi, M.; Miyata, T.; Kitamura, T.; et al. Endoplasmic reticulum stress-inducible protein, herp, enhances presenilin-mediated generation of amyloid β-protein. *J. Biol. Chem.* **2002**, *277*, 12915–12920. [CrossRef] [PubMed]

135. Zhuo, J.M.; Portugal, G.S.; Kruger, W.D.; Wang, H.; Gould, T.J.; Praticò, D. Diet-induced hyperhomocysteinemia increases amyloid-β formation and deposition in a mouse model of Alzheimer's disease. *Curr. Alzheimer Res.* **2010**, *7*, 140–149. [CrossRef] [PubMed]

136. Pacheco-Quinto, J.; Rodriguez de Turco, E.B.; DeRosa, S.; Howard, A.; Cruz-Sanchez, F.; Sambamurti, K.; Refolo, L.; Petanceska, S.; Pappolla, M.A. Hyperhomocysteinemic Alzheimer's mouse model of amyloidosis shows increased brain amyloid β peptide levels. *Neurobiol. Dis.* **2006**, *22*, 651–656. [CrossRef] [PubMed]

137. Sontag, E.; Nunbhakdi-Craig, V.; Sontag, J.-M.; Diaz-Arrastia, R.; Ogris, E.; Dayal, S.; Lentz, S.R.; Arning, E.; Bottiglieri, T. Protein phosphatase 2A methyltransferase links homocysteine metabolism with tau and amyloid precursor protein regulation. *J. Neurosci.* **2007**, *27*, 2751–2759. [CrossRef] [PubMed]

138. Hooshmand, B.; Polvikoski, T.; Kivipelto, M.; Tanskanen, M.; Myllykangas, L.; Erkinjuntti, T.; Mäkelä, M.; Oinas, M.; Paetau, A.; Scheltens, P.; et al. Plasma homocysteine, Alzheimer and cerebrovascular pathology: A population-based autopsy study. *Brain* **2013**, *136*, 2707–2716. [CrossRef] [PubMed]

139. Walsh, D.M.; Hartley, D.M.; Kusumoto, Y.; Fezoui, Y.; Condron, M.M.; Lomakin, A.; Benedek, G.B.; Selkoe, D.J.; Teplow, D.B. Amyloid beta-protein fibrillogenesis: Structure and biological activity of protofibrillar intermediates. *J. Biol. Chem.* **1999**, *274*, 25945–25952. [CrossRef] [PubMed]

140. Hardy, J.; Allsop, D. Amyloid deposition as the central event in the aetiology of Alzheimer's disease. *Trends Pharmacol. Sci.* **1991**, *12*, 383–388. [CrossRef]

141. Li, J.-G.; Praticò, D. High levels of homocysteine results in cerebral amyloid angiopathy in mice. *J. Alzheimer's Dis.* **2015**, *43*, 29–35.

142. Zhang, C.-E.; Wei, W.; Liu, Y.-H.; Peng, J.-H.; Tian, Q.; Liu, G.-P.; Zhang, Y.; Wang, J.-Z. Hyperhomocysteinemia increases β-amyloid by enhancing expression of γ-secretase and phosphorylation of amyloid precursor protein in rat brain. *Am. J. Pathol.* **2009**, *174*, 1481–1491. [CrossRef] [PubMed]

143. Agnati, L.F.; Genedani, S.; Leo, G.; Forni, A.; Woods, A.S.; Filaferro, M.; Franco, R.; Fuxe, K. Aβ peptides as one of the crucial volume transmission signals in the trophic units and their interactions with homocysteine. Physiological implications and relevance for Alzheimer's disease. *J. Neural Transm.* **2007**, *114*, 21–31. [CrossRef] [PubMed]

144. De Felice, F.G.; Velasco, P.T.; Lambert, M.P.; Viola, K.; Fernandez, S.J.; Ferreira, S.T.; Klein, W.L. Aβ oligomers induce neuronal oxidative stress through an *N*-methyl-D-aspartate receptor-dependent mechanism that is blocked by the Alzheimer drug memantine. *J. Biol. Chem.* **2007**, *282*, 11590–11601. [CrossRef] [PubMed]

145. Butterfield, D.A.; Boyd-Kimball, D. Amyloid β-peptide(1–42) contributes to the oxidative stress and neurodegeneration found in Alzheimer's disease brain. *Brain Pathol.* **2004**, *14*, 426–432. [CrossRef] [PubMed]

146. Troen, A.M.; Shea-Budgell, M.; Shukitt-Hale, B.; Smith, D.E.; Selhub, J.; Rosenberg, I.H. B-vitamin deficiency causes hyperhomocysteinemia and vascular cognitive impairment in mice. *Proc. Natl. Acad. Sci. USA* **2008**, *105*, 12474–12479. [CrossRef] [PubMed]

147. Upchurch, G.R., Jr.; Welch, G.N.; Fabian, A.J.; Freedman, J.E.; Johnson, J.L.; Keaney, J.F., Jr.; Loscalzo, J. Homocyst(e)ine decreases bioavailable nitric oxide by a mechanism involving glutathione peroxidase. *J. Biol. Chem.* **1997**, *272*, 17012–17017. [CrossRef] [PubMed]

148. Kruman, I.I.; Culmsee, C.; Chan, S.L.; Kruman, Y.; Guo, Z.; Penix, L.; Mattson, M.P. Homocysteine elicits a DNA damage response in neurons that promotes apoptosis and hypersensitivity to excitotoxicity. *J. Neurosci.* **2000**, *20*, 6920–6926. [PubMed]

149. Grieve, A.; Butcher, S.P.; Griffiths, R. Synaptosomal plasma membrane transport of excitatory sulphur amino acid transmitter candidates: Kinetic characterisation and analysis of carrier specificity. *J. Neurosci. Res.* **1992**, *32*, 60–68. [CrossRef] [PubMed]

150. Farkas, M.; Keskitalo, S.; Smith, D.E.; Bain, N.; Semmler, A.; Ineichen, B.; Smulders, Y.; Blom, H.; Kulic, L.; Linnebank, M. Hyperhomocysteinemia in Alzheimer's disease: The hen and the egg? *J. Alzheimers Dis.* **2013**, *33*, 1097–1104. [PubMed]

151. Fuchs, D.; Jaeger, M.; Widner, B.; Wirleitner, B.; Artner-Dworzak, E.; Leblhuber, F. Is hyperhomocysteinemia due to the oxidative depletion of folate rather than to insufficient dietary intake? *Clin. Chem. Lab. Med.* **2001**, *39*, 691–694. [CrossRef] [PubMed]

152. Widner, B.; Fuchs, D.; Leblhuber, F.; Sperner-Unterwege, B.; Reynolds, E.; Bottiglieri, T. Does disturbed homocysteine and folate metabolism in depression result from enhanced oxidative stress? *J. Neurol. Neurosurg. Psychiatry* **2001**, *70*, 419. [CrossRef] [PubMed]

153. Mudd, S.H.; Poole, J.R. Labile methyl balances for normal humans on various dietary regimens. *Metabolism* **1975**, *24*, 721–735. [CrossRef]

154. Obeid, R. The metabolic burden of methyl donor deficiency with focus on the betaine homocysteine methyltransferase pathway. *Nutrients* **2013**, *5*, 3481–3495. [CrossRef] [PubMed]

155. McKeever, M.P.; Weir, D.G.; Molloy, A.; Scott, J.M. Betaine-homocysteine methyltransferase: Organ distribution in man, pig and rat and subcellular distribution in the rat. *Clin. Sci.* **1991**, *81*, 551–556. [CrossRef] [PubMed]

156. Caudill, M.A.; Dellschaft, N.; Solis, C.; Hinkis, S.; Ivanov, A.A.; Nash-Barboza, S.; Randall, K.E.; Jackson, B.; Solomita, G.N.; Vermeylen, F. Choline intake, plasma riboflavin, and the phosphatidylethanolamine *N*-methyltransferase G5465A genotype predict plasma homocysteine in folate-deplete mexican-american men with the methylenetetrahydrofolate reductase 677TT genotype. *J. Nutr.* **2009**, *139*, 727–733. [CrossRef] [PubMed]

157. Ortbauer, M.; Ripper, D.; Fuhrmann, T.; Lassi, M.; Auernigg-Haselmaier, S.; Stiegler, C.; König, J. Folate deficiency and over-supplementation causes impaired folate metabolism: Regulation and adaptation mechanisms in caenorhabditis elegans. *Mol. Nutr. Food Res.* **2016**, *60*, 949–956. [CrossRef] [PubMed]

158. Field, M.S.; Kamynina, E.; Agunloye, O.C.; Liebenthal, R.P.; Lamarre, S.G.; Brosnan, M.E.; Brosnan, J.T.; Stover, P.J. Nuclear enrichment of folate cofactors and methylenetetrahydrofolate dehydrogenase 1 (MTHFD1) protect de novo thymidylate biosynthesis during folate deficiency. *J. Biol. Chem.* **2014**, *289*, 29642–29650. [CrossRef] [PubMed]

159. Morrison, L.D.; Smith, D.D.; Kish, S.J. Brain *S*-adenosylmethionine levels are severely decreased in Alzheimer's disease. *J. Neurochem.* **1996**, *67*, 1328–1331. [CrossRef] [PubMed]

160. Wang, S.-C.; Oelze, B.; Schumacher, A. Age-specific epigenetic drift in late-onset Alzheimer's disease. *PLoS ONE* **2008**, *3*, e2698. [CrossRef] [PubMed]

161. van Driel, L.M.J.W.; Eijkemans, M.J.C.; de Jonge, R.; de Vries, J.H.M.; van Meurs, J.B.J.; Steegers, E.A.P.; Steegers-Theunissen, R.P.M. Body mass index is an important determinant of methylation biomarkers in women of reproductive ages. *J. Nutr.* **2009**, *139*, 2315–2321. [CrossRef] [PubMed]

162. Axelrod, J. Methylation reaction in the formation and metabolism of catecholamines and other biogenic amines. *Pharmacol. Rev.* **1966**, *18*, 95–113. [PubMed]

163. Flynn, D.D.; Kloog, Y.; Potter, L.T.; Axelrod, J. Enzymatic methylation of the membrane-bound nicotinic acetylcholine receptor. *J. Biol. Chem.* **1982**, *257*, 9513–9517. [PubMed]

164. Kim, S.; Lim, I.K.; Park, G.-H.; Paik, W.K. Biological methylation of myelin basic protein: Enzymology and biological significance. *Int. J. Biochem. Cell Biol.* **1997**, *29*, 743–751. [CrossRef]

165. Strittmatter, W.J.; Hirata, F.; Axelrod, J. Regulation of the beta-adrenergic receptor by methylation of membrane phospholipids. *Adv. Cyclic Nucleotide Res.* **1981**, *14*, 83–91. [PubMed]

166. Sontag, J.-M.; Nunbhakdi-Craig, V.; Montgomery, L.; Arning, E.; Bottiglieri, T.; Sontag, E. Folate deficiency induces in vitro and mouse brain region-specific downregulation of leucine carboxyl methyltransferase-1 and protein phosphatase 2A Bα subunit expression that correlate with enhanced tau phosphorylation. *J. Neurosci.* **2008**, *28*, 11477–11487. [CrossRef] [PubMed]

167. Fuso, A.; Cavallaro, R.A.; Zampelli, A.; D'Anselmi, F.; Piscopo, P.; Confaloni, A.; Scarpa, S. Gamma-secretase is differentially modulated by alterations of homocysteine cycle in neuroblastoma and glioblastoma cells. *J. Alzheimers Dis.* **2007**, *11*, 275–290. [PubMed]

168. Fuso, A.; Nicolia, V.; Pasqualato, A.; Fiorenza, M.T.; Cavallaro, R.A.; Scarpa, S. Changes in presenilin 1 gene methylation pattern in diet-induced b vitamin deficiency. *Neurobiol. Aging* **2011**, *32*, 187–199. [CrossRef] [PubMed]

169. Fuso, A. The 'golden age' of DNA methylation in neurodegenerative diseases. *Clin. Chem. Lab. Med.* **2013**, *51*, 523–534. [CrossRef] [PubMed]

170. Li, W.; Liu, H.; Yu, M.; Zhang, X.; Zhang, M.; Wilson, J.X.; Huang, G. Folic acid administration inhibits amyloid β-peptide accumulation in app/ps1 transgenic mice. *J. Nutr. Biochem.* **2015**, *26*, 883–891. [CrossRef] [PubMed]

171. Liu, J.J.; Green, P.; Mann, J.J.; Rapoport, S.I.; Sublette, M.E. Pathways of polyunsaturated fatty acid utilization: Implications for brain function in neuropsychiatric health and disease. *Brain Res.* **2015**, *1597*, 220–246. [CrossRef] [PubMed]

172. Watkins, S.M.; Zhu, X.; Zeisel, S.H. Phosphatidylethanolamine-n-methyltransferase activity and dietary choline regulate liver-plasma lipid flux and essential fatty acid metabolism in mice. *J. Nutr.* **2003**, *133*, 3386–3391. [PubMed]

173. Vance, D.E.; Walkey, C.J.; Cui, Z. Phosphatidylethanolamine N-methyltransferase from liver. *Biochim. Biophys. Acta* **1997**, *1348*, 142–150. [CrossRef]

174. Astarita, G.; Jung, K.-M.; Berchtold, N.C.; Nguyen, V.Q.; Gillen, D.L.; Head, E.; Cotman, C.W.; Piomelli, D. Deficient liver biosynthesis of docosahexaenoic acid correlates with cognitive impairment in Alzheimer's disease. *PLoS ONE* **2010**, *5*, e12538. [CrossRef] [PubMed]

175. Beyer, K.; Lao, J.I.; Latorre, P.; Riutort, N.; Matute, B.; Fernandez-Figueras, M.T.; Mate, J.L.; Ariza, A. Methionine synthase polymorphism is a risk factor for Alzheimer's disease. *Neuroreport* **2003**, *14*, 1391–1394. [CrossRef] [PubMed]

176. Dorszewska, J.; Florczak, J.; Rozycka, A.; Kempisty, B.; Jaroszewska-Kolecka, J.; Chojnacka, K.; Trzeciak, W.H.; Kozubski, W. Oxidative DNA damage and level of thiols as related to polymorphisms of MTHFR, mtr, mthfd1 in Alzheimer's and Parkinson's diseases. *Acta Neurobiol. Exp.* **2007**, *67*, 113–129.

177. Shea, T.B.; Rogers, E.; Ashline, D.; Ortiz, D.; Sheu, M.-S. Original contribution: Apolipoprotein e deficiency promotes increased oxidative stress and compensatory increases in antioxidants in brain tissue. *Free Radic. Biol. Med.* **2002**, *33*, 1115–1120. [CrossRef]

178. Shea, T.B.; Rogers, E. Research report: Folate quenches oxidative damage in brains of apolipoprotein E-deficient mice: Augmentation by vitamin E. *Mol. Brain Res.* **2002**, *108*, 1–6. [CrossRef]

179. Huang, R.-F.S.; Hsu, Y.-C.; Lin, H.-L.; Yang, F.L. Folate depletion and elevated plasma homocysteine promote oxidative stress in rat livers. *J. Nutr.* **2001**, *131*, 33–38. [PubMed]

180. Fan, J.; Ye, J.; Kamphorst, J.J.; Shlomi, T.; Thompson, C.B.; Rabinowitz, J.D. Quantitative flux analysis reveals folate-dependent nadph production. *Nature* **2014**, *510*, 298–302. [CrossRef] [PubMed]

181. Wakutani, Y.; Kowa, H.; Kusumi, M.; Nakaso, K.; Yasui, K.I.; Isoe-Wada, K.; Yano, H.; Urakami, K.; Takeshima, T.; Nakashima, K. A haplotype of the methylenetetrahydrofolate reductase gene is protective against late-onset Alzheimer's disease. *Neurobiol. Aging* **2004**, *25*, 291–294. [CrossRef]

182. Kruman, II; Kumaravel, T.S.; Lohani, A.; Pedersen, W.A.; Cutler, R.G.; Kruman, Y.; Haughey, N.; Lee, J.; Evans, M.; Mattson, M.P. Folic acid deficiency and homocysteine impair DNA repair in hippocampal neurons and sensitize them to amyloid toxicity in experimental models of Alzheimer's disease. *J. Neurosci.* **2002**, *22*, 1752–1762. [PubMed]

183. Taoka, S.; Ohja, S.; Shan, X.; Kruger, W.D.; Banerjee, R. Evidence for heme-mediated redox regulation of human cystathionine β-synthase activity. *J. Biol. Chem.* **1998**, *273*, 25179–25184. [CrossRef] [PubMed]

184. Pfeiffer, C.M.; Sternberg, M.R.; Fazili, Z.; Lacher, D.A.; Zhang, M.; Johnson, C.L.; Hamner, H.C.; Bailey, R.L.; Rader, J.I.; Yamini, S.; et al. Folate status and concentrations of serum folate forms in the us population: National health and nutrition examination survey 2011–2. *Br. J. Nutr.* **2015**, *113*, 1965–1977. [CrossRef] [PubMed]

185. Regland, B.; Blennow, K.; Germgård, T.; Koch-Schmidt, A.C.; Gottfries, C.G. The role of the polymorphic genes apolipoprotein E and methylene-tetrahydrofolate reductase in the development of dementia of the Alzheimer type. *Dement. Geriatr. Cogn. Disord.* **1999**, *10*, 245–251. [CrossRef] [PubMed]

186. Bailey, R.L.; Carmel, R.; Green, R.; Pfeiffer, C.M.; Cogswell, M.E.; Osterloh, J.D.; Sempos, C.T.; Yetley, E.A. Monitoring of vitamin B-12 nutritional status in the united states by using plasma methylmalonic acid and serum vitamin B-12. *Am. J. Clin. Nutr.* **2011**, *94*, 552–561. [CrossRef] [PubMed]

187. Bailey, R.L.; Dodd, K.W.; Gahche, J.J.; Dwyer, J.T.; McDowell, M.A.; Yetley, E.A.; Sempos, C.A.; Burt, V.L.; Radimer, K.L.; Picciano, M.F. Total folate and folic acid intake from foods and dietary supplements in the united states: 2003–2006. *Am. J. Clin. Nutr.* **2010**, *91*, 231–237. [CrossRef] [PubMed]

188. Agarwal, S.; Reider, C.; Brooks, J.R.; Fulgoni, V.L. Comparison of prevalence of inadequate nutrient intake based on body weight status of adults in the united states: An analysis of nhanes 2001–2008. *J. Am. Coll. Nutr.* **2015**, *34*, 126–134. [CrossRef] [PubMed]

189. Roman Vinas, B.; Ribas Barba, L.; Ngo, J.; Gurinovic, M.; Novakovic, R.; Cavelaars, A.; de Groot, L.C.; Van't Veer, P.; Matthys, C.; Serra Majem, L. Projected prevalence of inadequate nutrient intakes in Europe. *Ann. Nutr. Metab.* **2011**, *59*, 84–95. [CrossRef] [PubMed]

190. Hopkins, S.M.; Gibney, M.J.; Nugent, A.P.; McNulty, H.; Molloy, A.M.; Scott, J.M.; Flynn, A.; Strain, J.J.; Ward, M.; Walton, J.; et al. Impact of voluntary fortification and supplement use on dietary intakes and biomarker status of folate and vitamin B-12 in irish adults. *Am. J. Clin. Nutr.* **2015**, *101*, 1163–1172. [CrossRef] [PubMed]

191. Herrmann, W.; Obeid, R. Cobalamin deficiency. In *Water Soluble Vitamins*; Stanger, O., Ed.; Springer: Dordrecht, The Netherlands, 2012; Volume 56, pp. 301–322.

192. Carmel, R. Current concepts in cobalamin deficiency. *Annu. Rev. Med.* **2000**, *51*, 357–375. [CrossRef] [PubMed]

193. Carmel, R. Efficacy and safety of fortification and supplementation with vitamin B12: Biochemical and physiological effects. *Food Nutr. Bull.* **2008**, *29*, S177–S187. [CrossRef] [PubMed]

194. Carmel, R. Nutritional anemias and the elderly. *Semin. Hematol.* **2008**, *45*, 225–234. [CrossRef] [PubMed]

195. Oulhaj, A.; Jerneren, F.; Refsum, H.; Smith, A.D.; de Jager, C.A. Omega-3 fatty acid status enhances the prevention of cognitive decline by B vitamins in mild cognitive impairment. *J. Alzheimers Dis.* **2016**, *50*, 547–557. [CrossRef] [PubMed]

196. Stark, K.D.; Van Elswyk, M.E.; Higgins, M.R.; Weatherford, C.A.; Salem, N., Jr. Global survey of the omega-3 fatty acids, docosahexaenoic acid and eicosapentaenoic acid in the blood stream of healthy adults. *Prog. Lipid Res.* **2016**. [CrossRef] [PubMed]

197. Nilsson, K.; Gustafson, L.; Hultberg, B. Improvement of cognitive functions after cobalamin/folate supplementation in elderly patients with dementia and elevated plasma homocysteine. *Int. J. Geriatr. Psychiatry* **2001**, *16*, 609–614. [CrossRef] [PubMed]

5

Novel Approaches to Investigate One-Carbon Metabolism and Related B-Vitamins in Blood Pressure

Amy McMahon, Helene McNulty, Catherine F. Hughes, J. J. Strain and Mary Ward *

Northern Ireland Centre for Food and Health, Ulster University, Coleraine BT52 1SA, UK;
McMahon-A13@email.ulster.ac.uk (A.M.); h.mcnulty@ulster.ac.uk (H.M.); c.hughes@ulster.ac.uk (C.F.H.);
JJ.Strain@ulster.ac.uk (J.J.S.)
* Correspondence: mw.ward@ulster.ac.uk

Abstract: Hypertension, a major risk factor for heart disease and stroke, is the world's leading cause of preventable, premature death. A common polymorphism (677C→T) in the gene encoding the folate metabolizing enzyme methylenetetrahydrofolate reductase (MTHFR) is associated with increased blood pressure, and there is accumulating evidence demonstrating that this phenotype can be modulated, specifically in individuals with the *MTHFR* 677TT genotype, by the B-vitamin riboflavin, an essential co-factor for MTHFR. The underlying mechanism that links this polymorphism, and the related gene-nutrient interaction, with hypertension is currently unknown. Previous research has shown that 5-methyltetrahydrofolate, the product of the reaction catalysed by MTHFR, appears to be a positive allosteric modulator of endothelial nitric oxide synthase (eNOS) and may thus increase the production of nitric oxide, a potent vasodilator. Blood pressure follows a circadian pattern, peaking shortly after wakening and falling during the night, a phenomenon known as 'dipping'. Any deviation from this pattern, which can only be identified using ambulatory blood pressure monitoring (ABPM), has been associated with increased cardiovascular disease (CVD) risk. This review will consider the evidence linking this polymorphism and novel gene-nutrient interaction with hypertension and the potential mechanisms that might be involved. The role of ABPM in B-vitamin research and in nutrition research generally will also be reviewed.

Keywords: riboflavin; methylenetetrahydrofolate reductase (MTHFR); hypertension; blood pressure; ABPM; DNA methylation

1. Introduction

Hypertension, defined as a systolic/diastolic blood pressure (BP) of 140/90 mmHg or greater, is the world's leading cause of preventable, premature death and is the most important risk factor for cardiovascular disease (CVD) and stroke. Hypertension is responsible for 7.5 million deaths worldwide and an estimated 12.8% of all deaths annually [1]. It is estimated that by 2025, 1.56 billion people worldwide will suffer with hypertension, and by 2030, costs to the global economy will soar to $274 billion [2–4]. Treating hypertension is highly effective in reducing CVD and mortality [5], with a decrease of as little as 2 mmHg in systolic BP reported to reduce CVD risk by 10% [6]. BP is normally treated using antihypertensive medication, but this is not always effective, and BP control rates can remain poor (even when three or more drugs are co-administered, i.e., polytherapy) [7,8]. Current guidelines to treat hypertension are aimed at achieving a BP of <140/90 mmHg [7]; however, recent evidence suggests that a more intensive treatment regime to reduce BP to as low as <120/80 may be significantly more beneficial, even when BP values fall within the normotensive range [8–10].

There are many well-known modifiable risk factors for hypertension, such as smoking, obesity, high salt intake and physical inactivity, and thus, addressing lifestyle factors is generally the first line of treatment recommended by medical practitioners to reduce BP [7]. Genome-wide association studies (GWAS) have however identified a number of areas in the genome related to the variability in BP, including a region near the *MTHFR* locus [11], a finding replicated by other GWAS [12–14]. Likewise, large meta-analyses of epidemiological studies have shown that adults with the homozygous variant (TT genotype) for the common *MTHFR* C677T polymorphism are at an increased risk of developing hypertension [15–19]. Riboflavin is required as a cofactor for MTHFR, and previous studies at this centre have shown that supplementation with riboflavin significantly reduces BP in adults with this genetic risk factor [20–22]. The mechanism by which riboflavin lowers BP in this genetically at-risk group is unknown; however, some mechanisms have been speculated, and these will be explored below [22,23].

All studies to date investigating this gene-nutrient interaction in hypertension have relied on clinic BP measurements. An alternative, more robust method of BP measurement is ambulatory blood pressure monitoring (ABPM), which can track the circadian pattern of BP, and it is reported to be a better predictor of mortality [24]. Despite the use of ABPM being first reported in the mid-1960s [25], it was not introduced into the relevant UK clinical guidelines to confirm the diagnosis of hypertension until 2011 [7].

2. One-Carbon Metabolism and Related B-Vitamins

In order to be biochemically active, folate needs to be in the fully reduced form as tetrahydrofolate (THF; Figure 1). Thus, folic acid, the synthetic vitamin form as found in supplements and fortified food, requires biological modification (via dihydrofolate reductase (DHFR)) to form THF [26]. This occurs in two consecutive NADPH-dependent reactions, to form dihydrofolate (DHF) and subsequently THF. The reduction of folic acid is, however, a slow process that is influenced by individual variation in DHFR activity [26]. It is possible therefore that exposure to high oral doses of folic acid may result in the appearance of unmetabolised folic acid in the circulation [27], which some have suggested may be associated with adverse health effects [28]. Once THF enters the folate cycle, it gains a methyl group from the conversion of serine to glycine in a vitamin B6-dependent (i.e., pyridoxal 5′-phosphate) reaction to form 5,10-methyleneTHF. Riboflavin also participates in one-carbon metabolism in its active co-factor forms flavin adenine dinucleotide (FAD) and flavin mononucleotide (FMN). Pyridoxine-phosphate oxidase requires FMN for the formation of the active form of vitamin B6, pyridoxal 5′-phosphate, from pyridoxine phosphate. MTHFR, which requires FAD as a co-factor, converts 5,10-methyleneTHF to 5-methylTHF which is subsequently converted to THF, in a reaction catalysed by methionine synthase, completing the cycle. The latter conversion also requires vitamin B12 (i.e., methylcobalamin) as a co-factor and simultaneously enables the remethylation of homocysteine to methionine and subsequently S-adenosylmethionine (SAM), the universal methyl donor, which is essential for a range of methylation processes, including DNA methylation. DNA methylation involves the addition of a methyl group to the DNA base cytosine, which can alter the transcription of the gene and potentially reduce enzyme production [29]. Thus, apart from folate, three other B-vitamins play essential roles in one-carbon metabolism, as they are required for the activity of the various enzymes within the folate cycle.

It is well established that the common *MTHFR* C677T polymorphism, which causes an amino acid change from alanine to valine in the protein, produces a thermolabile enzyme [30]. Individuals with the *MTHFR* 677TT genotype have 70% reduced activity of MTHFR in comparison to the *MTHFR* 677CC genotype, which in turn reduces the rate of 5-methylTHF production [30] and, potentially, SAM production in cells. The *MTHFR* 677TT genotype is thus associated with increased homocysteine concentration as the primary phenotype [30].

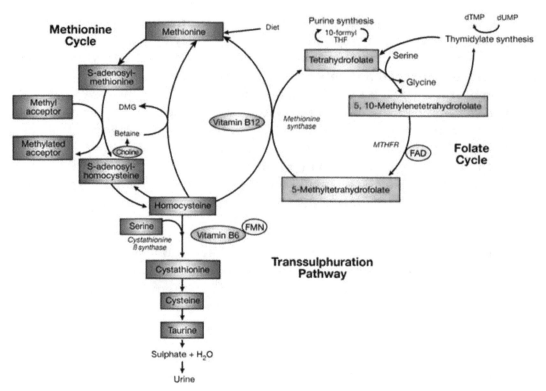

Figure 1. One-carbon metabolism pathway reproduced from Clarke et al. [31]. FAD, flavin adenine dinucleotide; FMN, flavin adenine dinucleotide.

3. B-Vitamins, Cardiovascular Disease and Blood Pressure

Increased plasma homocysteine and/or poor status of the metabolically-related B-vitamins have been linked with an increased risk of CVD over many years, albeit the literature is somewhat controversial [32]. It is well established that intervention with folate, along with vitamin B12 and vitamin B6, can reduce plasma homocysteine concentrations (by about 3 μmol/L) as reported in a large meta-analysis of randomised controlled trials [33]. Of the B-vitamins investigated, folic acid has been shown to be most effective, even at doses as low as 0.2 mg/day when maintained for a long enough period of intervention (i.e., 24 weeks) [33,34]. Separate meta-analyses estimated that a reduction in homocysteine by 25% could reduce the risk of stroke by up to 24% and heart disease by 16% [35,36]. To subsequently establish a cause and effect relationship between elevated homocysteine and CVD outcomes, a number of randomised controlled trials with B-vitamins were conducted; however, despite significant homocysteine lowering, the majority failed to show a reduction in CVD risk in response to intervention with B-vitamins (as extensively reviewed elsewhere; [32,37]). Of note however, a secondary analysis of the Heart Outcomes Prevention Evaluation 2 trial (HOPE 2) and two subsequent meta-analyses demonstrated that interventions with folic acid and related B-vitamins could substantially reduce the risk of stroke [38–40]. This effect was generally confined to trials that were three years in length or greater (suggesting that trials of shorter duration may have underestimated or missed this benefit) and in trials involving participants with no previous history of stroke. However, the vast majority of the previous trials were secondary prevention trials in patients with overt CVD, and as such, participants would be less likely to respond to B-vitamin intervention. Furthermore, it has been reported that antiplatelet drugs, such as aspirin (commonly prescribed to patients after a CVD event) might mask any CVD risk reduction [41]. Of note, a recent primary prevention trial in 20,702 hypertensive Chinese adults reported that folic acid supplementation (0.8 mg/day), for a median duration of 4.5 years, reduced the risk of stroke in those with elevated cholesterol by as much as 31% [42]. The balance of evidence therefore suggests that any beneficial effects of B-vitamins would be most relevant in the prevention rather than the treatment of CVD.

Although most of the previous studies in relation to CVD were designed to examine homocysteine lowering in relation to CVD risk, some also considered the relationship of B-vitamins with BP. One of the largest studies, the VISP (Vitamin Intervention for Stroke Prevention) trial, which involved supplementing 3649 cerebral infarct patients with high or low doses of folic acid for two years, successfully reduced homocysteine, but showed no corresponding effect on BP [43]. Likewise, McMahon and colleagues also reported a significant reduction in homocysteine in response to supplementation with folic acid, B6 and B12 for two years, but no effect on BP [44]. One small study of just 130 individuals who were supplemented with high dose folic acid (5 mg/day) and B6 (250 mg/day) for two years, reported a reduction in homocysteine by 7.8 μmol/L and did achieve a corresponding lowering of systolic BP (−3.7 mmHg) [45]. Somewhat surprisingly, a further study of only 24 male smokers reported a smaller, albeit significant, reduction in homocysteine (2.6 μmol/L) and found a greater lowering of systolic BP (−8 mmHg SBP); however this study was conducted in adults who smoke, and it is well known that smoking increases homocysteine and BP [46,47]. If homocysteine was causally linked with increased BP, intervention studies to lower homocysteine would invariably show a corresponding BP response; however, this is not the case [32,37], suggesting there is no mechanistic association between homocysteine and BP. All of the aforementioned studies reported BP using the clinic BP monitor and have not considered the influence of *MTHFR* genotypes on BP response.

The *MTHFR* 677TT genotype has been independently associated with increased CVD risk [35,48–51]. This association is generally assumed to be owed to homocysteine, which is invariably found to be highest in those with the TT genotype and lowest in the CC genotype, with CT individuals having intermediate concentrations [32,35]. More recently, emerging evidence suggests that the excess genetic risk of CVD owed to this polymorphism may be through an independent association with BP. Furthermore, meta-analyses that have investigated the association between the TT genotype and CVD risk generally show a stronger relationship for stroke [49,51], than for heart disease [35,48,50,52]. Moreover, in studies focusing on the risk of hypertension (as opposed to CVD outcomes), the relationship is stronger again [15–19]. This is of importance as hypertension is a major risk factor for stroke [15–19]. Apart from hypertension in the general population [15,17,19], this polymorphism has also been linked with hypertension in pregnancy [16,18]. Given that hypertension is such a major risk factor for stroke, it is possible that the onset of stroke could be prevented or delayed by modulating the blood pressure phenotype in individuals with the *MTHFR* 677TT genotype.

Among the studies investigating the association between MTHFR and BP, there are differences in the extent of risk linking this polymorphism with CVD including stroke [15–19]. Environmental factors affecting different populations, particularly B-vitamin status, could strongly influence the BP phenotype and thus stroke risk. Within these meta-analyses, the excess risk owed to the *MTHFR* 677TT genotype is found to be considerably higher in Asian populations for both CVD (OR 1.68, 95% CI 1.44–1.97) [51] and hypertension (OR 1.87, 95% CI 1.31–2.68) [16] and lower in North American populations.

Leading on from earlier work, which demonstrated that supplementation with riboflavin could improve MTHFR activity in vivo (evident by decreasing plasma homocysteine concentrations) [53], researchers at this centre investigated the BP lowering effect of riboflavin in adults with the *MTHFR* 677TT genotype. In the first study, Horigan et al. [20] conducted a randomised controlled trial of riboflavin supplementation at 1.6 mg/day in premature CVD patients stratified for the *MTHFR* C677T polymorphism (*n* = 181). At baseline, BP control rates were poor in the TT genotype group, with 63% failing to reach the target BP of <140/90 mmHg on treatment with antihypertensive drugs. Systolic and diastolic BP were also significantly higher at baseline in the TT compared to the CC or CT genotype groups. In response to intervention with riboflavin (1.6 mg/day for 16 weeks), riboflavin biomarker status improved in all three genotypes in response to intervention (*p* < 0.001; as measured using the erythrocyte glutathione reductase activation coefficient). However, BP was significantly reduced in the TT genotype group only, with one third of patients in this group achieving a reduction in systolic

BP by as much as 20 mmHg. When the *MTHFR* 677TT genotype participants from this first study were subsequently followed up four years later and assigned to further intervention in a cross-over design study (with the original treatments reversed), the BP lowering effects of riboflavin in the TT genotype group were replicated [21]. The BP lowering achieved in response to riboflavin occurred despite a major change in the UK clinical guidelines for the management of hypertension during the four-year follow-up period, resulting in a shift from monotherapy to polytherapy, thus additional medications being prescribed, and a change from β-blockers to angiotensin-converting enzyme (ACE) inhibitors as the drugs of first choice [7]. In a subsequent study, the genotype-specific BP lowering effects of riboflavin were also demonstrated in hypertensive adults without overt CVD [22]; albeit the extent of BP lowering was less pronounced (ranging from 5.6 to 13 mmHg systolic and 6–8 mmHg diastolic). It is not entirely clear why the extent of BP lowering was somewhat less in the last of these trials [22] compared to the previous ones [20,21], but recent evidence from our centre indicates that age and gender may strongly influence the BP phenotype [54]. To date, all studies investigating this gene-nutrient interaction in BP have intervened with riboflavin only. Given the close metabolic interplay between folate and riboflavin and the likelihood that enhancing MTHFR activity increases levels of 5-methylTHF, it is possible that supplementing with 5-methylTHF alone could have beneficial effects on BP in those with the *MTHFR* 677TT genotype, similar to that of riboflavin. Further research is required to investigate the role of 5-methylTHF in individuals with the *MTHFR* 677TT genotype. In any case, these findings have important implications for BP management for subpopulations worldwide given the high frequency of the *MTHFR* 677TT genotype (on average 10%, but as high as 32% in Mexico) [55]. Although biomarker status of riboflavin is rarely measured in populations, deficient and low status appears to commonly occur, especially in countries where intakes of riboflavin-rich food are low [56]. Further studies are clearly required to investigate this phenotype in younger adults in both genders and to consider the potential for preventing the development of hypertension through optimising riboflavin status. Of note, to date, all studies investigating the *MTHFR* C677T polymorphism and BP have utilized clinic BP. Ambulatory blood pressure monitoring (ABPM) offers an alternative method, which measures BP over a 24-h period and will be discussed later.

4. Biological Mechanisms Linking Blood Pressure with One-Carbon Metabolism

When the *MTHFR* C677T polymorphism was first described, Frosst et al. [30] reported that there is a 70% reduced activity in the mutated enzyme as measured in human lymphocytes. Further evidence from in vitro studies in *Escherichia coli* demonstrated that the mutated MTHFR enzyme loses its FAD cofactor at a much greater rate than the wild-type enzyme, reducing the overall functioning of the enzyme [57]. This was supported by a subsequent in vitro study in recombinant human MTHFR, which reported that in low folate compared to optimal folate conditions, the loss of FAD co-factor from the mutated enzyme was exacerbated [58]. As discussed previously, the FAD-dependent enzyme MTHFR is essential for the production of 5-methylTHF within the one-carbon metabolism cycle. Bagely and Selhub [59] observed decreased concentrations of 5-methylTHF and an accumulation of 10-formylTHF in red blood cells of individuals with the TT genotype, indicative of altered red blood cell folate distribution as a result of decreased MTHFR activity. It has also been postulated that the mutated enzyme has an altered active site, therefore reducing the efficacy of the binding of FAD [60]. It is not known how enzyme activity is enhanced by supplementation with riboflavin [53], but it is possible that this is achieved through stabilization of the variant enzyme and potentially increasing the enzyme-substrate binding, thereby improving its function [23].

The potential mechanism underlying the role of MTHFR in hypertension is currently unknown, but may involve endothelial nitric oxide synthase (eNOS). In one study involving patients undergoing cardiac bypass surgery, researchers found that vascular tissue concentrations of 5-methylTHF were positively associated with endothelial function (regardless of *MTHFR* C677T genotype) via the production of nitric oxide, a potent vasodilator [61]. A subsequent study from the same researchers reported that vascular 5-methylTHF is an important regulator of eNOS coupling and nitric oxide bioavailability [62]. It is possible therefore that supplementation with riboflavin (i.e., the MTHFR cofactor) in individuals with the *MTHFR* 677TT genotype could increase MTHFR enzyme activity in vivo, resulting in an increased cellular production of 5-methylTHF and, thus, lower BP by promoting vasodilation [22,23,61].

A further, and possibly complementary, mechanism to explain this novel gene-nutrient interaction in hypertension may involve epigenetic modification. Epigenetics can change the expression of a gene without altering the underlying DNA sequence by histone modification, RNA interference or DNA methylation [29]. The majority of research into epigenetic modifications is in relation to DNA methylation. Folate, owing to its importance in one-carbon metabolism and the production of SAM, plays a key role in modulating DNA methylation levels, of relevance to diseases, such as cancer [63], and folic acid supplementation during pregnancy has also been reported to alter DNA methylation in the offspring [64]. Furthermore, animal studies have shown that in folate-deficient mice, aberrant DNA methylation occurs at the promoter regions of the *MTHFR* gene, resulting in alterations in gene expression [65]. In support of these findings, the same researchers have found increased methylation in the promoter region of the *MTHFR* gene in paediatric cancerous tissues [65]. One study that investigated the *MTHFR* C677T polymorphism and folate status in relation to DNA methylation found that the TT genotype combined with low folate status was associated with low genomic DNA methylation levels [66]. A reduction in genomic DNA methylation levels could lead to altered gene expression, and optimizing folate status in these individuals could counteract this effect.

One meta-analysis of observational studies examined the relationship between *MTHFR* single nucleotide polymorphisms and genomic DNA methylation. Of the 16 studies included, 10 studies examined the role of the *MTHFR* C677T polymorphism on global DNA methylation and found no significant association. It is important to note however that the studies included in this meta-analysis were designed to examine a number of diseases and were not focused on hypertension alone [67]. Elsewhere, long interspersed element-1 (LINE-1) methylation (an indication of global methylation) has been reported to be significantly lower in individuals with the *MTHFR* 677TT genotype compared to those with the CC genotype [68]. Furthermore, adults with the TT genotype compared to the CC genotype had diminished genomic DNA methylation, and this correlated with folate status [66]. There is also some evidence linking pre-eclampsia (characterised by proteinuria and hypertension) with *MTHFR* gene hypermethylation [69]. However, DNA methylation at *MTHFR* has not been examined to any great extent in relation to hypertension generally. Aberrant LINE-1 and gene-specific DNA methylation profiles have been reported to improve the prediction accuracy of the occurrence of myocardial infarction, when other well-known risk factors for hypertension are taken into account [70]. One randomised controlled trial found that B-vitamin supplementation (folic acid, vitamins B6 and B12) in combination with vitamin D and calcium, increased LINE-1 DNA methylation, but this study did not account for different *MTHFR* genotypes [71].

As MTHFR is required for normal folate recycling and thus the generation of SAM, stabilization of the mutated enzyme by riboflavin supplementation may overcome any possible aberrant DNA methylation owing to this polymorphism. In any case, further studies are required to investigate DNA methylation in relation to MTHFR-mediated blood pressure and to ascertain whether DNA methylation is altered by riboflavin supplementation in the TT genotype group.

5. Ambulatory Blood Pressure Monitoring

BP can be measured in a number of ways in clinical and research settings. The most common and convenient method of BP measurement of patients in the clinic is with a standard sphygmomanometer; however, as a result of BP variability, a one-off clinic BP reading may be a poor representation of an individual's true BP [72]. Out-of-office BP measurement, such as home BP monitoring (HBPM) and ABPM, is recognised as a more accurate measure of BP, as it is not influenced by the clinical environment. ABPM is considered to be more superior to HBPM, as it is a non-invasive and a robust measure of BP owing to its ability to record BP over a defined period of time, usually 24-h. This continuous monitoring accounts for the daily variability in BP and, as such, is regarded as the gold standard in BP monitoring [73]. The 24-h window of BP monitoring can be further sub-divided into: the white coat window, daytime window, nighttime window and morning increase in BP [74], with each period being independently associated with CVD risk (as will be discussed further below). Despite being first reported in the early 1960s [25], ABPM has only recently been introduced into UK clinical guidelines as a method of confirming a diagnosis of hypertension [7]. The current guidelines recommend that hypertensive patients, once diagnosed, should be monitored on an annual basis using ABPM.

There are a number of important differences between clinic BP and ABPM, as summarised in Table 1, which are discussed in detail below. The most important advantage of ABPM is that it provides a minimum of 14-day time systolic and diastolic BP readings, allowing a more accurate diagnosis of hypertension to be made [75]. These multiple readings improve the prediction of CVD risk and stroke, as clinic BP only provides a 'snap-shot' of the BP [76,77]. Of note, different cut-off values are used for diagnosing hypertension, depending on whether clinic BP or ABPM is used. Clinical guidelines in the UK define hypertension as a clinic BP reading (systolic/diastolic) of $\geq$140/90 mmHg, whereas using ABPM, the corresponding cut-off values are $\geq$135/85 mmHg [7].

Table 1. Clinic BP vs. ABPM.

CLINIC BP	ABPM
• Defines hypertension as $\geq$140/90 mmHg *	• Defines hypertension as $\geq$135/85 mmHg * (daytime average)
• Convenient, quick, non-invasive method to measure blood pressure • One off measurement of: Systolic and Diastolic BP Pulse Rate	• Robust measure of BP over a 24-h period • Average 24-h/daytime/night-time measurement of: Systolic BP and Diastolic BP Mean Arterial Pressure Pulse Pressure Heart Rate
	• Identifies white-coat/masked/resistant hypertension; • A superior predictor of mortality; • Provides information on: Circadian pattern Morning surge % time in hypertensive state over 24-h Night-time dipping pattern

* Blood pressure is recorded as systolic BP/diastolic BP.

Along with providing multiple measurements of systolic and diastolic BP, continuous monitoring by ABPM provides a wealth of additional relevant information including mean arterial pressure, pulse pressure and heart rate, each of which are independently associated with CVD risk [78]. Although encompassing aspects of systolic and diastolic BP, the relevance of mean arterial pressure (i.e., defined as $\frac{2}{3}$ diastolic BP + $\frac{1}{3}$ systolic BP), is often underestimated as an independent risk factor for hypertension. In one large study of 11,150 adults, mean arterial pressure was linked with an increased risk of CVD, and this association was strongest in younger males (relative risk 2.52 95% CI 1.87–3.40 compared to 1.43 95% CI 1.07–1.92 in older males) [78]. The relevance of pulse pressure (i.e., defined as the difference between systolic BP and diastolic BP) as a predictor of CVD risk has been more extensively investigated, as it is an indicator of large arterial stiffness and isolated systolic hypertension. As people age, systolic BP increases, and diastolic BP remains steady or may even decrease, ultimately resulting in an increased pulse pressure, with estimates that each 10 mmHg increase in pulse pressure is associated with a 22%–35% increased risk of fatal stroke [79,80] and a 35% increased risk of cardiac events [80]. Thus, increased pulse pressure is now recognised by the European Society of Hypertension as an independent risk factor for cardiovascular events and is distinct from the risk associated with the increase in systolic BP with ageing [81]. Heart rate is another independent risk factor, which can be measured using ABPM. Increased heart rate has been associated with increasing BP independently of age and sex [82,83]. An increase in heart rate of 10 beats/min is associated with increased risk of cardiac death by as much as 20% and is also related to the severity of atherosclerosis at all ages [83,84]. In contrast, pulse pressure, which increases as people age, is more important for determining CVD risk in the later stages in life. Targeting heart rate could therefore potentially offer a therapeutic option when treating hypertension; however, results to date from trials are inconsistent [85].

5.1. White-Coat Hypertension

ABPM also offers the advantage of enabling the identification of a phenomenon first described by Pickering et al. in 1988, named white-coat hypertension (WCH). This occurs when a patient has BP readings in the hypertensive range as measured in the clinic, but normal BP when monitored throughout the day [86]. WCH is thought to affect up to 30% of the general population [87] and can only be detected by the use of HBPM or ABPM. The main advantage of identifying WCH is to ensure antihypertensive medication is only prescribed to individuals who require it. Furthermore, dietary and lifestyle changes may offer greater benefit to patients with WCH, at least initially [88].

Although earlier studies investigating WCH did not link it with additional CVD risk [89], more recent research has associated WCH with an increased risk of CVD [90,91]. A recent meta-analysis of 29,100 participants reported that patients with WCH (compared to normotensive controls) were at an increased risk of incidence of cardiovascular events (OR 1.73, 95% CI 1.27–2.36) and CVD mortality (OR 2.79, 95% CI 1.62–4.80), although not all-cause mortality or stroke [92]. Two recent studies have also shown that WCH is associated with subclinical arterial wall damage, including thickening of the arterial wall [93,94]. Whilst the association between WCH and CVD risk is not fully understood, it might be due to BP variability, which is associated with increased risk of CVD events and mortality [95]. Randomised controlled trials are required to determine if reducing the BP in WCH patients could reduce CVD risk. Aside from WCH, ABPM also has the ability to detect masked hypertension (i.e., normotensive clinic BP, but hypertensive ABPM) and resistant hypertension (i.e., difficult to treat hypertension). Masked hypertension is generally undetected owing to the appearance of normal BP in the clinic and is therefore associated with a higher risk of cardiovascular events as it remains untreated [90]. In relation to resistant hypertension, ABPM can identify patients that have true resistant hypertension (unresponsive to three or more antihypertensive medications), and is reviewed extensively elsewhere [96,97].

5.2. Circadian Pattern of Blood Pressure

The benefit of being able to trace the circadian pattern of BP is that it enables the identification of those who do not follow the expected pattern, in particular, where BP rises sharply in the morning and falls at night, while sleeping (a phenomenon known as 'dipping'). When first reported, individual patients were categorised into either a dipping or non-dipping pattern [98]. The non-dipping pattern has been independently associated with increased risk of CVD in many studies [99–104] and has also been associated with increased CVD risk in adults without hypertension [105]. It is now more common to further divide non-dippers into three groups; thus, four groups in total referred to as: dippers (considered to have a normal dipping pattern; ≥10%–20% fall at night), extreme dippers (≥20%), non-dippers (≥0%–10%) or risers (increase in BP), depending on how much their BP falls at night in comparison to the average daytime BP.

Meta-analyses of studies that have investigated the circadian pattern of BP in relation to CVD events are summarised in Table 2. Salles et al. conducted a large meta-analysis in over three continents to investigate the effect of various dipping patterns on cardiovascular events and stroke [106]. Compared to the normal dipping pattern, individuals with any other dipping pattern at night were found to be at an increased risk of cardiovascular events (OR 1.40, 95% CI 1.20–1.63) and in particular stroke (OR 1.43, 95% CI 1.15–1.77). When the non-dipping pattern was further subdivided, a rising pattern (increase in BP at night), in comparison to the normal dipping pattern, increased the risk of CVD by 79% and stroke by 89%. An increase in the morning surge of BP has also been associated with increased risk of coronary events [107], suggesting that varying circadian patterns of BP (daytime or nighttime) can increase the risk of CVD. Other large meta-analyses investigating the variation in circadian pattern in different populations support this finding, with estimates of excess CVD risk owing to atypical dipping ranging from 15% to 49% [102,108,109].

Table 2. Meta-analyses of circadian pattern abnormalities and cardiovascular events.

Author	Sample Size (n)	Populations	ABPM 24-h Profile	Odds Ratio (95% CI) for Cardiovascular Events
Salles et al. [106]	17,312 hypertensives	South America, Europe and Asia	Non-dippers vs. dippers *	1.40 (1.20–1.63)
Xie et al. [108]	14,133 hypertensives	Europe, South America and Asia	Morning surge	1.24 (0.60–2.53)
Hansen et al. [109]	23,856 hypertensives	Europe, South America and Asia	Non-dippers vs. dippers *	1.25 (1.02–1.52)
	9641 general population			1.15 (1.00–1.33)
Fagard et al. [102]	3468 hypertensives	Europe	Reverse dippers vs. other dipping patterns	1.49 (1.17–1.91)

Definition of dipping patterns (i.e., blood pressure fall at night comparted to daytime average): dippers ≥10%–20% fall in BP; non-dippers ≥0%–10% fall in BP; extreme dippers ≥20% fall in BP; reverse dippers, rise in BP; morning surge in BP is the increase in BP shortly after awakening. * These studies compare the normal dipping patterns of ≥10%–20% (dippers) and all other dipping patterns combined, collectively referred to as 'non-dippers'.

The mechanism for deviation in the circadian dipping pattern is unknown. Speculated mechanisms include increased sympathetic nervous system activity [110,111], decreased baroreceptor reflex sensitivity [112], increased arterial stiffness [113] and endothelial dysfunction [114]. Ageing is also known to play a role in the reduced decline in BP at night as there is an increase in the activity of the sympathetic nervous system and a decrease in baroreceptor reflex sensitivity. Poor quality of sleep has also been associated with increased BP readings at night and therefore could provide inaccurate reporting of dipping status [115]. Measures used to minimize the risk of inaccurate readings include ensuring that the right size of BP cuff is used, that the patient is fully informed of the procedure and a diary of events is kept (including any disturbed sleep). Although the reproducibility of nighttime dipping pattern (based on ABPM carried out on different days) has been questioned by some [116], Keren et al. reported that 71% of individuals reproduced the same dipping pattern when two 24-h readings were taken within 14 weeks [117].

In the clinical setting, ABPM can also be used to monitor the BP response to antihypertensive medication and to detect under- or over-treatment. Some patients present with resistant hypertension (the ineffective response to three or more antihypertensive medications) and chronotherapy can be introduced to potentially overcome this. Chronotherapy, in relation to hypertension treatment, is the administration of medication at a certain time of day, in line with the peaks in BP (as measured by ABPM) to improve the patient's response to treatment [118]. If the non-dipper or riser BP pattern at night is present, ingestion of medication at night, rather than in the morning, may be more beneficial [118,119]. One study reported that changing the time of administrating medication from morning to night significantly reduced BP ($p < 0.001$) in 250 hypertensive adults [118].

In summary, given these clear advantages, ABPM should be used in the clinical setting to diagnose hypertension accurately, to identify those at risk through abnormal circadian patterns and to help identify the optimum time for taking antihypertensive medication to maximise its effect. Further research is required to understand the effects of WCH and the potential effects of lowering BP in this at-risk group.

5.3. Nutrition, B-Vitamins and ABPM

As mentioned above, diet and lifestyle factors are usually suggested as the first line of treatment for the management of hypertension before pharmacological intervention is commenced, unless other CVD risk factors have been noted [7]. Many studies have investigated BP response to nutrition intervention; however, few studies have used ABPM to measure BP response. Those studies that have generally tend to report mean systolic BP and diastolic BP only, with many failing to consider the wealth of additional information that ABPM can contribute. The case for the use of ABPM in nutrition interventions is strong as ABPM has been reported to rule out the placebo effect after the first initial hours of recording BP, providing a more robust measure of potential BP reduction in intervention trials [120,121].

The relationship between obesity and BP as measured by ABPM has been investigated, confirming that BP increases with increasing BMI and showing that the non-dipping pattern is more prevalent in those with a BMI in the obese or severely obese range [122,123]. Micronutrients have also been investigated in relation to BP, and vitamin D deficiency has been associated with increased BP and with the non-dipping BP at night [124,125]. Other studies have reported that higher concentrations of serum calcium, phosphate and parathyroid hormone are associated with the non-dipping pattern in hypertensive patients without renal disease [126]. The majority of other studies failed to report the dipping pattern, mean arterial pressure, heart rate and/or pulse pressure despite the use of ABPM [127–139].

A limited number of randomised controlled trials have examined ABPM response to nutrition interventions, with somewhat inconsistent findings (Table 3). One of the first randomised controlled trials to investigate the ABPM response to a nutrition intervention (and the most comprehensive study to date) involved the Dietary Approaches to Stop Hypertension (DASH) trial [127]. The DASH diet incorporates low fat dairy products along with high intakes of fruit and vegetables and is characterised by being rich in protein and fibre, as well as potassium, magnesium and calcium, and low in saturated fat and cholesterol [140]. In an eight-week study investigating the ABPM response to the DASH diet versus a control diet or a diet rich in fruits and vegetables, the DASH diet was shown to result in the greatest BP lowering, achieving a mean systolic BP lowering of 4.5 mmHg [127]. Two additional DASH studies, also reporting ABPM, confirmed these findings and reported a lowering of systolic BP of between 9.5 and 15 mmHg in response to intervention [128,129]. The greatest lowering achieved (a mean reduction in systolic BP of 15 mmHg) reported by Paula et al. is likely to be explained by the inclusion of an exercise component within this intervention [129].

5.4. Blood Pressure Lowering by B-Vitamins as Measured by ABPM

Few studies to date have investigated the BP response to B-vitamin intervention specifically using ABPM. One small study of 30 postmenopausal women reported that high-dose folate supplementation (in the form of 5-methylTHF, the product of the reaction catalysed by MTHFR), significantly decreased nighttime systolic BP (-4.48 ± 1.8 mmHg; $p = 0.029$), diastolic BP (-5.33 ± 1.3 mmHg; $p < 0.001$) and mean arterial pressure (-5.10 ± 1.1 mmHg; $p = 0.005$), with no effect of daytime BP [141,142]. ABPM has been used in one study that investigated the effect of folic acid supplementation on BP by the *MTHFR* C677T genotype [143]. Although ABPM was reported, the study was confined to hypertensive males, and ABPM was not reported as a primary outcome measure. No BP lowering effect was noted in this study, although a significant decrease in brachial pulse pressure (PP) (4.7 ± 1.6 mmHg; $p < 0.05$) was observed across *MTHFR* genotype groups in response to intervention [143]. To date, the randomised controlled trials investigating this polymorphism in relation to BP have focused on folic acid/folate supplementation, and no previous ABPM studies have considered the BP lowering effects of riboflavin, arguably much more important, given its role in stabilizing MTHFR.

Table 3. Nutritional studies that report blood pressure response using ABPM in randomised controlled trials.

Author	Population	Sample Size	Average Systolic BP Change (mmHg)	Duration of Intervention	ABPM Parameters Reported			
					Dipping Status	Mean Arterial Pressure	Heart Rate	Pulse Pressure
DASH Diet Interventions								
Moore et al. [127]	USA	354	−4.5 ≠	8 weeks	Yes	No	No	No
Miller et al. [128]	USA	44	−9.5 ≠	9 weeks	No	No	No	No
Paula et al. * [129]	Brazil	40	−15.0 †	4 weeks	No	No	Yes	No
Dairy Product Interventions								
Drouin-Chartier et al. [130]	Canada	89	−2.0 †	4 weeks	No	No	No	No
Machin et al. [131]	USA	49	−8.0 ≠	4 weeks	No	No	No	Yes
Beetroot Interventions								
Hobbs et al. [132]	Europe	24	-	Acute	No	Yes	Yes	Yes
Jajja et al. [133]	Europe	24	-	3 weeks	No	No	Yes	No
Kapil et al. [134]	Europe	68	−7.7 ≠	4 weeks	No	No	Yes	No
Coles et al. [135]	Australia	30	−4.6 †	Acute	No	No	Yes	Yes
Vitamin D Intervention								
Larsen et al. [136]	Europe	112	−3 ≠	20 weeks	Yes	No	Yes	No
Pilz et al. [137]	Europe	200	-	8 weeks	No	No	No	No
Other								
Brull et al. [138]	Europe	70	−3.6 ≠	6 weeks	Yes	Yes	Yes	No
Sauder et al. * [139]	USA	30	−3.5 ≠	4 weeks	Yes	No	Yes	No

* Denotes studies in diabetic patients; acute studies refer to one-off ingestions of beetroot product and effects monitored over 6–24 h. ≠ Systolic BP response over 24h; † systolic BP response during daytime. Brull et al. supplemented adults with quercetin-rich onion skin extract; Sauder et al. supplemented adults with pistachio nuts.

6. Conclusions and Future Work

Evidence is accumulating to support the role of the *MTHFR* C677T polymorphism in hypertension and indicates that the BP phenotype may be much more relevant to CVD than the metabolite homocysteine. Riboflavin is an important modulator of the BP phenotype in individuals with the *MTHFR* 677TT genotype, but further work is required to investigate the influence of age and gender on this gene-nutrient interaction in BP. The biological mechanism by which riboflavin lowers BP in individuals with the variant *MTHFR* 677TT genotype is unknown; however, aberrant DNA methylation should be considered, along with other postulated mechanisms. Studies to date investigating the BP-lowering effect of riboflavin on genetically at-risk individuals and in nutrition studies generally have utilized clinic BP, but ABPM is now accepted as being a more robust measure of BP and a better indicator of cardiovascular health and disease risk. Its use in this area and in nutrition research generally should be considered. Given the global burden of hypertension, further research is required to understand the role of the *MTHFR* C677T polymorphism in BP, the modulating effect of riboflavin and the implications of this novel gene-nutrient interaction for the diagnosis and management of hypertension in different populations.

Acknowledgments: The PhD studentship of A.M. was funded by the Northern Ireland Department for Employment and Learning. DSM Nutritional Products Ltd. partly supported project costs associated with this work. The funders had no role in the design, analysis or writing of this paper.

Author Contributions: A.M. drafted the manuscript, and M.W., H.M., C.F.H. and J.J.S. critically revised the manuscript for important intellectual content. All authors have read and approved the final manuscript.

References

1. World Health Organisation—Global Health Observatory (GHO) Data for Raised Blood Pressure. Available online: http://www.who.int/gho/ncd/risk_factors/blood_pressure_prevalence_text/en/ (accessed on 19 September 2016).
2. Joffres, M.; Falaschetti, E.; Gillespie, C.; Robitaille, C.; Loustalot, F.; Poulter, N.; McAlister, F.A.; Johansen, H.; Baclic, O.; Campbell, N. Hypertension prevalence, awareness, treatment and control in national surveys from England, the USA and Canada, and correlation with stroke and ischaemic heart disease mortality: A cross-sectional study. *BMJ Open* **2013**, *3*, e003423. [CrossRef] [PubMed]
3. Kearney, P.M.; Whelton, M.; Reynolds, K.; Muntner, P.; Whelton, P.K.; He, J. Global burden of hypertension: Analysis of worldwide data. *Lancet* **2005**, *365*, 217–223. [CrossRef]
4. Mozaffarian, D.; Benjamin, E.J.; Go, A.S.; Arnett, D.K.; Blaha, M.J.; Cushman, M.; Das, S.R.; de Ferranti, S.; Després, J.-P.; Fullerton, H.J.; et al. Heart disease and stroke statistics-2016 update: A report from the american heart association. *Circulation* **2016**, *133*, e38–e360. [CrossRef] [PubMed]
5. Ettehad, D.; Emdin, C.A.; Kiran, A.; Anderson, S.G.; Callender, T.; Emberson, J.; Chalmers, J.; Rodgers, A.; Rahimi, K. Blood pressure lowering for prevention of cardiovascular disease and death: A systematic review and meta-analysis. *Lancet* **2016**, *387*, 957–967. [CrossRef]
6. Lewington, S.; Clarke, R.; Qizilbash, N.; Peto, R.; Collins, R. Age-specific relevance of usual blood pressure to vascular mortality: A meta-analysis of individual data for one million adults in 61 prospective studies. *Lancet* **2002**, *360*, 1903–1913. [CrossRef]
7. National Collaborating Centre for Chronic Conditions and the British Hypertension Society. *Hypertension in Adults: Diagnosis and Management Management*; Royal College of Physicians: London, UK, 2011.
8. Wright, J.T.; Williamson, J.D.; Whelton, P.S.K.; Snyder, J.K.; Sink, K.M.; Rocco, M.V.; Reboussin, D.C.E.M.; Rahman, M.; Oparil, S.; Lewis, C.E.; et al. A randomized trial of intensive versus standard blood-pressure control. *N. Engl. J. Med.* **2015**, *373*, 2103–2116. [PubMed]
9. Xie, X.; Atkins, E.; Lv, J.; Bennett, A.; Neal, B.; Ninomiya, T.; Woodward, M.; MacMahon, S.; Turnbull, F.; Hillis, G.S.; et al. Effects of intensive blood pressure lowering on cardiovascular and renal outcomes: Updated systematic review and meta-analysis. *Lancet* **2016**, *387*, 435–443. [CrossRef]

10. Williamson, J.D.; Supiano, M.A.; Applegate, W.B.; Berlowitz, D.R.; Campbell, R.C.; Chertow, G.M.; Fine, L.J.; Haley, W.E.; Hawfield, A.T.; Ix, J.H.; et al. Intensive vs. standard blood pressure control and cardiovascular disease outcomes in adults aged ≥75 years. *JAMA* **2016**, *315*, 2673–2682. [CrossRef] [PubMed]

11. Newton-Cheh, C.; Johnson, T.; Gateva, V.; Tobin, M.D.; Bochud, M.; Coin, L.; Najjar, S.S.; Zhao, J.H.; Heath, S.C.; Eyheramendy, S.A. Genome-wide association study identifies eight loci associated with blood pressure. *Nat. Genet.* **2009**, *41*, 666–676. [CrossRef] [PubMed]

12. Levy, D.; Ehret, G.B.; Rice, K.; Verwoert, G.C.; Launer, L.J.; Dehghan, A.; Glazer, N.L.; Morrison, A.C.; Johnson, A.D.; Aspelund, T. Genome-wide association study of blood pressure and hypertension. *Nat. Genet.* **2009**, *41*, 677–687. [CrossRef] [PubMed]

13. Ehret, G.B.; Munroe, P.B.; Rice, K.M.; Bochud, M.; Johnson, A.D.; Chasman, D.I.; Smith, A.V.; Tobin, M.D.; Verwoert, G.C.; Hwang, S.-J.; et al. Genetic variants in novel pathways influence blood pressure and cardiovascular disease risk. *Nature* **2011**, *478*, 103–109. [CrossRef] [PubMed]

14. Flister, M.J.; Tsaih, S.W.; O'Meara, C.C.; Endres, B.; Hoffman, M.J.; Geurts, A.M.; Dwinell, M.R.; Lazar, J.; Jacob, H.J.; Moreno, C. Identifying multiple causative genes at a single GWAS locus. *Genome Res.* **2013**, *23*, 1996–2002. [CrossRef] [PubMed]

15. Qian, X.; Lu, Z.; Tan, M.; Liu, H.; Lu, D. A meta-analysis of association between C677T polymorphism in the methylenetetrahydrofolate reductase gene and hypertension. *Eur. J. Hum. Genet.* **2007**, *15*, 1239–1245. [CrossRef] [PubMed]

16. Niu, W.-Q.; You, Y.-G.; Qi, Y. Strong association of methylenetetrahydrofolate reductase gene C677T polymorphism with hypertension and hypertension-in-pregnancy in Chinese: A meta-analysis. *J. Hum. Hypertens.* **2012**, *26*, 259–267. [CrossRef] [PubMed]

17. Wu, Y.L.; Hu, C.Y.; Lu, S.S.; Gong, F.F.; Feng, F.; Qian, Z.Z.; Ding, X.X.; Yang, H.Y.; Sun, Y.H. Association between methylenetetrahydrofolate reductase (MTHFR) C677T/A1298C polymorphisms and essential hypertension: A systematic review and meta-analysis. *Metabolism* **2014**, *63*, 1503–1511. [CrossRef] [PubMed]

18. Yang, B.; Fan, S.; Zhi, X.; Li, Y.; Liu, Y.; Wang, D.; He, M.; Hou, Y.; Zheng, Q.; Sun, G. Associations of MTHFR gene polymorphisms with hypertension and hypertension in pregnancy: A meta-analysis from 114 studies with 15411 cases and 21970 controls. *PLoS ONE* **2014**, *9*, e87497. [CrossRef] [PubMed]

19. Yang, K.-M.; Jia, J.; Mao, L.-N.; Men, C.; Tang, K.-T.; Li, Y.-Y.; Ding, H.-X.; Zhan, Y.-Y. Methylenetetrahydrofolate reductase C677T gene polymorphism and essential hypertension: A meta-analysis of 10,415 subjects. *Biomed. Rep.* **2014**, *2*, 699–708. [CrossRef] [PubMed]

20. Horigan, G.; McNulty, H.; Ward, M.; Strain, J.J.; Purvis, J.; Scott, J.M. Riboflavin lowers blood pressure in cardiovascular disease patients homozygous for the 677C→T polymorphism in MTHFR. *J. Hypertens.* **2010**, *28*, 478–486. [CrossRef] [PubMed]

21. Wilson, C.P.; Ward, M.; McNulty, H.; Strain, J.J.; Trouton, T.G.; Horigan, G.; Purvis, J.; Scott, J.M. Riboflavin offers a targeted strategy for managing hypertension in patients with the MTHFR 677TT genotype: A 4-y follow-up. *Am. J. Clin. Nutr.* **2012**, *95*, 766–772. [CrossRef] [PubMed]

22. Wilson, C.P.; McNulty, H.; Ward, M.; Strain, J.J.; Trouton, T.G.; Hoeft, B.A.; Weber, P.; Roos, F.F.; Horigan, G.; McAnena, L.; et al. Blood pressure in treated hypertensive individuals with the mthfr 677tt genotype is responsive to intervention with riboflavin: Findings of a targeted randomized trial. *Hypertension* **2013**, *61*, 1302–1308. [CrossRef] [PubMed]

23. Strain, J.; Hughes, C.F.; Mcnulty, H.; Ward, M. Riboflavin Lowers Blood Pressure: A Review of a Novel Gene-nutrient Interaction. *Nutr. Food Sci. Res.* **2015**, *2*, 3–6.

24. Verdecchia, P.; Porcellati, C.; Schillaci, G.; Borgioni, C.; Ciucci, A.; Battistelli, M.; Guerrieri, M.; Gatteschi, C.; Zampi, I.; Santucci, A.; et al. Ambulatory blood pressure. An independent predictor of prognosis in essential hypertension. *Hypertension (Dallas, TX, 1979)* **1994**, *24*, 793–801. [CrossRef]

25. Hinman, A.T.; Engel, B.T.; Bickford, A.F. Portable blood pressure recorder Accuracy and preliminary use in evaluating intradaily variations in pressure. *Am. Heart J.* **1962**, *63*, 663–668. [CrossRef]

26. Bailey, L.B.; Stover, P.J.; Mcnulty, H.; Fenech, M.F.; Iii, J.F.G.; Mills, J.L.; Pfeiffer, C.M.; Fazili, Z.; Zhang, M.; Ueland, P.M.; et al. Biomarkers of Nutrition for Development—Folate Review. *J. Nutr.* **2015**, 1–45. [CrossRef] [PubMed]

27. Kelly, P.; McPartlin, J.; Goggins, M.; Weir, D.G.; Scott, J.M. Unmetabolized folic acid in serum: Acute studies in subjects consuming fortified food and supplements. *Am. J. Clin. Nutr.* **1997**, *65*, 1790–1795. [PubMed]

28. Morris, M.S.; Jacques, P.F.; Rosenberg, I.H.; Selhub, J. Circulating unmetabolized folic acid and 5-methyltetrahydrofolate in relation to anemia, macrocytosis, and cognitive test performance in American seniors. *Am. J. Clin. Nutr.* **2010**, *91*, 1733–1744. [CrossRef] [PubMed]

29. Russo, V.; Martienssen, R.; Riggs, A. Epigenetic mechanisms of gene regulation. *Cold Spring Harb. Monogr.* **1996**, *13*, 425–437.

30. Frosst, P.; Blom, H.J.; Milos, R.; Goyette, P.; Sheppard, C.A.; Matthews, R.G.; Boers, G.J.; den Heijer, M.; Kluijtmans, L.A.; van den Heuvel, L.P. A candidate genetic risk factor for vascular disease: A common mutation in methylenetetrahydrofolate reductase. *Nat. Genet.* **1995**, *10*, 111–113. [CrossRef] [PubMed]

31. Clarke, M.; Ward, M.; Strain, J.J.; Hoey, L.; Dickey, W.; McNulty, H. B-vitamins and bone in health and disease: The current evidence. *Proc. Nutr. Soc.* **2014**, *73*, 330–339. [CrossRef] [PubMed]

32. McNulty, H.; Strain, J.J.; Pentieva, K.; Ward, M. C1 metabolism and CVD outcomes in older adults. *Proc. Nutr. Soc.* **2012**, *71*, 213–221. [CrossRef] [PubMed]

33. Homocysteine Lowering Trialists. Dose-dependent effects of folic acid on blood concentrations of homocysteine: A meta-analysis of the randomized trials 1–3. *Am. J. Clin. Nutr.* **2005**, *82*, 806–812.

34. Tighe, P.; Ward, M.; Mcnulty, H.; Finnegan, O.; Dunne, A.; Strain, J.J.; Molloy, A.M.; Duffy, M.; Pentieva, K.; et al. A dose-finding trial of the effect of long-term folic acid intervention: Implications for food fortification policy. *Am. J. Clin. Nutr.* **2011**, *93*, 11–18. [CrossRef] [PubMed]

35. Wald, D.S.; Law, M.; Morris, J.K. Homocysteine and cardiovascular disease: Evidence on causality from a meta-analysis. *BMJ* **2002**, *325*, 1202. [CrossRef] [PubMed]

36. Homocysteine Studies Collaboration. Homocysteine and risk of ischemic heart disease and stroke: A meta-analysis. *JAMA* **2002**, *288*, 2015–2022.

37. Wilson, C.P.; McNulty, H.; Scott, J.M.; Strain, J.J.; Ward, M. The MTHFR C677T polymorphism, B-vitamins and blood pressure. *Proc. Nutr. Soc.* **2010**, *69*, 156–165. [CrossRef] [PubMed]

38. The Heart Outcomes Prevention Evaluation Investigators (HOPE) 2 Investigators. Homocysteine lowering with folic acid and B vitamins in vascular disease. *N. Engl. J. Med.* **2006**, *354*, 1567–1577.

39. Wang, X.; Qin, X.; Demirtas, H.; Li, J.; Mao, G.; Huo, Y.; Sun, N.; Liu, L.; Xu, X. Efficacy of folic acid supplementation in stroke prevention: A meta-analysis. *Lancet* **2007**, *369*, 1876–1882. [CrossRef]

40. Lee, M.; Hong, K.-S.; Chang, S.-C.; Saver, J.L. Efficacy of homocysteine-lowering therapy with folic Acid in stroke prevention: A meta-analysis. *Stroke* **2010**, *41*, 1205–1212. [CrossRef] [PubMed]

41. Hankey, G.J.; Eikelboom, J.W.; Yi, Q.; Lees, K.R.; Chen, C.; Xavier, D.; Navarro, J.C.; Ranawaka, U.K.; Uddin, W.; Ricci, S.; et al. Antiplatelet therapy and the effects of B vitamins in patients with previous stroke or transient ischaemic attack: A post-hoc subanalysis of VITATOPS, a randomised, placebo-controlled trial. *Lancet Neurol.* **2012**, *11*, 512–520. [CrossRef]

42. Qin, X.; Li, J.; Spence, J.D.; Zhang, Y.; Li, Y.; Wang, X.; Wang, B.; Sun, N.; Chen, F.; Guo, J.; et al. Folic Acid Therapy Reduces the First Stroke Risk Associated With Hypercholesterolemia Among Hypertensive Patients. *Stroke* **2016**, *47*, 2805–2812. [CrossRef] [PubMed]

43. Toole, J.F.; Malinow, M.R.; Chambless, L.E.; Spence, J.D.; Pettigrew, L.C.; Howard, V.J.; Sides, E.G.; Wang, C.-H.; Stampfer, M. Lowering homocysteine in patients with ischemic stroke to prevent recurrent stroke, myocardial infarction, and death: The Vitamin Intervention for Stroke Prevention (VISP) randomized controlled trial. *JAMA* **2004**, *291*, 565–575. [CrossRef] [PubMed]

44. McMahon, J.A.; Skeaff, C.M.; Williams, S.M.; Green, T.J. Lowering homocysteine with B vitamins has no effect on blood pressure in older adults. *J. Nutr.* **2007**, *137*, 1183–1187. [PubMed]

45. Van Dijk, R.A.J.M.; Rauwerda, J.A.; Steyn, M.; Twisk, J.W.R.; Stehouwer, C.D.A. Long-term homocysteine-lowering treatment with folic acid plus pyridoxine is associated with decreased blood pressure but not with improved brachial artery endothelium-dependent vasodilation or carotid artery stiffness. *Arterioscler. Thromb. Vasc. Biol.* **2001**, *21*, 2072–2079. [CrossRef] [PubMed]

46. Mangoni, A.A.; Sherwood, R.A.; Swift, C.G.; Jackson, S.H.D. Folic acid enhances endothelial function and reduces blood pressure in smokers: A randomized controlled trial. *J. Intern. Med.* **2002**, *252*, 497–503. [CrossRef] [PubMed]

47. Kennedy, B.P.; Farag, N.H.; Ziegler, A.G.; Mills, P.J. Relationship of systolic blood pressure with plasma homocysteine: Importance of smoking status. *J. Hypertens.* **2003**, *21*, 1307–1312. [CrossRef] [PubMed]

48. Klerk, M.; Verhoef, P.; Clarke, R.; Blom, H.J.; Kok, F.J.; Schouten, E.G.; MTHFR Studies Collaboration Group. MTHFR 677C→T polymorphism and risk of coronary heart disease: A meta-analysis. *JAMA* **2002**, *288*, 2023–2031. [CrossRef] [PubMed]

49. Casas, J.P.; Bautista, L.E.; Smeeth, L.; Sharma, P.; Hingorani, A.D. Homocysteine and stroke: Evidence on a causal link from mendelian randomisation. *Lancet* **2005**, *365*, 224–232. [CrossRef]

50. Lewis, S.J.; Ebrahim, S.; Davey Smith, G. Meta-analysis of MTHFR 677C→T polymorphism and coronary heart disease: Does totality of evidence support causal role for homocysteine and preventive potential of folate? *BMJ* **2005**, *331*, 1053. [CrossRef] [PubMed]

51. Holmes, M.V.; Newcombe, P.; Hubacek, J.A.; Sofat, R.; Ricketts, S.L.; Cooper, J.; Breteler, M.M.B.; Bautista, L.E.; Sharma, P.; Whittaker, J.C. Effect modification by population dietary folate on the association between MTHFR genotype, homocysteine, and stroke risk: A meta-analysis of genetic studies and randomised trials. *Lancet* **2011**, *378*, 584–594. [CrossRef]

52. Clarke, R.; Bennett, D.A.; Parish, S.; Verhoef, P.; Dötsch-Klerk, M.; Lathrop, M.; Xu, P.; Nordestgaard, B.G.; Holm, H.; Hopewell, J.C.; et al. MTHFR Studies Collaborative Group Homocysteine and coronary heart disease: Meta-analysis of MTHFR case-control studies, avoiding publication bias. *PLoS Med.* **2012**, *9*, e1001177. [CrossRef] [PubMed]

53. McNulty, H.; Dowey, L.R.C.; Strain, J.J.; Dunne, A.; Ward, M.; Molloy, A.M.; McAnena, L.B.; Hughes, J.P.; Hannon-Fletcher, M.; Scott, J.M. Riboflavin lowers homocysteine in individuals homozygous for the MTHFR 677C→T polymorphism. *Circulation* **2006**, *113*, 74–80. [CrossRef] [PubMed]

54. Reilly, R.; Hopkins, S.; Ward, M.; McNulty, H.; McCann, A.; McNulty, B.; Walton, J.; Molloy, A.; Strain, J.J.; Flynn, A.; et al. MTHFR 677TT genotype and related B-vitamins: Novel determinants of hypertension in healthy Irish adults. *J. Inherit. Metab. Dis.* **2013**, *36*, 35.

55. Wilcken, B.; Bamforth, F.; Li, Z.; Zhu, H.; Ritvanen, A.; Renlund, M.; Stoll, C.; Alembik, Y.; Dott, B.; Czeizel, A.E.; et al. Geographical and ethnic variation of the 677C>T allele of 5,10 methylenetetrahydrofolate reductase (MTHFR): Findings from over 7000 newborns from 16 areas world wide. *J. Med. Genet.* **2003**, *40*, 619–625. [CrossRef] [PubMed]

56. McAuley, E.; McNulty, H.; Hughes, C.; Strain, J.J.; Ward, M. Riboflavin status, MTHFR genotype and blood pressure: Current evidence and implications for personalised nutrition. *Proc. Nutr. Soc.* **2016**, *75*, 405–414. [CrossRef] [PubMed]

57. Guenther, B.D.; Sheppard, C.A.; Tran, P.; Rozen, R.; Matthews, R.G.; Ludwig, M.L. The structure and properties of methylenetetrahydrofolate reductase from Escherichia coli suggest how folate ameliorates human hyperhomocysteinemia. *Nat. Struct. Biol.* **1999**, *6*, 359–365. [PubMed]

58. Yamada, K.; Chen, Z.; Rozen, R.; Matthews, R.G. Effects of common polymorphisms on the properties of recombinant human methylenetetrahydrofolate reductase. *Proc. Natl. Acad. Sci. USA* **2001**, *98*, 14853–14858. [CrossRef] [PubMed]

59. Bagley, P.J.; Selhub, J. A common mutation in the methylenetetrahydrofolate reductase gene is associated with an accumulation of formylated tetrahydrofolates in red blood cells. *Proc. Natl. Acad. Sci. USA* **1998**, *95*, 13217–13220. [CrossRef] [PubMed]

60. Shahzad, K.; Hai, A.; Ahmed, A.; Kizilbash, N.; Alruwaili, J. A structured-based model for the decreased activity of Ala222Val and Glu429Ala methylenetetrahydrofolate reductase (MTHFR) mutants. *Bioinformation* **2013**, *9*, 929–936. [CrossRef] [PubMed]

61. Antoniades, C.; Shirodaria, C.; Warrick, N.; Cai, S.; De Bono, J.; Lee, J.; Leeson, P.; Neubauer, S.; Ratnatunga, C.; Pillai, R.; et al. 5-Methyltetrahydrofolate rapidly improves endothelial function and decreases superoxide production in human vessels: Effects on vascular tetrahydrobiopterin availability and endothelial nitric oxide synthase coupling. *Circulation* **2006**, *114*, 1193–1201. [CrossRef] [PubMed]

62. Antoniades, C.; Shirodaria, C.; Leeson, P.; Baarholm, O.A.; Van-Assche, T.; Cunnington, C.; Pillai, R.; Ratnatunga, C.; Tousoulis, D.; Stefanadis, C.; et al. MTHFR 677C>T polymorphism reveals functional importance for 5-methyltetrahydrofolate, not homocysteine, in regulation of vascular redox state and endothelial function in human atherosclerosis. *Circulation* **2009**, *119*, 2507–2515. [CrossRef] [PubMed]

63. Crider, K.S.; Yang, T.P.; Berry, R.J.; Bailey, L.B. Folate and DNA methylation: A review of molecular mechanisms and the evidence for folate's role. *Adv. Nutr.* **2012**, *3*, 21–38. [CrossRef] [PubMed]

64. Haggarty, P.; Hoad, G.; Campbell, D.M.; Horgan, G.W.; Piyathilake, C.; McNeill, G. Folate in pregnancy and imprinted gene and repeat element methylation in the offspring. *Am. J. Clin. Nutr.* **2013**, *97*, 94–99. [CrossRef] [PubMed]

65. Lévesque, N.; Leclerc, D.; Gayden, T.; Lazaris, A.; De Jay, N.; Petrillo, S.; Metrakos, P.; Jabado, N.; Rozen, R. Murine diet/tissue and human brain tumorigenesis alter Mthfr/MTHFR 5′-end methylation. *Mamm. Genome* **2016**, *27*, 122–134. [CrossRef] [PubMed]

66. Friso, S.; Choi, S.-W.; Girelli, D.; Mason, J.B.; Dolnikowski, G.G.; Bagley, P.J.; Olivieri, O.; Jacques, P.F.; Rosenberg, I.H.; Corrocher, R.; et al. A common mutation in the 5,10-methylenetetrahydrofolate reductase gene affects genomic DNA methylation through an interaction with folate status. *Proc. Natl. Acad. Sci. USA* **2002**, *99*, 5606–5611. [CrossRef] [PubMed]

67. Wang, L.; Shangguan, S.; Chang, S.; Yu, X.; Wang, Z.; Lu, X.; Wu, L.; Zhang, T. Determining the association between methylenetetrahydrofolate reductase (MTHFR) gene polymorphisms and genomic DNA methylation level: A meta-analysis. *Birth Defects Res. A Clin. Mol. Teratol.* **2016**, *106*, 667–674. [CrossRef] [PubMed]

68. Lin, X.; Lu, Q.; Wang, T. Effect of MTHFR gene polymorphism impact on atherosclerosis via genome-wide methylation. *Med. Sci. Monit.* **2016**, *22*, 341–345. [CrossRef] [PubMed]

69. Ge, J.; Wang, J.; Zhang, F.; Diao, B.; Song, Z.F.; Shan, L.L.; Wang, W.; Cao, H.J.; Li, X.Q. Correlation between MTHFR gene methylation and pre-eclampsia, and its clinical significance. *Genet. Mol. Res.* **2015**, *14*, 8021–8028. [CrossRef] [PubMed]

70. Guarrera, S.; Fiorito, G.; Onland-Moret, N.C.; Russo, A.; Agnoli, C.; Allione, A.; Di Gaetano, C.; Mattiello, A.; Ricceri, F.; Chiodini, P. Gene-specific DNA methylation profiles and LINE-1 hypomethylation are associated with myocardial infarction risk. *Clin. Epigenet.* **2015**, *7*, 133. [CrossRef] [PubMed]

71. Pusceddu, I.; Herrmann, M.; Kirsch, S.H.; Werner, C.; Hübner, U.; Bodis, M.; Laufs, U.; Wagenpfeil, S.; Geisel, J.; Herrmann, W. Prospective study of telomere length and LINE-1 methylation in peripheral blood cells: The role of B vitamins supplementation. *Eur. J. Nutr.* **2016**, *55*, 1863–1873. [CrossRef] [PubMed]

72. Clement, D.L.; De Buyzere, M.L.; De Bacquer, D.A.; de Leeuw, P.W.; Duprez, D.A.; Fagard, R.H.; Gheeraert, P.J.; Missault, L.H.; Braun, J.J.; Six, R.O.; et al. Prognostic Value of Ambulatory Blood-Pressure Recordings in Patients with Treated Hypertension. *N. Engl. J. Med.* **2003**, *348*, 2407–2415. [CrossRef] [PubMed]

73. Hermida, R.C.; Smolensky, M.H.; Ayala, D.E.; Portaluppi, F.; Crespo, J.J.; Fabbian, F.; Haus, E.; Manfredini, R.; Mojón, A.; Moyá, A.; et al. 2013 Ambulatory blood pressure monitoring recommendations for the diagnosis of adult hypertension, assessment of cardiovascular and other hypertension-associated risk, and attainment of therapeutic goals. *Chronobiol. Int.* **2013**, *30*, 355–410. [CrossRef] [PubMed]

74. O'Brien, E.; Parati, G.; Stergiou, G.; Asmar, R.; Beilin, L.; Bilo, G.; Clement, D.; de la Sierra, A.; de Leeuw, P.; Dolan, E.; et al. European Society of Hypertension position paper on ambulatory blood pressure monitoring. *J. Hypertens.* **2013**, *31*, 1731–1768. [CrossRef] [PubMed]

75. Solak, Y.; Kario, K.; Covic, A.; Bertelsen, N.; Afsar, B.; Ozkok, A.; Wiecek, A.; Kanbay, M. Clinical value of ambulatory blood pressure: Is it time to recommend for all patients with hypertension? *Clin. Exp. Nephrol.* **2016**, *20*, 14–22. [CrossRef] [PubMed]

76. Dolan, E.; Stanton, A.V.; Thom, S.; Caulfield, M.; Atkins, N.; McInnes, G.; Collier, D.; Dicker, P.; O'Brien, E. Ambulatory blood pressure monitoring predicts cardiovascular events in treated hypertensive patients—An Anglo-Scandinavian cardiac outcomes trial substudy. *J. Hypertens.* **2009**, *27*, 876–885. [CrossRef] [PubMed]

77. Dolan, E.; Stanton, A.; Thijs, L.; Hinedi, K.; Atkins, N.; McClory, S.; Den Hond, E.; McCormack, P.; Staessen, J.A.; O'Brien, E. Superiority of ambulatory over clinic blood pressure measurement in predicting mortality: The Dublin outcome study. *Hypertension* **2005**, *46*, 156–161. [CrossRef] [PubMed]

78. Sesso, H.D.; Stampfer, M.J.; Rosner, B.; Hennekens, C.H.; Gaziano, J.M.; Manson, J.E.; Glynn, R.J. Systolic and Diastolic Blood Pressure, Pulse Pressure, and Mean Arterial Pressure as Predictors of Cardiovascular Disease Risk in Men. *Hypertension* **2000**, *36*, 801–807. [CrossRef] [PubMed]

79. Brown, D.W.; Giles, W.H.; Greenlund, K.J. Blood pressure parameters and risk of fatal stroke, NHANES II mortality study. *Am. J. Hypertens.* **2007**, *20*, 338–341. [CrossRef] [PubMed]

80. Verdecchia, P.; Schillaci, G.; Reboldi, G.; Franklin, S.S.; Porcellati, C. Different prognostic impact of 24-hour mean blood pressure and pulse pressure on stroke and coronary artery disease in essential hypertension. *Circulation* **2001**, *103*, 2579–2584. [CrossRef] [PubMed]

81. Mancia, G.; De Backer, G.; Dominiczak, A.; Cifkova, R.; Fagard, R.; Germano, G.; Grassi, G.; Heagerty, A.M.; Kjeldsen, S.E.; Laurent, S.; et al. 2007 Guidelines for the management of arterial hypertension. *Eur. Heart J* **2007**, *28*, 1462–1536. [CrossRef] [PubMed]

82. Morcet, J.F.; Safar, M.; Thomas, F.; Guize, L.; Benetos, A. Associations between heart rate and other risk factors in a large French population. *J. Hypertens.* **1999**, *17*, 1671–1676. [CrossRef] [PubMed]

83. Perret-Guillaume, C.; Joly, L.; Benetos, A. Heart rate as a risk factor for cardiovascular disease. *Prog. Cardiovasc. Dis.* **2009**, *52*, 6–10. [CrossRef] [PubMed]

84. Benetos, A.; Rudnichi, A.; Thomas, F.; Safar, M.; Guize, L. Influence of Heart Rate on Mortality in a French Population. *Hypertension* **1999**, *33*, 44–52. [CrossRef] [PubMed]

85. Reule, S.; Drawz, P.E. Heart rate and blood pressure: Any possible implications for management of hypertension? *Curr. Hypertens. Rep.* **2012**, *14*, 478–484. [CrossRef] [PubMed]

86. Pickering, T.G.; James, G.D.; Boddie, C.; Harshfield, G.A.; Blank, S.; Laragh, J.H. How common is white coat hypertension? *JAMA* **1988**, *259*, 225–228. [CrossRef] [PubMed]

87. Franklin, S.S.; Thijs, L.; Hansen, T.W.; O'Brien, E.; Staessen, J.A. White-coat hypertension: New insights from recent studies. *Hypertension* **2013**, *62*, 982–987. [CrossRef] [PubMed]

88. Mani, A. White-Coat Hypertension: A True Cardiovascular Risk? *J. Clin. Hypertens.* **2016**, *18*, 623–624. [CrossRef] [PubMed]

89. Pierdomenico, S.D.; Cuccurullo, F. Prognostic value of white-coat and masked hypertension diagnosed by ambulatory monitoring in initially untreated subjects: An updated meta analysis. *Am. J. Hypertens.* **2011**, *24*, 52–58. [CrossRef] [PubMed]

90. Tientcheu, D.; Ayers, C.; Das, S.R.; McGuire, D.K.; de Lemos, J.A.; Khera, A.; Kaplan, N.; Victor, R.; Vongpatanasin, W. Target organ complications and cardiovascular events associated with masked hypertension and white-coat hypertension: Analysis from the dallas heart study. *J. Am. Coll. Cardiol.* **2015**, *66*, 2159–2169. [CrossRef] [PubMed]

91. Gustavsen, P.H.; Høegholm, A.; Bang, L.E.; Kristensen, K.S. White coat hypertension is a cardiovascular risk factor: A 10-year follow-up study. *J. Hum. Hypertens.* **2003**, *17*, 811–817. [CrossRef] [PubMed]

92. Briasoulis, A.; Androulakis, E.; Palla, M.; Papageorgiou, N.; Tousoulis, D. White-coat hypertension and cardiovascular events: A meta-analysis. *J. Hypertens.* **2016**, *34*, 593–599. [CrossRef] [PubMed]

93. Wojciechowska, W.; Stolarz-Skrzypek, K.; Olszanecka, A.; Klima, Ł.; Gąsowski, J.; Grodzicki, T.; Kawecka-Jaszcz, K.; Czarnecka, D. Subclinical arterial and cardiac damage in white-coat and masked hypertension. *Blood Press.* **2016**, *25*, 249–256. [CrossRef] [PubMed]

94. Scuteri, A.; Morrell, C.H.; Orru', M.; AlGhatrif, M.; Saba, P.S.; Terracciano, A.; Ferreli, L.A.P.; Loi, F.; Marongiu, M.; Pilia, M.G.; et al. Gender specific profiles of white coat and masked hypertension impacts on arterial structure and function in the SardiNIA study. *Int. J. Cardiol.* **2016**, *217*, 92–98. [CrossRef] [PubMed]

95. Stevens, S.L.; Wood, S.; Koshiaris, C.; Law, K.; Glasziou, P.; Stevens, R.J.; McManus, R.J. Blood pressure variability and cardiovascular disease: Systematic review and meta-analysis. *BMJ* **2016**, *354*, i4098. [CrossRef] [PubMed]

96. Franklin, S.S.; O'Brien, E.; Thijs, L.; Asayama, K.; Staessen, J.A. Masked hypertension a phenomenon of measurement. *Hypertension* **2015**, *65*, 16–20. [CrossRef] [PubMed]

97. Lazaridis, A.A.; Sarafidis, P.A.; Ruilope, L.M. Ambulatory blood pressure monitoring in the diagnosis, prognosis, and management of resistant hypertension: Still a matter of our resistance? *Curr. Hypertens. Rep.* **2015**, *17*, 78. [CrossRef] [PubMed]

98. O'Brien, E.; Sheridan, J.; O'Malley, K. Dippers and non-dippers. *Lancet* **1988**, *332*, 397. [CrossRef]

99. Mezue, K.; Isiguzo, G.; Madu, C.; Nwuruku, G.; Rangaswami, J.; Baugh, D.; Madu, E. Nocturnal non-dipping blood pressure profile in black normotensives is associated with cardiac target organ damage. *Ethn. Dis.* **2016**, *26*, 279–284. [CrossRef] [PubMed]

100. Ohkubo, T.; Hozawa, A.; Yamaguchi, J.; Kikuya, M.; Ohmori, K.; Michimata, M.; Matsubara, M.; Hashimoto, J.; Hoshi, H.; Araki, T.; et al. Prognostic significance of the nocturnal decline in blood pressure in individuals with and without high 24-h blood pressure: The Ohasama study. *J. Hypertens.* **2002**, *20*, 2183–2189. [CrossRef] [PubMed]

101. Verdecchia, P.; Angeli, F.; Mazzotta, G.; Garofoli, M.; Ramundo, E.; Gentile, G.; Ambrosio, G.; Reboldi, G. Day-night dip and early-morning surge in blood pressure in hypertension: Prognostic implications. *Hypertension* **2012**, *60*, 34–42. [CrossRef] [PubMed]

102. Fagard, R.H.; Thijs, L.; Staessen, J.A.; Clement, D.L.; De Buyzere, M.L.; De Bacquer, D.A. Night-day blood pressure ratio and dipping pattern as predictors of death and cardiovascular events in hypertension. *J. Hum. Hypertens.* **2009**, *23*, 645–653. [CrossRef] [PubMed]

103. Eguchi, K.; Hoshide, S.; Ishikawa, J.; Pickering, T.G.; Schwartz, J.E.; Shimada, K.; Kario, K. Nocturnal nondipping of heart rate predicts cardiovascular events in hypertensive patients. *J. Hypertens.* **2009**, *27*, 2265–2270. [CrossRef] [PubMed]

104. Kario, K.; Pickering, T.G.; Matsuo, T.; Hoshide, S.; Schwartz, J.E.; Shimada, K. Stroke prognosis and abnormal nocturnal blood pressure falls in older hypertensives. *Hypertension* **2001**, *38*, 852–857. [CrossRef] [PubMed]

105. Hermida, R.C.; Ayala, D.E.; Mojón, A.; Fernández, J.R. Blunted sleep-time relative blood pressure decline increases cardiovascular risk independent of blood pressure level—The "normotensive non-dipper" paradox. *Chronobiol. Int.* **2013**, *30*, 87–98. [CrossRef] [PubMed]

106. Salles, G.F.; Reboldi, G.; Fagard, R.H.; Cardoso, C.R.L.; Pierdomenico, S.D.; Verdecchia, P.; Eguchi, K.; Kario, K.; Hoshide, S.; Polonia, J.; et al. Prognostic effect of the nocturnal blood pressure fall in hypertensive patients: The ambulatory blood pressure collaboration in patients with hypertension (ABC-H) meta-analysis. *Hypertension* **2016**, *67*, 693–700. [CrossRef] [PubMed]

107. Pierdomenico, S.D.; Pierdomenico, A.M.; Di Tommaso, R.; Coccina, F.; Di Carlo, S.; Porreca, E.; Cuccurullo, F. Morning blood pressure surge, dipping, and risk of coronary events in elderly treated hypertensive patients. *Am. J. Hypertens.* **2016**, *29*, 39–45. [CrossRef] [PubMed]

108. Xie, J.C.; Yan, H.; Zhao, Y.X.; Liu, X.Y. Prognostic value of morning blood pressure surge in clinical events: A meta-analysis of longitudinal studies. *J. Stroke Cerebrovasc. Dis.* **2015**, *24*, 362–369. [CrossRef] [PubMed]

109. Hansen, T.W.; Li, Y.; Boggia, J.; Thijs, L.; Richart, T.; Staessen, J.A. Predictive role of the nighttime blood pressure. *Hypertension* **2011**, *57*, 3–10. [CrossRef] [PubMed]

110. Grassi, G.; Seravalle, G.; Quarti-Trevano, F.; Dell'Oro, R.; Bombelli, M.; Cuspidi, C.; Facchetti, R.; Bolla, G.; Mancia, G. Adrenergic, metabolic, and reflex abnormalities in reverse and extreme dipper hypertensives. *Hypertension* **2008**, *52*, 925–931. [CrossRef] [PubMed]

111. Di Raimondo, D.; Miceli, G.; Casuccio, A.; Tuttolomondo, A.; Buttà, C.; Zappulla, V.; Schimmenti, C.; Musiari, G.; Pinto, A. Does sympathetic overactivation feature all hypertensives? Differences of sympathovagal balance according to night/day blood pressure ratio in patients with essential hypertension. *Hypertens. Res.* **2016**, *39*, 1–9. [CrossRef] [PubMed]

112. Kuo, T.B.J.; Chen, C.-Y.; Wang, Y.P.; Lan, Y.-Y.; Mak, K.-H.; Lee, G.-S.; Yang, C.C.H. The role of autonomic and baroreceptor reflex control in blood pressure dipping and nondipping in rats. *J. Hypertens.* **2014**, *32*, 806–816. [CrossRef] [PubMed]

113. Saeed, S.; Wajea-Andreassen, U.; Fromm, A.; Øygarden, H.; Naess, H.; Gerdts, E. Blunted nightly blood pressure reduction is associated with increased arterial stiffness in ischemic stroke patients: A Norwegian stroke in the young study. *J. Hypertens.* **2015**, *33*, e41. [CrossRef] [PubMed]

114. Fontes-Guerra, P.C.A.; Cardoso, C.R.L.; Muxfeldt, E.S.; Salles, G.F. Nitroglycerin-mediated, but not flow-mediated vasodilation, is associated with blunted nocturnal blood pressure fall in patients with resistant hypertension. *J. Hypertens.* **2015**, *33*, 1666–1675. [CrossRef] [PubMed]

115. Verdecchia, P.; Angeli, F.; Borgioni, C.; Gattobigio, R.; Reboldi, G. Ambulatory blood pressure and cardiovascular outcome in relation to perceived sleep deprivation. *Hypertension* **2007**, *49*, 777–783. [CrossRef] [PubMed]

116. Monte, M.; Cambão, M.; Mesquita Bastos, J.; Polónia, J. Reproducibility of ambulatory blood pressure values and circadian blood pressure patterns in untreated subjects in a 1–11 month interval. *Rev. Port. Cardiol.* **2015**, *34*, 643–650. [CrossRef] [PubMed]

117. Keren, S.; Leibowitz, A.; Grossman, E.; Sharabi, Y. Limited reproducibility of 24-h ambulatory blood pressure monitoring. *Clin. Exp. Hypertens.* **2015**, *37*, 599–603. [PubMed]

118. Hermida, R.C.; Ayala, D.E.; Fernández, J.R.; Calvo, C. Chronotherapy improves blood pressure control and reverts the nondipper pattern in patients with resistant hypertension. *Hypertension* **2008**, *51*, 69–76. [CrossRef] [PubMed]

119. Hermida, R.C.; Ayala, D.E.; Mojón, A.; Fernández, J.R. Influence of circadian time of hypertension treatment on cardiovascular risk: Results of the MAPEC study. *Chronobiol. Int.* **2010**, *27*, 1629–1651. [CrossRef] [PubMed]

120. Gould, B.A.; Mann, S.; Davies, A.B.; Altman, D.G.; Raftery, E.B. Does placebo lower blood-pressure? *Lancet* **1981**, *2*, 1377–1381. [CrossRef]

121. Mancia, G.; Omboni, S.; Parati, G.; Ravogli, A.; Villani, A.; Zanchetti, A. Lack of placebo effect on ambulatory blood pressure. *Am. J. Hypertens.* **1995**, *8*, 311–315. [CrossRef]

122. Kotsis, V.; Stabouli, S.; Bouldin, M.; Low, A.; Toumanidis, S.; Zakopoulos, N. Impact of obesity on 24-hour ambulatory blood pressure and hypertension. *Hypertension* **2005**, *45*, 602–607. [CrossRef] [PubMed]

123. Cuspidi, C.; Meani, S.; Valerio, C.; Negri, F.; Sala, C.; Maisaidi, M.; Giudici, V.; Zanchetti, A.; Mancia, G. Body mass index, nocturnal fall in blood pressure and organ damage in untreated essential hypertensive patients. *Blood Press. Monit.* **2008**, *13*, 318–324. [CrossRef] [PubMed]

124. Demir, M.; Günay, T.; Özmen, G.; Melek, M. Relationship between vitamin D deficiency and nondipper hypertension. *Clin. Exp. Hypertens.* **2013**, *35*, 45–49. [CrossRef] [PubMed]

125. Yilmaz, S.; Sen, F.; Ozeke, O.; Temizhan, A.; Topaloglu, S.; Aras, D.; Aydogdu, S. The relationship between vitamin D levels and nondipper hypertension. *Blood Press. Monit.* **2015**, *20*, 330–334. [CrossRef] [PubMed]

126. Kanbay, M.; Isik, B.; Akcay, A.; Ozkara, A.; Karakurt, F.; Turgut, F.; Alkan, R.; Uz, E.; Bavbek, N.; Yigitoglu, R.; et al. Relation between serum calcium, phosphate, parathyroid hormone and "nondipper" circadian blood pressure variability profile in patients with normal renal function. *Am. J. Nephrol.* **2007**, *27*, 516–521. [CrossRef] [PubMed]

127. Moore, T.J.; Vollmer, W.M.; Appel, L.J.; Sacks, F.M.; Svetkey, L.P.; Vogt, T.M.; Conlin, P.R.; Simons-Morton, D.G.; Carter-Edwards, L.; Harsha, D.W. Effect of dietary patterns on ambulatory blood pressure: Results from the dietary approaches to stop hypertension (DASH) trial. DASH collaborative research group. *Hypertension* **1999**, *34*, 472–477. [CrossRef] [PubMed]

128. Miller, E.R.; Erlinger, T.P.; Young, D.R.; Jehn, M.; Charleston, J.; Rhodes, D.; Wasan, S.K.; Appel, L.J. Results of the diet, exercise, and weight loss intervention trial (DEW-IT). *Hypertension* **2002**, *40*, 612–618. [CrossRef] [PubMed]

129. Paula, T.P.; Viana, L.V.; Neto, A.T.Z.; Leitão, C.B.; Gross, J.L.; Azevedo, M.J. Effects of the DASH diet and walking on blood pressure in patients with type 2 diabetes and uncontrolled hypertension: A randomized controlled trial. *J. Clin. Hypertens.* **2015**, *17*, 895–901. [CrossRef] [PubMed]

130. Drouin-Chartier, J.-P.; Gigleux, I.; Tremblay, A.J.; Poirier, L.; Lamarche, B.; Couture, P. Impact of dairy consumption on essential hypertension: A clinical study. *Nutr. J.* **2014**, *13*, 83. [CrossRef] [PubMed]

131. Machin, D.R.; Park, W.; Alkatan, M.; Mouton, M.; Tanaka, H. Hypotensive effects of solitary addition of conventional nonfat dairy products to the routine diet: A randomized controlled trial. *Am. J. Clin. Nutr.* **2014**, *100*, 80–87. [CrossRef] [PubMed]

132. Hobbs, D.A.; Goulding, M.G.; Nguyen, A.; Malaver, T.; Walker, C.F.; George, T.W.; Methven, L.; Lovegrove, J.A. Acute ingestion of beetroot bread increases endothelium-independent vasodilation and lowers diastolic blood pressure in healthy men: A randomized controlled trial. *J. Nutr.* **2013**, *143*, 1399–1405. [CrossRef] [PubMed]

133. Jajja, A.; Sutyarjoko, A.; Lara, J.; Rennie, K.; Brandt, K.; Qadir, O.; Siervo, M. Beetroot supplementation lowers daily systolic blood pressure in older, overweight subjects. *Nutr. Res.* **2014**, *34*, 868–875. [CrossRef] [PubMed]

134. Kapil, V.; Khambata, R.S.; Robertson, A.; Caulfield, M.J.; Ahluwalia, A. Dietary nitrate provides sustained blood pressure lowering in hypertensive patients: A randomized, phase 2, double-blind, placebo-controlled study. *Hypertension* **2015**, *65*, 320–327. [CrossRef] [PubMed]

135. Coles, L.T.; Clifton, P.M. Effect of beetroot juice on lowering blood pressure in free-living, disease-free adults: A randomized, placebo-controlled trial. *Nutr. J.* **2012**, *11*, 1–6. [CrossRef] [PubMed]

136. Larsen, T.; Mose, F.H.; Bech, J.N.; Hansen, A.B.; Pedersen, E.B. Effect of cholecalciferol supplementation during winter months in patients with hypertension: A randomized, placebo-controlled trial. *Am. J. Hypertens.* **2012**, *25*, 1215–1222. [CrossRef] [PubMed]

137. Pilz, S.; Gaksch, M.; Kienreich, K.; Grübler, M.; Verheyen, N.; Fahrleitner-Pammer, A.; Treiber, G.; Drechsler, C.; Ó Hartaigh, B.; Obermayer-Pietsch, B.; et al. Effects of vitamin D on blood pressure and cardiovascular risk factors: A randomized controlled trial. *Hypertension* **2015**, *65*, 1195–1201. [CrossRef] [PubMed]

138. Brüll, V.; Burak, C.; Stoffel-Wagner, B.; Wolffram, S.; Nickenig, G.; Müller, C.; Langguth, P.; Alteheld, B.; Fimmers, R.; Naaf, S.; et al. Effects of a quercetin-rich onion skin extract on 24 h ambulatory blood pressure and endothelial function in overweight-to-obese patients with (pre-)hypertension: A randomised double-blinded placebo-controlled cross-over trial. *Br. J. Nutr.* **2015**, *14*, 1263–1277. [CrossRef] [PubMed]

139. Sauder, K.A.; McCrea, C.E.; Ulbrecht, J.S.; Kris-Etherton, P.M.; West, S.G. Pistachio nut consumption

modifies systemic hemodynamics, increases heart rate variability, and reduces ambulatory blood pressure in well-controlled type 2 diabetes: A randomized trial. *J. Am. Heart Assoc.* **2014**, *3*, 1–9. [CrossRef] [PubMed]

140. Appel, L.J.; Moore, T.J.; Obarzanek, E.; Vollmer, W.M.; Svetkey, L.P.; Sacks, F.M.; Bray, G.A.; Vogt, T.M.; Cutler, J.A.; Windhauser, M.M.; et al. A clinical trial of the effects of dietary patterns on blood pressure. *N. Engl. J. Med.* **1997**, *336*, 1117–1124. [CrossRef] [PubMed]

141. Cagnacci, A.; Cannoletta, M.; Xholli, A.; Piacenti, I.; Palma, F.; Palmieri, B. Folate administration decreases oxidative status and blood pressure in postmenopausal women. *Eur. J. Nutr.* **2015**, *54*, 429–435. [CrossRef] [PubMed]

142. Cagnacci, A.; Cannoletta, M.; Volpe, A. High-dose short-term folate administration modifies ambulatory blood pressure in postmenopausal women. A placebo-controlled study. *Eur. J. Clin. Nutr.* **2009**, *63*, 1266–1268. [CrossRef] [PubMed]

143. Williams, C.; Kingwell, B.A.; Burke, K.; McPherson, J.; Dart, A.M. Folic acid supplementation for 3 weeks reduces pulse pressure and large artery stiffness independent of MTHFR genotype. *Am. J. Clin. Nutr.* **2005**, *82*, 26–31. [PubMed]

6

Voluntary Folic Acid Fortification Levels and Nutrient Composition of Food Products from the Spanish Market: A 2011–2015 Update

María Lourdes Samaniego-Vaesken, Elena Alonso-Aperte and Gregorio Varela-Moreiras *

Department of Pharmaceutical and Health Sciences, Faculty of Pharmacy, CEU San Pablo University, Madrid 28668, Spain; l.samaniego@ceu.es (M.L.S.-V.); eaperte@ceu.es (E.A.-A.)
* Correspondence: gvarela@ceu.es

Abstract: Introduction. Folic acid (FA) is a synthetic compound commonly added for voluntary fortification of food products in many European countries. In our country, food composition databases (FCDB) lack comprehensive data on FA fortification practices and this is considered a priority research need when undergoing nutritional assessment of the population. Methods. A product inventory was collected and updated by visiting retail stores in Madrid Region, conducting online supermarket searches, and by the provision of food label information by manufacturers. Euro-FIR FCDB guidelines for data compilation and harmonization were used. Results. The FCDB, compiled between 2011 and 2015, includes FA as well as macro and micronutrient data from 338 fortified foodstuffs. As compared to previous FCDB updates (May 2010), 37 products have ceased to declare added FA in their labels, mainly yogurt and fermented milk products. The main food subgroup is 'breakfast cereals' (n = 95, 34% of total). However, the highest average FA fortification levels per recommended serving were observed in the 'milk, milk products, and milk substitutes' group at $\geq$35% FA Nutrient Reference Values (NRV, 200 µg, EU Regulation 1169 of 2011) (60–76.3 µg FA per 200 mL). Average contribution to the FA NRV per food group and serving ranged between 16%–35%. Conclusion. Our data show a minor decrease in the number of FA fortified products, but vitamin levels added by manufacturers are stable in most food groups and subgroups. This representative product inventory comprises the main FA food source from voluntary fortification in our country. It is therefore a unique compilation tool with valuable data for the assessment of dietary intakes for the vitamin.

Keywords: folic acid; voluntary fortification; food composition database

1. Introduction

Folic acid (FA) is the synthetic form of an essential water-soluble vitamin generically regarded as folates or B9. It is involved in one-carbon metabolism, and it has been linked to lowering Neural Tube Defect (NTD) risk when taken as a supplement around the time of conception [1]. Folates are also naturally present in foods such as green vegetables, fruits, liver, legumes, and nuts. Women of childbearing age are strongly recommended to maintain an adequate folate status through diet and supplementation, although the strategy has been proven to be somewhat ineffective in lowering the risk of NTD in Europe due to a high percentage of unplanned pregnancies and the relatively low compliance with FA pharmacological supplementation [2]. With an aim to increasing women's FA intakes because of its public health relevance, fortification policies have been implemented worldwide. At present, only voluntary fortification of food products with FA takes place in Spain and the rest of Europe, whereas more than 60 countries add FA to wheat flour and other cereal products in a mandatory fortification scheme, according to data from the Food Fortification Initiative [3]. Voluntary fortification, also known as "discretionary fortification", is the addition of vitamins or minerals to foods at the discretion of the manufacturer in order to restore micronutrients, ensure the nutritional equivalence of substitute foods, and/or to enhance the nutritive value of a product. In this regard, FA addition is endorsed by the European Regulation 1925/2006 of the European Parliament and of the Council of 20 December 2006, on the addition of vitamins and minerals and of certain other substances to food [4], and Regulation 1169/2011 of the European Parliament and of the Council of 25 October 2011, on the provision of food information to consumers [5]. This last regulation lays down the levels of "significant" vitamin addition, the requirements for nutritional and health claims, as well as the Nutrient Reference Values (NRV) for different vitamins, including folate.

In the last few years, an increasing number of researchers have questioned whether Europe should consider implementing mandatory fortification with FA, since current strategies, such as supplementation campaigns, have not been successful in reducing NTD prevalence [2,6]. On the other hand, concerns about the effects of extra FA intakes in children and the elderly are still a major issue that delays the implementation of this population-wide measure [7,8]. Although the Mediterranean diet is naturally a good folate source, data show that the Spanish population is folate deficient [9] and, most remarkably, the Mediterranean Diet is moving towards a less healthy pattern. Traditionally, the Mediterranean diet is characterized by a high consumption of vegetable foods (fresh fruit, vegetables, legumes, wheat bread, and olive oil) and fish, and a low intake of meats (mainly poultry). The latest national data indicate that fresh fruit, legume, and vegetable intakes are decreasing [9], which is in agreement with the data from the Spanish Food Consumption Survey Panel. Approximately only 50%–58% of the adult population reach current FA recommended intakes [10].

Food Composition Tables and Databases (FCDB) are key tools for nutritional assessment of the population's diet. However, they are usually outdated in terms of inclusion of fortified products [11]. Important efforts have been made so far in developing specialized and standardized FCDB such as the one for the EPIC Project (European Prospective Investigation into Cancer and Nutrition) [12], and the Spanish FCDB BEDCA (Base Española de Datos de Composición de Alimentos) [13], both in line with the EuroFIR (European Food Information Resource Network) guidelines for harmonization and interchangeability [14]. However, the number of fortified food items included remains somewhat limited. It has been estimated that fortified foods provide only 5%–8% of the total energy intake of the European population [8], even though, market availability in the last 10 years has been consistently increasing [11]. Interestingly, data from surveys on total intakes of micronutrients (including fortified foods) in Europe and the US show that small proportions of the population, particularly children, may exceed the Upper Intake Levels (UL) for FA [15,16]. However, current fortification practices do not appear to contribute appreciably to the risk of adverse effects derived from nutrient intake [17]. Many researchers have outlined the importance of monitoring fortification practices and consumption of fortified foods in order to continuously assess the efficacy and safety of vitamin and mineral addition to foodstuffs [18–22]. At present, voluntary fortification practices are not being strictly monitored. An important number of brands commercialize fortified products in Spain [23], and continuous market evolution (new product launches and formulation changes) implies fortification level variations for specific vitamins. Food consumption surveys rarely assess fortified food products' potential impact because of the absence of updated data on these products in most commonly used food composition tables and databases [11]. Nonetheless, important efforts have been made to include them, namely the Enkid study, which assessed consumption of fortified products such as breakfast cereals in children and adolescents [24].

For all the aforementioned, since December 2007 we have been actively working on the development of a comprehensive FCDB including all available FA fortified products from the Spanish market [23]. Enhanced reliability and comprehensiveness of food composition tables has been identified as a key research need worldwide in the context of a rapidly changing food supply [25]. Therefore, in this article we present the main findings and trends from the latest database update comprising FA fortified products commercialized in Spain.

2. Materials and Methods

Database design and structure has been previously described [23]. Briefly, Microsoft Office Access® 2003 software (Microsoft Co., Redmond, Washington, DC, USA) was used for designing a tailor-made relational database. The LanguaL™ food description thesaurus and EuroFIR guidelines were adopted, including food group classification schemes [26]. The FCDB update was conducted through a market and online survey from January 2011 to June 2015 based in the Madrid Region. The consumption of fortified foodstuffs in the Madrid Region is higher as compared to the national average consumption [27], and the region includes the Capital City and a highly urbanized area (Metropolitan Madrid). Therefore, food availability in Madrid may be considered to include all fortified food products that would be available throughout different regions of the country. Retail centres such as hypermarkets, supermarkets, and convenience stores were visited over a four week period each year of the study and were selected in accordance with their sales data [28]. In addition, commercial online stores were accessed for product search, which includes food product availability nationwide. Foods that declared FA on the ingredient list by the following terms: B_9, folate, folacin, or FA were identified and listed as potential FCDB inclusions. Compiled data included macro and micronutrients per 100 g or mL, recommended serving size, nutritional and health claims, and a photograph of the product package. Once completed, quality control checks were applied to the FCDB numerical data to assess potential errors and inconsistencies in recorded data. FA fortification levels were assessed as percentage of FA NRV (200 µg, [5]) provided per recommended serving for each food group as described in our previous studies [21]. All values are expressed per 100 g of edible portion on a fresh weight basis, unless otherwise stated. Food and Agriculture Organization (FAO) Guidelines for checking food composition prior to publication of a user database were followed when applicable [29].

Results of macro- and micronutrient contents are presented as median and interquartile range for skewed variables. Variables were tested for normality using a Kolmogorov-Smirnov test. All statistical analyses were performed using SPSS Software (SPSS 20.0, SPSS Inc., Chicago, IL, USA).

3. Results

A total of 338 FA fortified products were compiled and assessed. 37 products were removed from the FCDB as they are no longer available for purchase or because FA is no longer included in their composition (Figure 1), mainly breakfast cereals, cereal bars, flours or starch, foods for weight reduction, milk, yogurts (fermented milks), cheese, juice or nectar, margarine and vegetable fats and oils, and chocolate products. A total of 25 products were new to the database, mainly foods for infants, coffee, tea, cocoa or infusions, soft drinks, pastries and cakes, and bread. Four food groups and 13 subgroups were included in the FCBD and their distribution is presented in Table 1. 'Grain and grain products' (50%, n = 169), and 'products for special nutritional uses or dietary supplements' (31%, n = 105) represented the highest proportion of available fortified products, while 'milk, milk products, or milk substitutes' (15%, n = 52) and 'beverages (non-milk)' (4%, n = 12) were minor. Total number of brands was 39, of which 31 were traditional manufacturer's brands and 8 were from distribution (supermarket own brand). Ten products declared FA content on labels (ingredients list) but did not specify the quantity per 100 g or serving in the nutritional information label. Median declared FA contents ranged from 15 µg per 100 g (30 µg per 200 mL serving) in 'nectar and juices' and 'soft drinks' to 199 µg per 100 g (39.8 µg per 20 g serving) in 'coffee, tea, cocoa, or infusions' (Table 2). 'Breakfast cereals' is the subgroup that represented the highest proportion of FA fortified products (n = 95, 28% of total), with median declared FA levels of 170 µg per 100 g (51 µg per 30 g serving). Secondly, 'foods for infants' accounted for 20% (n = 70) of fortified products, with median declared FA levels of 65 µg per 100 g (16.25 µg per 25 g serving). Median energy content provided by each FA fortified food group ranged from 22.5 kcal per 100 mL in the case of 'soft drinks', to 406 kcal per 100 g in 'cereal bars'. Carbohydrates were the main declared macronutrient in all groups, ranging from 5 to 80 g per 100 mL or g; of these, added sugars accounted for 5 to 72 g per 100 mL or g, and fibre content was 0.5 to 12 g per 100 g. Starch content, however, was not declared in most products. Total fat contents were 1.6 to

10 g per 100 g and the lipid profile (proportion of monounsaturated, polyunsaturated, and saturated fatty acids) was not declared in most food groups. Protein contents were 0.2 to 14 g per 100 mL or g.

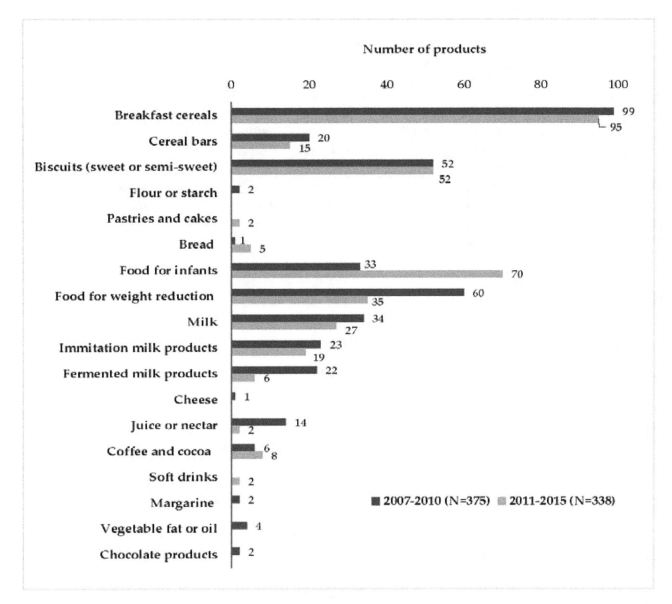

Figure 1. Food subgroup distribution in the Voluntary Folic Acid Fortification Food Composition Database: comparison between first (2007–2010) and second (2011–2015) compilation.

A general outlook of the Access® relational database, as well as an example of two database tables compiling fortified food data can be found at the Supplementary Material section. Most frequently added vitamins and minerals to FA fortified food formulations are shown in Tables 2 and 3. All data are presented as medians and interquartile ranges. 'Foods for infants' and 'foods for weight reduction' were the groups that presented the highest proportion of simultaneous addition of vitamins other than FA, containing nearly all vitamins with the exception of vitamin K in 'foods for weight reduction'. 'Milk products' declared to contain vitamins C, B1, B2, B3, B6, B12, pantothenic acid, and biotin; 'imitation milk products' contained vitamins A, D, E, and B6; 'coffee, tea, cocoa or infusions' declared vitamins A, E, D, C, B1, B2, B3, B6, B12, and pantothenic acid; and 'breakfast cereals' included mainly vitamins D, B1, B2, B3, B6, B12 and pantothenic acid, together with FA. In the case of added minerals, again 'foods for infants' and 'foods for weight reduction' were those that declared a higher number as compared to the other subgroups. All 'grain products' declared Iron addition, and specifically 'cereal bars' and 'bread products' also declared the addition of calcium and sodium, respectively; some 'milk products' included calcium, phosphorus, and zinc addition. This shows that in most analysed products mineral addition was limited when compared to vitamins.

FA fortification levels from compiled products were calculated from labelled FA values and recommended servings per each product, using the FA Nutrient Reference Value (200 µg/day, NRV) as guidance (Figure 2). In the major food group of the FCDB, 'grain and grain products', 56% of items presented fortification at level 2 which accounts for 16.1% to 25.9% of FA NRV per recommended serving. Fortification at level 1 (≤16% FA NRV) was observed in 63% of 'products for special nutritional uses' ('foods for infant' and 'weight reduction') and 72% of 'milk, milk products or milk substitutes' were fortified at the highest level available (level 4, ≥35% FA NRV). Finally, the 'beverages' group showed a higher proportion of level 1 fortification, as 42% of products provided less than 16% of FA NRV per recommended serving. These data should be interpreted with care in terms of FA contribution since NRV are set at 200 µg/day of FA according to EU Regulation, while in Spain, recommended FA intakes for women of childbearing age are 400 µg/day. Accordingly, the actual contribution of these products is well below half of this group's needs.

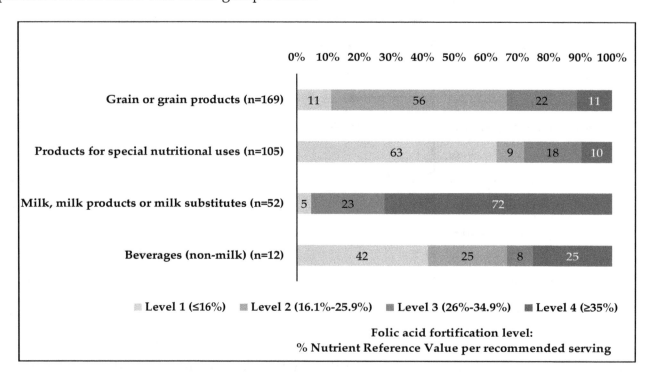

Figure 2. Folic acid fortification levels calculated per manufacturer's recommended serving in compiled food groups from the Voluntary Folic Acid Fortification Food Composition Database.

Table 1. Macronutrient distribution, fibre and salt content in folic acid-fortified food products from the Spanish market.

Food Groups and Subgroups	N	Energy (kcal)	Declared Serving (g or mL)	Fats (Total) (g)	SFA (g)	MUFA (g)	PUFA (g)	Carbohydrates (g)	Sugars (g)	Starch (g)	Fibre (g)	Protein (g)	Salt (g)
Grain or grain products	169												
Breakfast cereals	95	386 (378–403)	30 (25–30)	3 (1–7)	1 (0–3)	ND	ND	76 (67–81)	24 (20–30)	ND	5 (3–8.25)	8 (6–8)	0 (0–1)
Biscuits, sweet and semi-sweet	52	444 (423.2–462.7)	25 (25–29.5)	15.5 (12–17.5)	2 (1–4)	ND	ND	66.5 (63–71.5)	21 (17.5–23)	ND	4 (2–7.75)	7 (6–8)	0.41 (0.23–0.83)
Cereal bars	15	406 (380–416.5)	25 (23–30)	10 (7–13)	4 (3–9)	ND	ND	67 (61–74)	30 (23–35)	0 (0–36.5)	4 (3–6)	6 (5–7)	ND
Bread and similar products	5	375 (368–389)	ND	4 (3–5.5)	0.6 (0.45–1.65)	1.25 (0.75–2.2)	2.5 (0.87–4.05)	63 (59–70)	2 (1–4)	ND	12 (6.5–14)	14 (12–15)	1 (0.5–1)
Pastries and cakes	2	383 (383–389)	40	13 (13–13.5)	ND	ND	ND	58	34 (34–36)	ND	8 (8–8.5)	4	0.51 (0.45–0.58)
Products for special nutritional uses or dietary supplements	105												
Foods for infants	70	387 (90–483.2)	25 (20–24.75)	3 (2–21.2)	1.3 (0.47–7.72)	7.9 (1.7–9.7)	3.2 (0.5–5.1)	60 (13–78)	25 (7.7–39.2)	ND	0.5 (0–4.25)	9 (2–10)	0.1 (0.025–0.3)
Foods for weight reduction	35	383 (368–462)	45 (20–63)	12 (10–17)	5 (3–11)	ND	ND	45 (37–55)	29 (14–34)	ND	5 (2–8)	24 (6–26)	ND
Milk, milk products, or milk substitutes	52												
Milk	27	46 (38–52)	250	1.6 (0.3–1.95)	1 (0.275–1.1)	0.1 (0–0.6)	0 (0–0.3)	4 (4–5)	4 (4–5)	ND	ND	3 (3–3)	0.13 (0.13–0.2)
Imitation milk products	19	52 (49–60)	250	1.9 (1.6–2.5)	0.56 (0.41–1.05)	1.2 (0.4–1.4)	0.2 (0.2–0.3)	5 (4–6)	5 (4–6)	ND	0 (0–0.225)	3 (2–3)	0.13 (0.1–0.18)
Fermented milk products	6	49 (45–77)	65 (65–100)	1.85 (0.32–2.2)	0.2 (0.17–0.37)	1.15 (0.17–1.4)	0.6	3 (3–12.7)	3 (3–12)	ND	1.1	2 (2–2.25)	0.1 (0.1–0.12)
Beverages (non-milk)	12												
Coffee, tea, cocoa, or infusion	8	386.5 (371–548.5)	20 (15.25–30)	3.5 (2.5–16)	1 (1–8)	ND	ND	80 (73.5–81)	72 (61.5–75)	ND	6.5 (4–8.5)	5.5 (4.25–35.25)	0 (0–2.25)
Juice or nectar	2	24	200	ND	ND	ND	ND	5.5	5.2	ND	0.4	0.2	0.025
Soft drinks	2	22.5 (22–22.5)	310	ND	ND	ND	ND	5	5	ND	ND	ND	ND
TOTAL	338												

N = number of products. Values are expressed as median and interquartile range per 100 g or mL. ND = not declared; SFA = saturated fatty acids; MUFA = monounsaturated fatty acids; PUFA = polyunsaturated fatty acids.

Table 2. Vitamin content distribution in folic acid-fortified food products from the Spanish market.

Food Groups and Subgroups	N	A (µg)	D (µg)	E (mg)	K (µg)	C (mg)	B1 (mg)	B2 (mg)	B3 (mg)	B6 (mg)	Folic Acid (µg)	B12 (µg)	Biotin (µg)	Pantothenic Acid (mg)
Grain or grain products	169													
Breakfast cereals	95	ND	0 (0–1)	0 (0–10)	ND	ND	0 (0–1)	1 (1–1)	13 (13–14)	1 (1–1)	170 (166–200)	2 (0–2)	ND	0 (0–5)
Biscuits, sweet and semi-sweet	52	ND	ND	ND	ND	ND	ND	ND	ND	ND	100 (71.5–100)	ND	ND	0 (0–1)
Cereal bars	15	ND	0 (0–2)	0 (0–4)	ND	ND	0 (0–1)	1 (1–1)	13 (11–16)	1 (1–1)	170 (140–200)	2 (0–2)	ND	2 (0–5)
Bread and similar products	5	ND	ND	ND	ND	ND	ND	ND	0 (0–4.5)	0 (0–0.5)	100 (0–100)	ND	ND	0 (0–1.5)
Pastries and cakes	2	ND	ND	ND	ND	ND	ND	ND	10	ND	126	1	ND	ND
Products for special nutritional uses or dietary supplements	105													
Foods for infants	70	375 (101–459)	7.5 (1.7–8.9)	4 (1.3–6.2)	5.8 (0–33)	25 (14–71.5)	0.4 (0.15–0.58)	0.6 (0.11–0.87)	4.5 (1.7–6.95)	0.34 (0.1–0.6)	65 (15–70)	0.5 (0.1–1.18)	12 (1.9–15)	2.8 (0.4–3)
Foods for weight reduction	35	375 (105–467)	2 (1–3)	5 (4–7)	ND	25 (0–36)	0.7 (0.44–0.97)	0.76 (0.37–1.1)	8.4 (5.5–12)	0.9 (0.7–1.2)	120 (76–150)	0.38 (0.7–1.2)	12 (8–33)	1.9 (0.9–3)
Milk, milk products, or milk substitutes	52													
Milk	27	120 (120–120)	0.75 (0.75–0.76)	1.8 (1.5–1.8)	ND	0 (0–4.5)	0 (0–0.085)	0 (0–0.105)	0 (0–0.8)	0 (0–0.105)	30 (30–30)	ND	ND	0 (0–0.45)
Imitation milk products	19	120 (120–120)	0.75 (0.75–0.8)	1.8 (1.5–1.8)	ND	0 (0–12)	0 (0–0.21)	0 (0–0.23)	0 (0–2.4)	0.24 (0.2–0.3)	30 (30–30)	0.38 (0–0.4)	0 (0–4.9)	0 (0–0.8)
Fermented milk products	6	ND	0 (0–0.75)	ND	ND	ND	ND	ND	ND	0.85 (0.2–0.9)	90 (30–145)	0 (0–0.38)	ND	ND
Beverages (non-milk)	12													
Coffee, tea, cocoa, or infusion	8	0 (0–716)	5 (5–7)	0 (0–13.75)	ND	48 (46–78)	1 (0–1)	0 (0–1)	18 (16.25–21)	1.5 (1–2)	199 (190–283)	0 (0–1.5)	ND	3 (1–5.5)
Juice or nectar	2	60 (0–60)	ND	ND	ND	6 (0–6)	ND	ND	1 (0–1)	ND	15 (0–15)	ND	3 (0–3)	ND
Soft drinks	2	ND	ND	ND	ND	ND	ND	ND	ND	ND	15 (0–15)	ND	ND	ND
TOTAL	338													

N = number of products. Values are expressed as median and interquartile range per 100 g or mL. ND = not declared.

Table 3. Mineral content distribution in folic acid-fortified food products from the Spanish market.

Food Groups and Subgroups	N	Sodium (mg)	Potassium (mg)	Calcium (mg)	Phosphorus (mg)	Magnesium (mg)	Iron (mg)	Zinc (mg)	Copper (mg)	Manganese (mg)	Selenium (µg)	Iodine (µg)
Grain or grain products	169											
Breakfast cereals	95	ND	ND	ND	ND	ND	7 (7–8)	ND	ND	ND	ND	ND
Biscuits, sweet and semi-sweet	52	ND	ND	ND	ND	ND	ND	ND	ND	ND	ND	ND
Cereal bars	15	ND	ND	0 (0–760)	ND	ND	7 (0–10)	ND	ND	ND	ND	ND
Bread and similar products	5	400 (0–480)	ND	ND	ND	ND	0 (0–3.5)	ND	ND	ND	ND	ND
Pastries and cakes	2	ND	ND	ND	ND	ND	6	ND	ND	ND	ND	ND
Products for special nutritional uses or dietary supplements	105											
Foods for infants	70	0 (0–139)	0 (0–507.7)	175 (121–372)	59 (0–228)	0 (0–38.2)	6 (2.1–7.5)	0.8 (0–3.8)	0 (0–0.3)	0 (0–0.525)	0 (0–8.95)	12 (0–74.7)
Foods for weight reduction	35	29 (0–91.5)	781 (267.5–1091)	328 (0–436)	367 (0–469)	88 (0–110)	8 (0–10)	5 (0–6)	0 (0–0.65)	0.47 (0–0.8)	28 (0–31.5)	61 (0–86)
Milk, milk products, or milk substitutes	52											
Milk	27	ND	ND	120 (110–160)	0 (0–120)	ND	ND	ND	ND	ND	ND	ND
Imitation milk products	19	ND	ND	120 (105–132)	0 (0–67)	ND	ND	0 (0–1)	ND	ND	ND	ND
Fermented milk products	6	ND	ND	ND	ND	ND	ND	ND	ND	ND	ND	ND
Beverages (non-milk)	12											
Coffee, tea, cocoa, or infusion	8	ND	0 (0–3132)	260 (145.2–1079)	301.5 (0–1091.5)	170 (0–236)	7.5 (0–24)	0 (0–11)	0 (0–0.75)	0 (0–0.75)	0 (0–45)	0 (0–139.5)
Juice or nectar	2	ND	ND	ND	ND	ND	ND	ND	ND	ND	ND	ND
Soft drinks	2	ND	ND	ND	ND	ND	ND	ND	ND	ND	ND	ND
TOTAL	338											

N = number of products. Values are expressed as median and interquartile range per 100 g or mL. ND = not declared.

4. Discussion

To our best knowledge, this is a unique updated food composition data compilation and assessment of FA fortified products available in the Spanish market. The Spanish fortified food supply is widespread through almost all available food groups. However, staple food products such as breads are only fortified to a limited extent when compared to other European countries such as Ireland and the UK, where breads, fat spreads, and fruit juices are commonly fortified [30]. In our country, fat spreads do not have added FA anymore, while only five years ago, up to six products containing FA were available [23]. Although it was not a main aim of our study, a limitation pertaining the use of the label-declared FA values is that we found fortification overages (higher than declared values added to products) in a number of products in previous studies [21]. The use of analytical FA contents from foodstuffs is always advisable, but the present work includes such a high number of products and types of food matrixes, that it would be a highly expensive and unaffordable task to undertake.

In order to assess the potential impact of FA-fortified products on a population's nutritional status, it is also necessary to evaluate if product market availability is in line with the most-consumed products in our country. Although data on fortified food consumption in Spain are scarce, in 2011 a study by the Spanish Nutrition Foundation showed that fortified milks were the most consumed fortified product amongst the population (49.61 g/person/day) followed by fortified yogurt (14.22 g/person/day) [27] by using data of the Food Consumption Panel. Our data indicates that voluntary FA fortification strategies do not follow this trend as fortified 'milk and milk products' are decreasing over time, whilst 'breakfast cereal' availability remains constant.

The main challenges of voluntary food fortification are reaching target populations such as women of childbearing age, which should be the main objective, and avoiding extra FA intakes in non-target groups. In Spain, women of childbearing age are at risk of insufficient folate intakes since only 50% of recommended folate intake is ingested through diet at present [10]. The daily inclusion of fortified products could provide this population group with 20%–60% of FA recommended intake, when fortification level 4 products are consumed [31]. On the other hand, there is concern that population subgroups, including children and the elderly, may be at risk of consuming usual intakes above the UL. In a previous study we assessed the potential intake of the main FA fortified products by children aged 2–13 years and the ULs were exceeded in no case [32]. In addition, the composition of these foodstuffs has also been discussed previously, as a high percentage of them contain high levels of added simple sugars, salt, and fat [33]. According to our results, fortified groups contain between 2–24 g of sugar per 100 g in 'bread and similar products' and 'breakfast cereals'. However, these quantities should be considered on the serving basis, since 'breads' may contain 1.2 g of sugar per 60 g serving and 'breakfast cereals', 7.2 g of sugar per 30 g serving (Table 1). Taking into consideration the World's Health Organization (WHO) and the European Food Safety Authority (EFSA) recommendations to keep simple sugar intake below 10% of daily Total Energy Intake [34], especially amongst the child population, specific fortified food products could be included with moderation in the context of a varied diet. The nutritional benefits of increased vitamin intakes should not be outweighed, however, by the risks according to the present results. Whether voluntary fortification is beneficial depends on which foods manufacturers fortify, which nutrients are chosen as fortificants, how much of the fortificant is added, and what portion of the population consumes the fortified products.

For research purposes, databases must be constantly updated to reflect the rapidly evolving marketplace, so that the contribution of both added and intrinsic micronutrients may provide accurate estimates of population intakes. In 2007, Irish researchers examined the effect of voluntary food fortification on dietary intake and biomarker status of folate and other homocysteine-related B vitamins in a healthy adult population (aged 18–92 years) using an updated FCDB [22]. They found that red blood cell folate concentrations were 387 nmol/L higher and plasma total homocysteine concentrations were 2 μmol/L lower in the group with the highest fortified food intake (median FA intake: 208 μg/day), as compared to the non-consumers of fortified foods, showing a substantial increase in dietary intakes as well as biomarkers of folate status. Regardless the widespread availability of FA fortified products, this type of assessment has not been performed to date in a representative sample of the Spanish population. It would be advisable to have detailed food consumption data at a brand level from the Spanish population in order to evaluate the actual impact of the observed fortification practices with FA. Data is scarce and therefore quantification of the underestimation of FA intake due to the non-consideration of fortified products is still speculative. According to our previous studies, the non-consideration of FA fortification may underestimate as much as 40% of actual folate and folic acid intake in women [31] and children [32]. In the Irish study [22] the difference in total folate and FA intake between consumers and non-consumers of fortified products is above 50%. These observations should be taken into account if the availability of FA fortified food items prevails and may be consumed by a significant number of individuals.

5. Conclusions

This newly updated and representative database reflects the energy and nutrient composition data of FA voluntarily fortified foods from four main categories commercialized in Spain. There is an important number and variety of available products. Our data show a minor decrease in FA fortified products, but vitamin levels added by manufacturers are stable in most food groups and subgroups. It is therefore a unique compilation tool with valuable data for the monitoring and assessment of dietary intakes of this vitamin.

Acknowledgments: This work was funded by the Spanish Ministry of Education and Science, Project AGL2005-06957: "Folic acid content and bioavailability in fortified foods in Spain. Impact on folate intake in population groups at risk and evaluation as potential functional foods".

Author Contributions: All authors conceived and designed the study. Mª de L. Samaniego-Vaesken compiled and analyzed the data, and wrote the manuscript. E. Alonso-Aperte and G. Varela-Moreiras corrected manuscript drafts. All authors have read and approved the final manuscript.

References

1. MRC Vitamin Study Research Group. Prevention of neural tube defects: Results of the Medical Research Council Vitamin Study. *Lancet* **1991**, *338*, 131–137.
2. Obeid, R.; Pietrzik, K.; Oakley, G.P., Jr.; Kancherla, V.; Holzgreve, W.; Wieser, S. Preventable spina bifida and anencephaly in Europe. *Birth Defects Res. Part A Clin. Mol. Teratol.* **2015**, *103*, 763–771. [CrossRef] [PubMed]
3. FFI, Wheat Flour Fortification Status—December 2014. Map of Global Progress. Countries with Mandatory Wheat Flour Fortification Regulations. Flour Fortification Innitiative (FFI). Available online: http://www.ffinetwork.org/global_progress/index.php (accessed on 16 January 2016).
4. European Union. *Regulation (EC) No 1925/2006 of the European Parliament and of the Council of 20 December 2006 on the Addition of Vitamins and Minerals and of Certain Other Substances to Foods*; Official Journal of the European Union 404/26; EU Law and Publications: Luxembourg, 2006.
5. European Union. *Regulation (EU) No 1169/2011 of the European Parliament and of the Council of 25 October 2011 on the provision of food information to consumers, amending Regulations (EC) No 1924/2006 and (EC) No 1925/2006 of the European Parliament and of the Council, and repealing Commission Directive 87/250/EEC, Council Directive 90/496/EEC, Commission Directive 1999/10/EC, Directive 2000/13/EC of the European Parliament and of the Council, Commission Directives 2002/67/EC and 2008/5/EC and Commission Regulation (EC) No 608/2004*; Official Journal of the European Union 22.11.2011; EU Law and Publications: Luxembourg, 2011.
6. Mills, J.L.; Dimopoulos, A. Folic acid fortification for Europe? *Br. Med. J.* **2015**, *351*. [CrossRef] [PubMed]
7. Selhub, J.; Rosenberg, I.H. Excessive folic acid intake and relation to adverse health outcome. *Biochimie* **2016**, *126*, 71–78. [CrossRef] [PubMed]
8. EFSA, ESCO Report Prepared by the EFSA Scientific Cooperation Working Group on Analysis of Risks and Benefits of Fortification of Food with Folic Acid. 2009. Available online: http://www.efsa.europa.eu/fr/supporting/pub/3e.htm (accessed on 17 May 2010).

9.   Informe del Consumo de Alimentación en España 2015. (2015). Ministerio de Agricultura, Alimentación y Medio Ambiente. Available online: http://www.magrama.gob.es/es/alimentacion/temas/consumo-y-comercializacion-y-distribucion-alimentaria/informeconsumoalimentacion2015_tcm7--422694.pdf (accessed on 10 May 2016).

10. Del Pozo, S.; García, V.; Cuadrado, C.; Ruiz, E.; Valero, T.; Ávila J y Varela-Moreiras, G. Valoración Nutricional de la Dieta Española de acuerdo al Panel de Consumo Alimentario. Ministerio de Agricultura, Alimentación y Medio Ambiente. Fundación Española de la Nutrición, 2008. Available online: http://www.fen.org.es/imgPublicaciones/30092012125258.pdf (accessed on 17 May 2013).

11. Bouckaert, K.; Slimani, N.; Nicolas, G.; Vignat, J.; Wright, A.J.; Roe, M.; Witthöft, C.M.; Finglas, P.M. Critical evaluation of folate data in European and international databases: Recommendations for standardization in international nutritional studies. *Mol. Nutr. Food Res.* **2011**, *55*, 166–180. [CrossRef] [PubMed]

12. Nicolas, G.; Witthöft, C.M.; Vignat, J.; Knaze, V.; Huybrechts, I.; Roe, M.; Finglas, P.; Slimani, N. Compilation of a standardised international folate database for EPIC. *Food Chem.* **2016**, *193*, 134–140. [CrossRef] [PubMed]

13. AESAN/BEDCA, Base de Datos Española de Composición de Alimentos v1.0. 2010. Available online: http://www.bedca.net/bdpub/index.php (accessed on 21 September 2015).

14. Westenbrink, S.; Marine, O.; Isabel, C.; Mark, R. Food composition databases: The EuroFIR approach to develop tools to assure the quality of the data compilation process. *Food Chem.* **2009**, *113*, 759–767. [CrossRef]

15. Pfeiffer, C.M.; Sternberg, M.R.; Fazili, Z.; Yetley, E.A.; Lacher, D.A.; Bailey, R.L.; Johnson, C.L. Unmetabolized Folic Acid Is Detected in Nearly All Serum Samples from US Children, Adolescents, and Adults. *J. Nutr.* **2015**. [CrossRef]

16. Vaish, S.; White, M.; Daly, L.; Molloy, A.M.; Staines, A.; Sweeney, M.R. Synthetic folic acid intakes and status in children living in Ireland exposed to voluntary fortification. *Am. J. Clin. Nutr.* **2016**. [CrossRef] [PubMed]

17. Hennessy, Á.; Walton, J.; Flynn, A. The impact of voluntary food fortification on micronutrient intakes and status in European countries: A review. *Proc. Nutr. Soc.* **2013**, *72*, 433–440. [CrossRef] [PubMed]

18. Hennessy, Á.; Hannon, E.M.; Walton, J.; Flynn, A. Impact of voluntary food fortification practices in Ireland: Trends in nutrient intakes in Irish adults between 1997–9 and 2008–10. *Br. J. Nutr.* **2015**, *113*, 310–320. [CrossRef]

19. Dwyer, J.T.; Wiemer, K.L.; Dary, O.; Keen, C.L.; King, J.C.; Miller, K.B.; Philbert, M.A.; Tarasuk, V.; Taylor, C.L.; Gaine, P.C.; et al. Fortification and Health: Challenges and Opportunities. *Adv. Nutr.* **2015**, *6*, 124–131. [CrossRef] [PubMed]

20. Smith, A.D.; Kim, Y.-I.; Refsum, H. Is folic acid good for everyone? *Am. J. Clin. Nutr.* **2008**, *87*, 517–533. [PubMed]

21. Samaniego-Vaesken, M.L.; Alonso-Aperte, E.; Varela-Moreiras, G. Voluntary fortification with folic acid in Spain: An updated food composition database. *Food Chem.* **2016**, *193*, 148–153. [CrossRef] [PubMed]

22. Hoey, L.; McNulty, H.; Askin, N.; Dunne, A.; Ward, M.; Pentieva, K.; Strain, J.; Molloy, A.M.; Flynn, C.A.; Scott, J.M. Effect of a voluntary food fortification policy on folate, related B vitamin status, and homocysteine in healthy adults. *Am. J. Clin. Nutr.* **2007**, *86*, 1405–1413. [PubMed]

23. Samaniego-Vaesken, M.L.; Alonso-Aperte, E.; Varela-Moreiras, G. Folic acid fortified foods available in Spain: Type of products, level of fortification and target population groups. *Nutr. Hosp.* **2009**, *24*, 459–466. [PubMed]

24. Aranceta Bartrina, J.; Serra-Majem, L. Hábitos alimentarios y consumo de alimentos en la población infantil y juvenil española (1998–2000). In *Estudio enKid*; Masson: Barcelona, Spain, 2000.

25. National Toxicology Program. NTP Monograph: Identifying Research Needs for Assessing Safe Use of High Intakes of Folic Acid. 1 August 2015; 51p. Available online: http://ntp.niehs.nih.gov/ntp/ohat/folicacid/final_monograph_508.pdf (accessed on 10 April 2016).

26. Møller, A.; Ireland, J. LanguaL™ 2014—The LanguaL™ Thesaurus. Technical Report. Danish Food Informatics, 2015. Available online: http://www.langual.org/download/LanguaL2014/LanguaL%202014%20Thesaurus%20-%20Final.pdf (accessed on 28 February 2015).

27. Varela-Moreiras, G.; del Pozo, S.; Ávila, J.M.; Cuadrado, C.; Ruiz, E.; Moreiras, O. *Evaluación del Consumo de Alimentos Enriquecidos/Fortificados en España a Través del Panel de Consumo Alimentario*; Fundación Española de la Nutrición (FEN), Ministerio de Medio Ambiente y Medio Rural y Marino (MARM): Madrid, Spain, 2011; Available online: http://www.fen.org.es/storage/app/media/imgPublicaciones/31082011130802.pdf (accessed on 3 March 2017).

28. Alimentación en España 2010. Producción, Industria, Distribución y Consumo. Available online: http: //www.munimerca.es/mercasa/alimentacion_2010/3_info_sectores.html (accessed on 15 May 2011).
29. FAO/INFOODS Guidelines for Checking Food Composition Data prior to the Publication of a User Table/Database—Version 1.0. FAO: Rome, 2012. Available online: http://www.fao.org/fileadmin/ templates/food_composition/documents/Guidelines_data_checking_02.pdf (accessed on 20 January 2016).
30. Kelly, F.; Gibney, E.R.; Boilson, A.; Staines, A.; Sweeney, M.R. Folic acid levels in some food staples in Ireland are on the decline: Implications for passive folic acid intakes? *J. Public Health* **2016**, *38*, 265–269. [CrossRef] [PubMed]
31. Samaniego-Vaesken, M.d.L.; Alonso-Aperte, E.; Varela-Moreiras, G. Contribution of folic acid-fortified foods to fertile women's folate Recommended Nutrient Intake through breakfast simulation models. *Public Health Nutr.* **2015**, *18*, 1960–1968. [CrossRef] [PubMed]
32. Samaniego-Vaesken, M.L.; Alonso-Aperte, E.; Varela-Moreiras, G. Voluntary food fortification with folic acid in Spain: Predicted contribution to children's dietary intakes as assessed with new food folate composition data. *Food Chem.* **2013**, *140*, 526–532. [CrossRef] [PubMed]
33. Rauber, F.; Campagnolo, P.D.; Hoffman, D.J.; Vitolo, M.R. Consumption of ultra-processed food products and its effects on children's lipid profiles: A longitudinal study. *Nutr. Metab. Cardiovasc. Dis.* **2015**, *25*, 116–122. [CrossRef] [PubMed]
34. European Food Safety Authority. Scientific Opinion on Dietary Reference Values for carbohydrates and dietary fibre. EFSA Panel on Dietetic Products, Nutrition, and Allergies (NDA). *EFSA J.* **2010**, *8*, 1462.

7

Vitamin B12 Status among Pregnant Women in the UK and its Association with Obesity and Gestational Diabetes

Nithya Sukumar [1,2], Hema Venkataraman [1], Sean Wilson [3], Ilona Goljan [2], Selvin Selvamoni [2], Vinod Patel [1,2] and Ponnusamy Saravanan [1,2,*]

[1] Warwick Medical School, University of Warwick, Coventry CV2 2DX, UK;
     N.Sukumar@warwick.ac.uk (N.S.); H.Venkataraman@warwick.ac.uk (H.V.);
     Vinod.Patel@warwick.ac.uk (V.P.)
[2] Academic Department of Diabetes, Endocrinology and Metabolism, George Eliot Hospital,
     Nuneaton CV10 7DJ, UK; ilona.goljan@geh.nhs.uk (I.G.); selvamonis@geh.nhs.uk (S.S.)
[3] Hull York Medical School, Hertford Building, University of Hull, Hull HU6 7RX, UK; hysdw3@hyms.ac.uk
*   Correspondence: P.Saravanan@warwick.ac.uk

Abstract: Background: To evaluate vitamin B12 and folate status in pregnancy and their relationship with maternal obesity, gestational diabetes mellitus (GDM), and offspring birthweight. Methods: A retrospective case-control study of 344 women (143 GDM, 201 no-GDM) attending a district general hospital and that had B12 and folate levels measured in the early 3rd trimester was performed. Maternal history including early pregnancy body mass index (BMI) and neonatal data (birthweight, sex, and gestational age) was recorded for all subjects. Results: 26% of the cohort had B12 levels <150 pmol/L (32% vs. 22% in the two groups respectively, $p < 0.05$) while 1.5% were folate deficient. After adjusting for confounders, 1st trimester BMI was negatively associated with 3rd trimester B12 levels. Women with B12 insufficiency had higher odds of obesity and GDM (aOR (95% CI) 2.40 (1.31, 4.40), $p = 0.004$, and 2.59 (1.35, 4.98), $p = 0.004$, respectively), although the latter was partly mediated by BMI. In women without GDM, the lowest quartile of B12 and highest quartile of folate had significantly higher adjusted risk of fetal macrosomia (RR 5.3 (1.26, 21.91), $p = 0.02$ and 4.99 (1.15, 21.62), $p = 0.03$ respectively). Conclusion: This is the first study from the UK to show that maternal B12 levels are associated with BMI, risk of GDM, and additionally may have an independent effect on macrosomia. Due to the increasing burden of maternal obesity and GDM, longitudinal studies with B12 measurements in early pregnancy are needed to explore this link.

Keywords: vitamin B12; gestational diabetes; obesity; macrosomia

---

1. Introduction

The burden of maternal obesity (defined as body mass index (BMI) greater than 30 kg/m^2) is rapidly increasing, affecting nearly 20% of pregnant women in the UK [1]. High BMI is associated with adverse pregnancy outcomes including recurrent miscarriages and maternal deaths [2]. In parallel, the incidence of gestational diabetes mellitus (GDM) has also risen affecting 5%–18% of all pregnancies depending on the diagnostic criteria applied [3,4].

Vitamin B12 (B12) and folate are essential micronutrients required for the synthesis of DNA, protein, and lipids, in a series of cellular reactions collectively known as one-carbon metabolism [5,6]. One step in this process is the conversion of homocysteine (Hcy) to a methyl donor, methionine, for which B12 and folate are necessary cofactors. Additionally, the mitochondrial conversion of methylmalonyl-CoA to succinyl-CoA requires B12 as a coenzyme and in its absence, accumulation of the former compound inhibits fatty acid oxidation, thereby promoting lipogenesis [7,8]. Therefore it can be postulated that low B12, at a cellular level, may be linked to adipocyte dysfunction and obesity-related complications by modulating lipid metabolism, cellular inflammation [9], and causing hypomethylation of cholesterol biosynthesis pathways [10].

A recent systematic review showed that B12 insufficiency among pregnant women across the world was common in all trimesters (20%–30%) [11]. Low B12 during pregnancy has implications for materno-fetal health including maternal adiposity, maternal and offspring insulin resistance [12–14], and adverse lipid profile in neonates [10,15]. The first two observations were replicated in a cohort of women without GDM from South West England [16] but there are no data available on the role of B12 in GDM in the UK.

Low B12 can have an impact on fetal birthweight by influencing placental development [17], although evidence for association with low birthweight (LBW) is equivocal [18–20]. At the other end of the spectrum, maternal obesity and insulin resistance are well-known to be associated with higher fetal birthweight [21,22]. Since B12 may be inversely associated with maternal BMI [12,16], it is possible that B12 is an independent mediator or a confounder for high birthweight.

The primary aim of our study is to investigate the B12 and folate status of pregnant women in the UK and their relationship with obesity and GDM, and secondarily to assess their relationship with fetal birthweight.

2. Methods

A retrospective case-control study of pregnant women attending the antenatal clinic in a district general hospital in the West Midlands, UK, between 2010 and 2013 was conducted. Using the hospital information database which had routine materno-fetal records of all deliveries during this period, we identified women who had a diagnosis of GDM and those who did not (labelled as no-GDM) and had their B12 levels measured in the 2nd or 3rd trimesters of their pregnancies. The no-GDM group consisted predominantly of women attending the medical obstetrics clinic for varying medical conditions. B12 and folate levels were measured routinely for screening for anaemia by the medical obstetric lead (VP), in addition to haemoglobin and ferritin. The physician (PS) running the antenatal-diabetes clinic measured these micronutrient levels for similar reasons in their first visit after the diagnosis of GDM. The following women were excluded from our analysis: pre-gestational diabetes (Type 1 and 2), multiple pregnancies, and those on vitamin B12 supplements at the time of blood sampling.

Clinical information about the women including medical and pregnancy history, smoking status, and BMI at booking was recorded from the database. Fetal outcomes such as birthweight, sex, and gestation were obtained for the secondary outcome analysis. Analysis of glucose was done by a hexokinase enzymatic method in the hospital laboratory and serum B12 and folate by an electrochemiluminescent immunoassay using a Roche Cobas immunoassay analyser (Roche Diagnostics UK, Burgess Hill, UK).

2.1. Definitions

A selective screening approach was used to screen high-risk women for GDM according to the National Institute for Health and Care Excellence (NICE) guidelines [23] (i.e., BMI > 30 kg/m^2, previous GDM, previous macrosomia, first degree relative with diabetes, and ethnic minority race). This consisted of a 2-h 75 g glucose tolerance test (GTT) between 26 and 28 weeks of gestation. The modified World Health Organisation (WHO) 1999 criteria was used to diagnose GDM (fasting glucose $\geq$ 6.1 mmol/L or 2-h glucose $\geq$ 7.8 mmol/L) during the study period. The reference range for serum B12 was 150–489 pmol/L and for serum folate was 7.0–42.4 nmol/L, respectively. Insufficiency of the two micronutrients were defined as <150 pmol/L and <7 nmol/L, respectively [12,16]. Birthweight percentiles and z-scores were calculated using gestational age at delivery and sex-specific reference standards published by the Intergrowth calculator 21st Project [24]. Macrosomia was defined as birthweight > 4000 g, large for gestational age (LGA) as >90th percentile for sex and gestational age, LBW as <2500 g, and small for gestational age (SGA) as <10th percentile for sex and gestational age.

2.2. Statistical Analysis

Based on the pilot data, the required sample size in each group to demonstrate a 15% difference in mean B12 with 90% power and at 5% significance was calculated to be 144. Statistical analysis was performed using SPSS version 22.0 [25]. Since BMI, serum B12, and folate were not normally distributed, they were log-transformed for statistical purposes. For comparison of GDM and no-GDM mothers, the Student's t-test was used for continuous variables (e.g., B12, folate, and BMI) and the Chi-square test for categorical variables. Stepwise multiple linear regression was performed with B12 and folate as the dependent variables with the predictors entered or removed from the model according to the following criteria: Probability-of-F-to-enter ≤ 0.050, Probability-of-F-to-remove ≥ 0.100. Logistic regression was performed to determine the odds of maternal obesity and GDM according to B12/folate insufficiency status and the risk of macrosomia, LGA, LBW, and SGA according to quartiles of B12/folate. The regression models included the following co-variates: age, parity, ethnic origin, smoking, gestation of bloods, BMI, B12, and folate (where appropriate). For macrosomia and LBW, sex and gestational age were additionally added to the models.

Our institution has obtained ethics approval to collect B12 and folate data from pregnant women in an anonymised form (NHS ethics committee reference number 12/LO/0239).

3. Results

Out of approximately 8400 deliveries in the hospital between 2010 and 2013 that were screened, 344 women (143 GDM, 201 no-GDM) who met the inclusion criteria and had B12 levels measured in the 3rd trimester of pregnancy were included. The clinical characteristics of the whole cohort and by GDM status are provided in Table 1. Of the 201 no-GDM women, 45% had GTT as per NICE selective screening criteria [23] and the characteristics of these women are summarised in the Supplementary Materials Table S1.

Table 1. Maternal characteristics according to GDM status.

Variables	Total	GDM	No GDM
Number (%)	344 (100)	143 (41.6)	201 (58.4)
Age (years)	30.3 ± 5.88	31.4 + 5.8	29.6 ± 5.9 **,a
BMI (kg/m^2) §	28.8 ± 7.46	31.7 ± 7.0	26.7 ± 7.1 ***
Obesity (BMI > 30 kg/m^2) (%)	38.0	60.6	22.0 ***
Current smokers (%)	18.7	15.2	19.9
Parity	1.1 ± 1.18	1.2 ± 1.18	1.0 ± 1.18
Ethnicity (%)			
European	86.9	86.0	87.6
South Asian	9.3	11.2	8.0
Afro-Caribbean	1.2	0.7	1.5
Other	1.2	1.4	1.0
Gestation of GTT (weeks) [b]	26.6 ± 3.95	26.4 ± 4.40	26.8 ± 3.10
Mean fasting glucose (mmol/L) §	4.9 ± 1.01	5.2 ± 1.15	4.4 ± 0.39 ***
Mean 2 h glucose (mmol/L) §	7.5 ± 1.94	8.7 ± 1.26	5.6 ± 1.13 ***
Gestation of B12 bloods (weeks)	26.9 ± 5.3	28.0 ± 4.3	26.2 + 5.7 **
Vitamin B12 (pmol/L) §	187.5 (146.9, 235.4)	169.0 (140.2, 217.7)	195.6 (157.9, 244.6) **
Vitamin B12 deficiency (<150 pmol/L), n (%)	90 (26.2)	46 (32.2)	44 (21.9) *
Serum folate (nmol/L) §	21.3 (14.0, 34.4)	21.5 (13.5, 34.5)	20.8 (14.5, 34.4)
Serum folate deficiency (<7 nmol/L), n (%)	5 (1.5)	3 (2.1)	2 (1.0)
Folic acid supplements taken (%)	91.4	90.9	91.5

Continuous variables are mean ± SD (or median (IQR)), categorical variables are percentages; [a] p-value as compared to the GDM group, * $p < 0.05$, ** $p < 0.01$, *** $p < 0.001$; [b] GTT results available in 90/201 (44.8%) of no-GDM women; § Log-transformed for statistical comparison, GDM: gestational diabetes mellitus, BMI: body mass index, GTT: glucose tolerance test.

For the whole cohort, the mean gestation of serum vitamin B12 and folate measurements was at 26.9 weeks and GTT was at 26.6 weeks. B12 levels were lower in women with GDM (169.0 vs. 195.6 pmol/L, $p < 0.001$) and a significantly higher proportion of women with GDM had B12 insufficiency compared to non-GDM (Table 1). Folate deficiency was rare and 91% of the whole cohort was taking folate supplements. Serum folate levels were not different in the two groups.

3.1. Vitamin B12, Folate Status, Maternal BMI, and GDM

Women with B12 insufficiency had higher 1st trimester BMI than those without (30.9 ± 7.56 vs. 28.0 ± 7.30 kg/m², $p < 0.05$). After adjusting for age, parity, ethnicity, smoking status, and gestation of blood tests, BMI was a significant negative predictor of B12 (β coefficient −0.21; 95% CI: −0.47, −0.13; $p = 0.001$) whilst serum folate showed a positive association with B12 (Table 2, Figure 1). BMI was also negatively associated with serum folate after adjustment although the strength of association was weaker (β coefficient −0.12; 95% CI: 0.00, 0.33; $p = 0.05$). Third trimester vitamin B12 insufficiency was additionally associated with a 2.4 times higher odds of first trimester obesity (Table 3).

Table 2. Predictors of vitamin B12 and folate.

Variables	Serum B12 §		Serum Folate §	
	β-Coefficient	p-Value	β-Coefficient	p-Value
Age	-	NS	0.32	<0.001
Parity	-	NS	−0.24	<0.001
BMI §	−0.21	0.001	−0.12	0.05
Ethnicity	-	NS	-	NS
Smoking	-	NS	-	NS
Gestation of B12/folate bloods	-	NS	−0.28	<0.001
Serum B12 §			0.12	0.05
Serum folate §	0.23	<0.001		
Folic acid supplements	-	NS	-	NS

§ Log-transformed for statistical calculations; NS: non-significant.

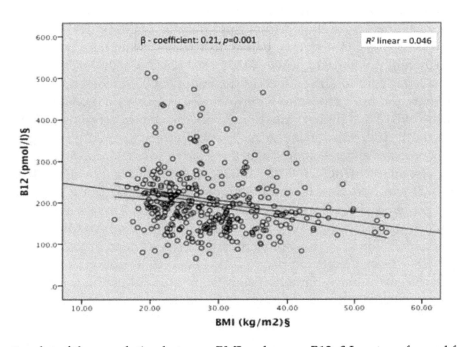

Figure 1. Scatterplot of the correlation between BMI and serum B12. § Log-transformed for statistical comparisons; Regression model included age, parity, ethnicity, smoking, gestation of bloods, folic acid supplements, and serum folate.

Table 3. Relationship of maternal B12 and folate with obesity and gestational diabetes.

	n (%)	Obesity, *n* (%)	GDM, *n* (%)
Vitamin B12 deficiency			
Yes	90	44 (49.4)	46 (51.1)
No	254	86 (34.0)	97 (38.2)
Model 1 OR (95% CI) [a]		2.40 (1.31, 4.40)	2.59 (1.35, 4.98)
adjusted *p*		0.004	0.004
Model 2 OR (95% CI) [b]		N/A	2.05 (1.03, 4.10)
adjusted *p*		N/A	0.042
Folate deficiency			
Yes	5	4 (80.0)	3 (60.0)
No	332	125 (37.9)	139 (41.9)
Model 1 OR (95% CI) [a]		6.29 (0.48, 82.79)	1.93 (0.17, 22.23)
adjusted *p*		NS	NS
Model 2 OR (95% CI) [b]		N/A	0.89 (0.07, 11.38)
adjusted *p*		N/A	NS

Table showing the proportions and odds ratio of obesity and development of GDM according to the thresholds of B12 and folate (reference categories are 'No B12/folate deficiency'); [a] Model 1 adjusted for age, parity, ethnic origin, smoking, gestation of bloods, and serum folate (or B12, respectively); [b] as for Model 1 plus gestational BMI; N/A: not applicable; NS: non-significant.

B12 deficient women were at 2.59-times higher odds of having a diagnosis of GDM after adjusting for age, parity, ethnic origin, smoking, gestation of bloods, and serum folate (Table 3). The effect size was weaker when maternal BMI was added into the model (aOR 2.05, $p = 0.04$). Folate deficiency was not significantly associated with a risk of GDM. There was also no association seen between folate thresholds and obesity.

3.2. Vitamin B12, Folate, and Birth Outcomes

Birth outcome data were available in 335 women (97% of total cohort) and one baby born at less than 32 weeks gestation was excluded from this analysis. 54.5% of the babies were male and the mean birthweight was 3353 g. GDM women delivered 10 days earlier than no-GDM women and their mean offspring birthweight was 180 g lower (3250 vs. 3428 g, $p < 0.01$) (Supplementary Materials Table S2). Due to the likely confounding effects of treatment in GDM women, the relationship between maternal B12 and folate and birth outcomes were analysed only in no-GDM women (Table 4). Women in the lowest quartile of B12 had higher rates of macrosomic babies compared to the highest quartile (22.9% vs. 8.0%) (Table 4). After adjustment for age, parity, ethnicity, smoking, serum folate, gestation of B12 bloods, and newborn sex and gestational age, the relative risk (RR) of fetal macrosomia was higher in women in the lowest quartile (RR 5.26, 95% CI: 1.26, 21.91, $p = 0.02$). The significance was attenuated when gestational BMI was added to the model (Table 4). A similar trend for the risk of LGA was observed although the result did not reach statistical significance. There was no association between B12 thresholds and the outcomes of LBW or SGA. The impact of serum folate on fetal macrosomia showed the reverse pattern for all of these outcome measures. Women in the highest quartile of folate had significantly higher risk of fetal macrosomia compared to those in the lowest quartile (RR 4.99, 95% CI: 1.15, 21.62, $p = 0.03$), which remained significant after adjusting for maternal BMI (RR 6.60, 95% CI: 1.42, 30.71, $p = 0.02$) (Table 4).

Table 4. Relationship between maternal B12 on birth outcome measures in no-GDM women.

	n	Range of Values (pmol/L)	Macrosomia, n (%)	LGA, n (%)	LBW, n (%)	SGA, n (%)
Vitamin B12 (quartiles)						
1	48	71.6, 157.2	11 (22.9)	12 (25.0)	1 (2.1)	4 (8.3)
2	48	158.7, 195.6	10 (20.8)	12 (25.0)	2 (4.2)	2 (4.2)
3	47	196.3, 244.3	9 (19.1)	10 (21.3)	3 (6.4)	3 (6.4)
4	50	245.0, 512.2	4 (8.0)	5 (10.0)	3 (6.0)	5 (10.0)
Relative risk (95% CI) [a]			5.26 (1.26, 21.91)	3.18 (0.96, 10.56)	0.10 (0.002, 5.75)	1.35 (0.28, 6.47)
p [b]			0.02	0.06	0.27	0.71
p [c]			0.05	0.13	0.37	0.52
Folate (quartiles)						
1	44	4.5, 14.3	5 (11.4)	7 (15.9)	4 (9.1)	4 (9.1)
2	47	14.5, 20.6	7 (14.9)	9 (19.1)	1 (2.1)	2 (4.3)
3	48	20.8, 34.2	11 (22.9)	10 (20.8)	1 (2.1)	3 (6.3)
4	48	34.4, 45.3	10 (20.8)	12 (25.0)	3 (6.3)	5 (10.4)
Relative risk (95% CI) [a]			4.99 (1.15, 21.62)	2.32 (0.74, 7.34)	0.21 (0.01, 9.64)	1.52 (0.26, 8.93)
p [b]			0.03	0.15	0.42	0.64
p [c]			0.02	0.06	0.41	0.90

[a] Relative risk of birthweight outcome in quartile 1 vs. quartile 4 of B12 and quartile 4 vs. quartile 1 of folate; [b] adjusted for age, parity, ethnic origin, smoking, gestation of bloods, and serum folate (or B12, respectively), plus sex and gestational age for macrosomia and LBW; [c] as for Model b plus gestational BMI; LGA: large for gestational age; LBW: low birthweight; SGA: small for gestational age.

4. Discussion

Our study, although retrospective in nature, showed three key findings. Firstly, it is the first study to show that low B12 status in pregnancy is associated with a higher risk of GDM in a UK population. Secondly, higher first trimester BMI was an independent predictor of later B12 insufficiency. Thirdly, low B12 levels were associated with macrosomia in the subgroup of no-GDM women, which seems to be partly mediated by maternal BMI.

The only other study that examined the link between B12 and GDM by Krishnaveni et al. was in an Indian cohort [12]. The magnitude of association found in that study was similar to ours, but the significance was lost after adjusting for maternal BMI. In our study, although the effect size was reduced when adjusted for BMI (aOR 2.59 vs. 2.05; Table 3), the significance persisted, suggesting a potential independent effect of B12. Higher numbers of women with GDM in our cohort and a 'case-control' design might explain the larger effect size. The recent finding by Knight et al., albeit in no-GDM women, also supports the inverse link between B12 levels and insulin resistance in pregnant White Caucasian women [16]. Indeed, higher insulin resistance in the context of low B12 has been shown by other authors in obese adolescents [26], non-pregnant adults [27,28], as well as in women with polycystic ovarian syndrome [28]. Prospective longitudinal studies are needed to investigate whether the presence of low B12 status in early pregnancy independently increases the risk of incident GDM.

The aetiology of the inverse relationship between B12 and BMI found in our study is an intriguing one. While confounding factors such as dietary habits, socioeconomic status, and hemodilution may be present, other studies that have corrected for these still show an independent link between B12 and BMI [12,16]. Interestingly, the frying and roasting of meat products reduces the bioavailability of B12 by 20%–40% [29], so higher consumption of processed foods may increase the risk of both B12 insufficiency and metabolic diseases. Additionally, B12 has been shown to be negatively associated with other markers of obesity such as triglycerides [7], blood pressure [30], and the metabolic syndrome [31], which lends support to a possible pathological association between them. In one trial, the supplementation of B12 and folate in adults with metabolic syndrome improved insulin resistance by ameliorating endothelial dysfunction, providing further insight into how these conditions may be linked [32]. Further studies are needed to determine the direction of association and a potential reverse causality.

This is the first study that has demonstrated a relationship between maternal B12 and macrosomia, which seem to be mediated in part by maternal obesity. We demonstrated this only in no-GDM women as the treatment of GDM is a major confounder for macrosomia. Unfortunately, we did not have adiposity measures or a bigger sample size to assess the interactions between B12 status and maternal BMI/adiposity with offspring size and adiposity.

The rates of B12 insufficiency observed in our no-GDM population was similar to that observed by Knight et al. [16] (22% vs. 20%), suggesting that such higher rates of insufficiency are not limited to Indian populations [11]. It must be noted that a fall in B12 during pregnancy may be physiological due to a decrease in the fraction bound to inactive haptocorrin [33], but the evidence is equivocal with regards to whether there is also a fall in the active form, holotranscobalamin [34,35]. In the absence of specific cut-off values to define B12 deficiency in pregnancy, we used the non-pregnant reference range (<150 pmmol/L). It is noteworthy that associations with adverse maternal metabolic outcomes [12] and elevation in Hcy during pregnancy [36] were found by other authors at B12 thresholds similar to this.

It was reassuring to see that folate deficiency was rare, albeit in this selected hospital-based cohort. However, the combination of low B12 and high folate has been shown to be associated with lower neonatal birthweight [37] as well as central adiposity and insulin resistance in 6-year old offspring [14]. Whilst our sample size was not large enough to perform a detailed subgroup analysis, we observed that women in the lowest quartile of B12 and highest quartile of folate had similar risks of macrosomia (aRR of 5.3 and 4.99; Table 4). Therefore, it is possible that the women with such a B12-folate imbalance are particularly at high risk of having larger babies. This phenomenon (high folate/low B12), is increasingly common in populations with mandatory folic acid fortification such as in the USA and Canada [38,39], and is related to adverse clinical outcomes in the elderly population [40].

Although we have identified associations between B12, maternal obesity, risk of GDM, and fetal macrosomia, our study does not prove causation or the direction of the relationship between these factors. Some of the important limitations were that this was a single-centre, retrospective study involving pregnant women attending a hospital clinic. Therefore it was not possible to obtain early pregnancy B12/folate levels. We adjusted for the gestation of bloods in all the regression analyses, to reduce some of the bias due to longitudinal changes in B12 during pregnancy. We did not have markers of adiposity, and therefore it was not possible to study the potential differential association of low B12 status with obesity and adiposity in pregnant women as well as their offspring. Lack of functional measures of B12 insufficiency, such as Hcy and methylmalonic acid (MMA), or holotranscobalamin, which is the active fraction of B12 available for uptake by tissues, limits the ability to study the thresholds of B12 sufficiency during pregnancy and should be measured in future studies.

5. Conclusions

We have shown for the first time in a UK population that B12 deficiency in pregnancy is common particularly in obese women, is independently associated with GDM, and may contribute to macrosomia. As the prevalence of maternal obesity and GDM is rapidly increasing, our findings warrant longitudinal cohort studies to understand the interplay between B12 and these outcomes. If early pregnancy B12 status is found to be independently predictive of incident GDM, such findings could potentially offer simple interventions to improve the metabolic health of pregnant women and their offspring.

Acknowledgments: The authors would like to acknowledge Paul Rushton (IT Site coordinator and Information Manager, Pathology, George Eliot Hospital) and Sonia Hayre (Maternity Data Clerk, George Eliot Hospital) who helped with collating the anonymous data from routinely collected maternity records.

Author Contributions: V.P. and P.S. conceptualised the study and reviewed the manuscript for intellectual content; N.S. collected the data, performed the statistical analysis, and wrote the manuscript; H.V., S.W., I.G. and S.S. contributed to data collection. All authors approved the final manuscript as submitted. P.S. is the guarantor of this work and had full access to all the data presented in the study and takes full responsibility for the integrity and the accuracy of the data analysis.

References

1. Heslehurst, N.; Rankin, J.; Wilkinson, J.R.; Summerbell, C.D. A nationally representative study of maternal obesity in England, UK: Trends in incidence and demographic inequalities in 619,323 births, 1989–2007. *Int. J. Obes. (Lond.)* **2010**, *34*, 420–428. [CrossRef] [PubMed]

2. Lewis, G. The Confidential Enquiry into Maternal and Child Health (CEMACH). In *Saving Mothers' Lives: Reviewing Maternal Deaths to Make Motherhood Safer—2003–2005. The Seventh Report on Confidential Enquiries into Maternal Deaths in the United Kingdom*; CEMACH: London, UK, 2007.

3. Buckley, B.S.; Harreiter, J.; Damm, P.; Corcoy, R.; Chico, A.; Simmons, D.; Vellinga, A.; Dunne, F.; DALI Core Investigator Group. Gestational diabetes mellitus in Europe: Prevalence, current screening practice and barriers to screening. A review. *Diabet. Med.* **2012**, *29*, 844–854. [CrossRef] [PubMed]

4. Cundy, T.; Ackermann, E.; Ryan, E.A. Gestational diabetes: New criteria may triple the prevalence but effect on outcomes is unclear. *BMJ* **2014**, *348*, g1567. [CrossRef] [PubMed]

5. Saravanan, P.; Yajnik, C.S. Role of maternal vitamin B12 on the metabolic health of the offspring: A contributor to the diabetes epidemic? *Br. J. Diabetes Vasc. Dis.* **2010**, *10*, 109–114. [CrossRef]

6. Finer, S.; Saravanan, P.; Hitman, G.; Yajnik, C. The role of the one-carbon cycle in the developmental origins of type 2 diabetes and obesity. *Diabet. Med.* **2014**, *31*, 263–272. [CrossRef] [PubMed]

7. Adaikalakoteswari, A.; Jayashri, R.; Sukumar, N.; Venkataraman, H.; Pradeepa, R.; Gokulakrishnan, K.; Anjana, R.M.; McTernan, P.G.; Tripathi, G.; Patel, V.; et al. Vitamin B12 deficiency is associated with adverse lipid profile in Europeans and Indians with type 2 diabetes. *Cardiovasc. Diabetol.* **2014**, *13*, 129. [CrossRef] [PubMed]

8. Brindle, N.P.; Zammit, V.A.; Pogson, C.I. Regulation of carnitine palmitoyltransferase activity by malonyl-CoA in mitochondria from sheep liver, a tissue with a low capacity for fatty acid synthesis. *Biochem. J.* **1985**, *232*, 177–182. [CrossRef] [PubMed]

9. Kumar, K.A.; Lalitha, A.; Pavithra, D.; Padmavathi, I.J.; Ganeshan, M.; Rao, K.R.; Venu, L.; Balakrishna, N.; Shanker, N.H.; Reddy, S.U.; et al. Maternal dietary folate and/or vitamin B12 restrictions alter body composition (adiposity) and lipid metabolism in wistar rat offspring. *J. Nutr. Biochem.* **2013**, *24*, 25–31. [CrossRef] [PubMed]

10. Adaikalakoteswari, A.; Finer, S.; Voyias, P.D.; McCarthy, C.M.; Vatish, M.; Moore, J.; Smart-Halajko, M.; Bawazeer, N.; Al-Daghri, N.M.; McTernan, P.G.; et al. Vitamin B12 insufficiency induces cholesterol biosynthesis by limiting s-adenosylmethionine and modulating the methylation of SREBF1 and LDLR genes. *Clin. Epigenet.* **2015**, *7*, 14. [CrossRef] [PubMed]

11. Sukumar, N.; Rafnsson, S.B.; Kandala, N.B.; Bhopal, R.; Yajnik, C.S.; Saravanan, P. Prevalence of vitamin B-12 insufficiency during pregnancy and its effect on offspring birth weight: A systematic review and meta-analysis. *Am. J. Clin. Nutr.* **2016**, *103*, 1232–1251. [CrossRef] [PubMed]

12. Krishnaveni, G.V.; Hill, J.C.; Veena, S.R.; Bhat, D.S.; Wills, A.K.; Karat, C.L.; Yajnik, C.S.; Fall, C.H. Low plasma vitamin B12 in pregnancy is associated with gestational 'diabesity' and later diabetes. *Diabetologia* **2009**, *52*, 2350–2358. [CrossRef] [PubMed]

13. Stewart, C.P.; Christian, P.; Schulze, K.J.; Arguello, M.; LeClerq, S.C.; Khatry, S.K.; West, K.P., Jr. Low maternal vitamin B-12 status is associated with offspring insulin resistance regardless of antenatal micronutrient supplementation in rural Nepal. *J. Nutr.* **2011**, *141*, 1912–1917. [CrossRef] [PubMed]

14. Yajnik, C.S.; Deshpande, S.S.; Jackson, A.A.; Refsum, H.; Rao, S.; Fisher, D.J.; Bhat, D.S.; Naik, S.S.; Coyaji, K.J.; Joglekar, C.V.; et al. Vitamin B12 and folate concentrations during pregnancy and insulin resistance in the offspring: The pune maternal nutrition study. *Diabetologia* **2008** *51*, 29–38. [CrossRef] [PubMed]

15. Adaikalakoteswari, A.; Vatish, M.; Lawson, A.; Wood, C.; Sivakumar, K.; McTernan, P.G.; Webster, C.; Anderson, N.; Yajnik, C.S.; Tripathi, G.; et al. Low maternal vitamin B12 status is associated with lower cord blood HDL cholesterol in white caucasians living in the UK. *Nutrients* **2015**, *7*, 2401–2414. [CrossRef] [PubMed]

16. Knight, B.A.; Shields, B.M.; Brook, A.; Hill, A.; Bhat, D.S.; Hattersley, A.T.; Yajnik, C.S. Lower circulating B12 is associated with higher obesity and insulin resistance during pregnancy in a non-diabetic white British population. *PLoS ONE* **2015**, *10*, e0135268. [CrossRef] [PubMed]

17. Koukoura, O.; Sifakis, S.; Spandidos, D.A. DNA methylation in the human placenta and fetal growth (review). *Mol. Med. Rep.* **2012**, *5*, 883–889. [PubMed]

18. Hogeveen, M.; Blom, H.J.; van der Heijden, E.H.; Semmekrot, B.A.; Sporken, J.M.; Ueland, P.M.; den Heijer, M. Maternal homocysteine and related B vitamins as risk factors for low birthweight. *Am. J. Obstet. Gynecol.* **2010**, *202*, 572. [CrossRef] [PubMed]

19. Muthayya, S.; Kurpad, A.V.; Duggan, C.P.; Bosch, R.J.; Dwarkanath, P.; Mhaskar, A.; Mhaskar, R.; Thomas, A.; Vaz, M.; Bhat, S.; et al. Low maternal vitamin B12 status is associated with intrauterine growth retardation in urban south Indians. *Eur. J. Clin. Nutr.* **2006**, *60*, 791–801. [CrossRef] [PubMed]

20. Sukumar, N.; Adaikalakoteswari, A.; Venkataraman, H.; Maheswaran, H.; Saravanan, P. Vitamin B12 status in women of childbearing age in the UK and its relationship with national nutrient intake guidelines: Results from two national diet and nutrition surveys. *BMJ Open* **2016**, *6*, e011247. [CrossRef] [PubMed]

21. Gaudet, L.; Ferraro, Z.M.; Wen, S.W.; Walker, M. Maternal obesity and occurrence of fetal macrosomia: A systematic review and meta-analysis. *BioMed Res. Int.* **2014**, *2014*, 640291. [CrossRef] [PubMed]

22. He, X.J.; Qin, F.Y.; Hu, C.L.; Zhu, M.; Tian, C.Q.; Li, L. Is gestational diabetes mellitus an independent risk factor for macrosomia: A meta-analysis? *Arch. Gynecol. Obstet.* **2015**, *291*, 729–735. [CrossRef] [PubMed]

23. National Institute for Health and Care Excellence. Diabetes in pregnancy: Management of diabetes and its complications from pre-conception to the postnatal period. In *NICE Clinical Guideline 63*; National Institute for Health and Care Excellence: Manchester, UK, 2008; pp. 1–42.

24. Villar, J.; Cheikh Ismail, L.; Victora, C.G.; Ohuma, E.O.; Bertino, E.; Altman, D.G.; Lambert, A.; Papageorghiou, A.T.; Carvalho, M.; Jaffer, Y.A.; et al. International standards for newborn weight, length, and head circumference by gestational age and sex: The newborn cross-sectional study of the intergrowth-21st project. *Lancet* **2014**, *384*, 857–868. [CrossRef]

25. IBM Corp. *IBM Spss Statistics for Windows*, version 22.0; IBM Corp: Armonk, NY, USA, 2013.

26. Ho, M.; Halim, J.H.; Gow, M.L.; El-Haddad, N.; Marzulli, T.; Baur, L.A.; Cowell, C.T.; Garnett, S.P. Vitamin B12 in obese adolescents with clinical features of insulin resistance. *Nutrients* **2014**, *6*, 5611–5618. [CrossRef] [PubMed]

27. Baltaci, D.; Kutlucan, A.; Turker, Y.; Yilmaz, A.; Karacam, S.; Deler, H.; Ucgun, T.; Kara, I.H. Association of vitamin B12 with obesity, overweight, insulin resistance and metabolic syndrome, and body fat composition; primary care-based study. *Med. Glas. (Zenica)* **2013**, *10*, 203–210. [PubMed]

28. Kaya, C.; Cengiz, S.D.; Satiroglu, H. Obesity and insulin resistance associated with lower plasma vitamin B12 in PCOS. *Reprod. Biomed. Online* **2009**, *19*, 721–726. [CrossRef] [PubMed]

29. United States Department of Agriculture. USDA Table of Nutrient Retention Factors, Release 6. Available online: https://www.ars.usda.gov/ARSUserFiles/80400525/Data/retn/retn06.pdf (accessed on 5 November 2016).

30. Karatela, R.A.; Sainani, G.S. Plasma homocysteine in obese, overweight and normal weight hypertensives and normotensives. *Indian Heart J.* **2009**, *61*, 156–159. [PubMed]

31. Guven, A.; Inanc, F.; Kilinc, M.; Ekerbicer, H. Plasma homocysteine and lipoprotein (a) levels in Turkish patients with metabolic syndrome. *Heart Vessels* **2005**, *20*, 290–295. [CrossRef] [PubMed]

32. Setola, E.; Monti, L.D.; Galluccio, E.; Palloshi, A.; Fragasso, G.; Paroni, R.; Magni, F.; Sandoli, E.P.; Lucotti, P.; Costa, S.; et al. Insulin resistance and endothelial function are improved after folate and vitamin B12 therapy in patients with metabolic syndrome: Relationship between homocysteine levels and hyperinsulinemia. *Eur. J. Endocrinol.* **2004**, *151*, 483–489. [CrossRef] [PubMed]

33. Koebnick, C.; Heins, U.A.; Dagnelie, P.C.; Wickramasinghe, S.N.; Ratnayaka, I.D.; Hothorn, T.; Pfahlberg, A.B.; Hoffmann, I.; Lindemans, J.; Leitzmann, C. Longitudinal concentrations of vitamin B(12) and vitamin B(12)-binding proteins during uncomplicated pregnancy. *Clin. Chem.* **2002**, *48*, 928–933. [PubMed]

34. Greibe, E.; Andreasen, B.H.; Lildballe, D.L.; Morkbak, A.L.; Hvas, A.M.; Nexo, E. Uptake of cobalamin and

markers of cobalamin status: A longitudinal study of healthy pregnant women. *Clin. Chem. Lab. Med.* **2011**, *49*, 1877–1882. [CrossRef] [PubMed]

35.   Murphy, M.M.; Molloy, A.M.; Ueland, P.M.; Fernandez-Ballart, J.D.; Schneede, J.; Arija, V.; Scott, J.M. Longitudinal study of the effect of pregnancy on maternal and fetal cobalamin status in healthy women and their offspring. *J. Nutr.* **2007**, *137*, 1863–1867. [PubMed]

36.   Guerra-Shinohara, E.M.; Morita, O.E.; Peres, S.; Pagliusi, R.A.; Neto, L.F.S.; D'Almeida, V.; Irazusta, S.P.; Allen, R.H.; Stabler, S.P. Low ratio of *S*-adenosylmethionine to *S*-adenosylhomocysteine is associated with vitamin deficiency in Brazilian pregnant women and newborns. *Am. J. Clin. Nutr.* **2004**, *80*, 1312–1322. [PubMed]

37.   Gadgil, M.; Joshi, K.; Pandit, A.; Otiv, S.; Joshi, R.; Brenna, J.T.; Patwardhan, B. Imbalance of folic acid and vitamin B12 is associated with birth outcome: An Indian pregnant women study. *Eur. J. Clin. Nutr.* **2014**, *68*, 726–729. [CrossRef] [PubMed]

38.   Ray, J.G.; Vermeulen, M.J.; Langman, L.J.; Boss, S.C.; Cole, D.E. Persistence of vitamin B12 insufficiency among elderly women after folic acid food fortification. *Clin. Biochem.* **2003**, *36*, 387–391. [CrossRef]

39.   Wyckoff, K.F.; Ganji, V. Proportion of individuals with low serum vitamin B-12 concentrations without macrocytosis is higher in the post folic acid fortification period than in the pre folic acid fortification period. *Am. J. Clin. Nutr.* **2007**, *86*, 1187–1192. [PubMed]

40.   Morris, M.S.; Jacques, P.F.; Rosenberg, I.H.; Selhub, J. Folate and vitamin B-12 status in relation to anemia, macrocytosis, and cognitive impairment in older Americans in the age of folic acid fortification. *Am. J. Clin. Nutr.* **2007**, *85*, 193–200. [PubMed]

8

Prevalence and Predictors of Low Vitamin B6 Status in Healthy Young Adult Women in Metro Vancouver

Chia-ling Ho [1,2], Teo A. W. Quay [1,2,†], Angela M. Devlin [2,3] and Yvonne Lamers [1,2,4,*]

[1] Food Nutrition and Health, Faculty of Land and Food Systems, The University of British Columbia, 2205 East Mall, Vancouver, BC V6T 1Z4, Canada; jennifer.ho@ubc.ca (C.-L.H.); quayt@mail.ubc.ca (T.A.W.Q.)
[2] Research Institute, British Columbia Children's Hospital, 950 West 28th Ave, Vancouver, BC V5Z 4H4, Canada; adevlin@cfri.ubc.ca
[3] Department of Pediatrics, The University of British Columbia, 4480 Oak Street, Vancouver, BC V6H 3V4, Canada
[4] Fraser Health Authority, 10334 152A St, Surrey, BC V3R 7P8, Canada
[*] Correspondence: yvonne.lamers@ubc.ca
[†] Currently affiliated with Canadian Agency for Drugs and Technologies in Health, 865 Carling Ave, Ottawa, ON K1S 5S8, Canada

Abstract: Low periconceptional vitamin B6 (B6) status has been associated with an increased risk of preterm birth and early pregnancy loss. Given many pregnancies are unplanned; it is important for women to maintain an adequate B6 status throughout reproductive years. There is limited data on B6 status in Canadian women. This study aimed to assess the prevalence of B6 deficiency and predictors of B6 status in young adult women in Metro Vancouver. We included a convenience sample of young adult non-pregnant women (19–35 years; $n = 202$). Vitamin B6 status was determined using fasting plasma concentrations of pyridoxal 5'-phosphate (PLP). Mean (95% confidence interval) plasma PLP concentration was 61.0 (55.2, 67.3) nmol/L. The prevalence of B6 deficiency (plasma PLP < 20 nmol/L) was 1.5% and that of suboptimal B6 status (plasma PLP = 20–30 nmol/L) was 10.9%. Body mass index, South Asian ethnicity, relative dietary B6 intake, and the use of supplemental B6 were significant predictors of plasma PLP. The combined 12.4% prevalence of B6 deficiency and suboptimal status was lower than data reported in US populations and might be due to the high socioeconomic status of our sample. More research is warranted to determine B6 status in the general Canadian population.

Keywords: vitamin B6; pyridoxal 5'-phosphate; suboptimal status; deficiency; ethnicity; dietary intake; supplement use; women; periconceptional

1. Introduction

Vitamin B6 (B6) has an obligatory role in the endocrine system, immune competence, and heme biosynthesis. In the form of pyridoxal 5'-phosphate (PLP), B6 serves as a coenzyme for >140 reactions in human metabolism, including in the interconversion of amino acids, synthesis of neurotransmitters, regulation of energy homeostasis, and formation of heme [1]. In one-carbon metabolism, PLP acts as a coenzyme for the glycine cleavage system, the interconversion of glycine and serine, and the transsulfuration pathway [2,3]. Other coenzyme functions of PLP include reactions in the kynurenine pathway that catabolizes tryptophan [4].

Maternal B6 adequacy is crucial at conception and throughout pregnancy to ensure healthy pregnancy outcomes. In a meta-analysis of maternal B6 interventions ($n = 247$), maternal B6 supplementation (2.6 to ≥ 50 mg/day) was associated with a 217 g higher infant birth weight [5]. A lower incidence of preeclampsia was reported in women supplementing with 10 mg/day of

B6 during pregnancy compared to those who did not use supplements [6]. Low maternal B6 status has been associated with a lower Apgar score, an indicator of infant birth health assessed within minutes after delivery [7,8]. In a prospective cohort of 458 young Chinese women, women who experienced an early pregnancy loss had significantly lower periconceptional plasma PLP concentration compared to women with a healthy pregnancy outcome [9]. Also, low periconceptional B6 status (plasma PLP < 30 nmol/L) has been associated with a reduced probability of conception [10]. Given an estimated 50% of pregnancies are unplanned [11], it is important for women to maintain an adequate B6 status throughout reproductive years.

Despite the crucial role of B6 in health, there is no nationally representative data on biochemical B6 status of Canadian women. The Canadian Community Health Survey (CCHS), Cycle 2.2, Nutrition Focus, in 2004 reported that 18% of Canadian adult women did not meet the Estimated Average Requirement (EAR; 1.1 mg/day) of B6 from dietary sources; however, there was no biochemical measurement of B6 status [12]. In the US National Health and Nutrition Examination Survey (NHANES), over 40% of young adult women (21–44 years) had B6 deficiency (defined as having plasma PLP concentration < 20 nmol/L; [13]). In light of these findings, there is an urgent need to investigate the B6 status of Canadian women.

In several other countries (US, Ireland, Norway), various socioeconomic and lifestyle factors have been associated with plasma PLP concentrations, including oral contraceptive use [13], use of supplemental B6 [13,14], smoking [15,16], physical inactivity, and poverty [17]. Finding predictors of low B6 status in a Canadian population will contribute to the identification of vulnerable populations groups for low B6 status and related health consequences in Canada.

This study aimed to determine the prevalence of suboptimal B6 status and B6 deficiency in a convenience sample of young adult women in Metro Vancouver, using plasma PLP, a biochemical marker of B6 status. Demographic, dietary, and lifestyle predictors associated with plasma PLP were also assessed.

2. Experimental Section

2.1. Participants

This study used data from a descriptive cross-sectional study conducted between 2012 and 2013. The original study was designed to determine the prevalence and predictors of low vitamin B12 status in a convenience sample of young adult women of South Asian and European descent. The recruitment and methods of the original study have been described in detail [18]. In brief, a total of 207 healthy, non-pregnant women aged 19 to 35 years of either South Asian or European descent living in Metro Vancouver were recruited by active and passive recruitment using paper and internet-based advertising, community outreach, and word of mouth. Eligibility of the potential research participants was determined by using a screening questionnaire that assessed multiple factors, including age, ethnicity, residence, and health condition to identify individuals who fit the target demographic. Informed written consent was obtained from all participants in the study. The UBC Clinical Research Ethics Board (H11-01216), Vancouver Coastal Health Research Ethics Board, and Fraser Health Research Ethics Board granted human ethics approval.

2.2. Blood Collection and Analysis

Fasting venous blood samples were obtained from all participants during a single clinic visit. Samples were collected into lithium heparin vacutainers. Plasma was separated using centrifugation and stored at −80 °C until analyses. Blood samples of 202 subjects were available for plasma PLP analysis. Plasma PLP was measured by quantification of its semicarbazide derivative using high-performance liquid chromatography (HPLC) with fluorescence detection [19]. The assay showed good agreement and high precision when measuring external controls at low, medium, and high PLP concentrations, with intra- and inter-assay coefficients of variation of 2.6%, 2.2%, and 2.3%, and 15.7%, 9.5%, and 10.2%, respectively. The cut-off values used for plasma PLP were: Plasma PLP > 30 nmol/L for adequate B6 status, plasma PLP = 20–30 nmol/L for suboptimal B6 status [20], plasma PLP < 20 nmol/L for B6 deficiency [20,21].

2.3. Demographic, Anthropometric, Exercise and Dietary Data

A demographic questionnaire, the "International Physical Activity Questionnaire (IPAQ)—Short Last 7 Day Self-Administered Format" [22,23], and a semi-quantitative Food Frequency Questionnaire (FFQ) "Your dietary intake" [24] were administered under the supervision of research staff during the clinic visit.

The demographic questionnaire collected information on age, ethnicity, immigration, education, household income, oral contraceptive use, and supplement use. South Asian and European ethnicities were defined as having at least three grandparents from a single ethnic group. South Asian ethnicity included Bangladeshi, Bengali, East Indian, Goan, Gujarati, Hindu, Ismaili, Kashmiri, Nepali, Pakistani, Punjabi, Sikh, Sinhalese, Sri Lankan, and Tamil ethnic groups. Because of the low number of participants ($n = 8$) indicating secondary school education or less than secondary school education, education was dichotomized. Low education was considered as below a bachelor's degree, and high education as equal or higher than bachelor's degree. Due to the low number of participants ($n = 36$) in the lowest household income bracket, household income was dichotomized into the following categories: Low income, total annual household income < $30,000 if 1–2 people, <$40,000 if 3–4 people, <$60,000 if ≥5 people, and high income, total annual household income ≥ $30,000 if 1–2 people, ≥$40,000 if 3–4 people, ≥$60,000 if ≥5 people. Participants who reported use of oral contraceptives were classified as oral contraceptive (OC) users. Duration and frequency of OC use were recorded. Participants who reported current consumption of any nutritional vitamin or mineral supplements were classified as nutritional supplement users. Participants were asked to bring in nutritional supplement bottles. Brand names and frequencies of intake were recorded and B6 content (yes/no) was obtained retrospectively by researchers from web-based product information. Participants who were taking supplements containing B6 were classified as supplemental B6 users. Subjects were asked about their smoking habit and categorized as non-smoker, former smoker, current occasional smoker (1–9 cigarettes/day), current regular smoker (10–19 cigarettes/day) or current frequent smoker (≥20 cigarettes/day). Due to the high number of non-smokers ($n = 174$), smoking data were dichotomized to non-smoker and smoker (including current smokers and former smokers).

The IPAQ asked the participants to recall their physical activities in the past seven days categorized as: Walking, moderate-intensity activities, and vigorous intensity activities. Each activity was recorded with its frequency (days per week) and duration (time per day). Participants were categorized into three physical activity levels; low, medium, and high, according to the IPAQ analysis protocol [22].

A semi-quantitative FFQ was used to determine dietary B6 intake. The questionnaire contained 78 food items and has been validated to assess micronutrient intakes in the Canadian population [24,25].

Anthropometric measurements, including height, weight, and waist circumference, were taken by research staff during the clinic visit. Body mass index (BMI) was calculated based on weight and height.

2.4. Statistical Analyses

The primary outcome of the presented analyses is B6 status and described using the direct biomarker plasma PLP and established cut-offs for adequate B6 status, suboptimal B6 status [20], and B6 deficiency [21]. Data were examined for normality by visual histogram assessment. Plasma PLP concentration was log-transformed to carry out statistical analyses and was presented as geometric mean (95% confidence interval (CI)). Relative dietary B6 intakes were presented as quartile ranges.

Bivariate analysis was conducted to identify variables associated with plasma PLP concentration (as continuous variable and as categorical variable using B6 status cutoffs) and relative dietary B6 intake. Two sample t tests were used for dichotomous variables, one-way ANOVA followed by

Tukey's Honest Significance test for categorical variables with more than two levels, and simple linear regression for continuous variables. If the P value from bivariate analysis was ≤ 0.2, the variable was carried forward to the stepwise multiple linear regression model. The full model with plasma PLP concentration as the dependent variable was controlled for relative dietary B6 intake, South Asian ethnicity, first generation immigrant status, BMI, education status, household income status, smoking status, and supplemental B6 use. Backward elimination procedure was used to establish the best fit multiple linear regression model. The estimated percentage change in plasma PLP concentration was presented for each variable after adjustment for other variables. Statistical significance was set at a two-sided p value of <0.05. All statistical analyses were performed using R software (3.1.2 windows version; R Foundation for Statistical Computing: Vienna, Austria).

3. Results

3.1. Participant Characteristics

Overall, subjects (n = 202) were highly educated, with 71% having a bachelor's degree or higher (Table 1). The rate of supplemental B6 use was 28% and did not differ based on age, BMI, ethnicity, household income, level of education, level of physical activity, OC use, or smoking status.

Table 1. Demographic and lifestyle characteristics of 202 healthy young adult women in Metro Vancouver.

Variables	Total (n = 202)
Age *, years	26.7 ± 4.2
Body mass index †, kg/m²	22.7 (22.2, 23.1)
Waist circumference †, cm	74.9 (73.7, 76.1)
Total energy intakes †,‡, kcal/day	1566 (1504, 1629)
Relative dietary vitamin B6 intake ‡, mg/day	
Q1	0–1.1
Q2	1.1–1.4
Q3	1.4–1.7
Q4	>1.7
Ethnicity, n (%)	
European	147 (73)
South Asian	55 (27)
Education, n (%)	
Less than secondary school education	2 (1)
Secondary school diploma	5 (3)
Post-secondary education	51 (25)
Bachelor's degree	87 (43)
University degree or >bachelor's degree	57 (28)
Household income §, n (%)	
Lowest	36 (20)
Lower-middle	44 (24)
Upper-middle	52 (28)
Highest	51 (28)
Physical activity level ||, n (%)	
Low	8 (4)
Medium	110 (55)
High	82 (41)
Use of oral contraceptives, n (%)	58 (29)
Use of nutritional supplements, n (%)	97 (48)
Use of supplemental vitamin B6, n (%)	56 (28)
Current or former smoker, n (%)	28 (14)

* Values presented as arithmetic mean ± SD. † Values presented as geometric mean (95% confidence interval). ‡ 18 samples were excluded due to plausible misreports in the food frequency questionnaire (n = 184). § Income quartiles are: Lowest: <$15,000 if 1–2 people, <$20,000 if 3–4 people, <$30,000 if ≥5 people, Lower-middle: $15,000–29,999 if 1–2 people, $20,000–39,999 if 3 or 4 people, $30,000 to 50,000 if ≥5 people, Upper-middle: $30,000–59,999 if 1–2 people, $40,000–79,999 if 3–4 people, $60,000–79,999 if ≥5 people, Highest: >$60,000 if 1–2 people, >$80,000 if ≥3 people. Only 183 subjects provided household income information. || Only 200 subjects completed physical activity questionnaire.

3.2. Blood Analyses

Mean (95% CI) concentration of plasma PLP was 61.0 (55.2, 67.3) nmol/L (Table 2). The prevalence of B6 deficiency (plasma PLP < 20 nmol/L) was 1.5% and that of suboptimal B6 status (plasma PLP = 20–30 nmol/L) was 10.9%.

Table 2. Differences in plasma pyridoxal 5′-phosphate (PLP) concentration in 202 healthy young adult women by categories of demographic and lifestyle factors.

Variables	Subjects n	Plasma PLP concentration			
		Mean (95% CI) nmol/L	<20 nmol/L n (%) *	20–30 nmol/L n (%) *	>30 nmol/L n (%)
Overall	202	61.0 (55.2, 67.3)	3 (1.5)	22 (11)	177 (88)
Anemia					
Hb > 12 g/dL	166	62.0 (55.5, 69.2)	3 (1.8)	17 (10)	146 (88)
Hb < 12 g/dL	36	56.4 (45.0, 70.8)	0	5 (14)	31 (86)
Ethnicity					
European ‡	147	66.9 (59.2, 75.6) †	2 (1.4)	14 (10)	131 (89)
South Asian	55	47.6 (41.2, 54.8)	1 (1.8)	8 (15)	46 (84)
Education					
Low	7	57.7 (28.5, 116.9)	0	2 (29)	5 (71)
High	195	61.1 (55.3, 67.5)	3 (1.5)	20 (10)	172 (88)
Household income					
Low	80	59.5 (52.1, 68.0)	1 (1.3)	7 (9)	72 (90)
High	103	63.6 (55.3, 73.0)	2 (1.9)	15 (13)	86 (83)
Physical activity level					
Low	8	44.4 (37.8, 52.3)	0	0	8 (100)
Medium	110	60.6 (53.0, 69.4)	2 (1.8)	13 (12)	95 (86)
High	82	63.8 (54.5, 74.8)	1 (1.2)	9 (11)	72 (88)
Oral contraceptive use					
Non-user	144	59.9 (53.5, 67.1)	2 (1.4)	17 (12)	125 (87)
User	58	63.6 (52.0, 77.8)	1 (1.7)	5 (9)	52 (90)
Supplemental vitamin B6 use					
Non-user ‡	146	48.5 (45.0, 52.3)	3 (2.1)	18 (12)	125 (86)
User	56	111.5 (87.2, 139.9) †	0	4 (7)	52 (93)
Smoker					
No	174	61.1 (55.0, 67.8)	2 (1.2)	18 (10)	154 (89)
Yes	28	60.2 (44.0, 82.3)	1 (3.6)	4 (14)	23 (82)

Plasma PLP concentration was presented as geometric mean (95% confidence interval (CI)) and was log-transformed to carry out the following statistical analyses. Hb, hemoglobin. * Chi-squared test revealed no significant difference in the prevalence of B6 deficiency and suboptimal B6 status in all the variables. † p value < 0.05 for two-sample t test comparing the indicated category with the referent category. ‡ Referent category.

Users of supplemental B6 had significantly higher plasma PLP concentration compared to non-users of supplemental B6; mean (95% CI) plasma PLP concentrations were 48.5 (45.0, 52.3) and 111.5 (87.2, 139.9), respectively ($p < 0.001$). Women of South Asian descent had significantly lower plasma PLP concentration (47.6 (41.2, 54.8)) compared with women of European descent (66.9 (59.2, 75.6), $p = 0.002$). There was no significant difference in plasma PLP concentration based on education level, household income, physical activity level, OC use, or smoking status in bivariate analyses. There was no significant difference in the prevalence of B6 deficiency, suboptimal B6 status or both combined (plasma PLP < 30 nmol/L) compared to adequate B6 status based on any demographic or lifestyle factors.

3.3. Dietary Analyses

Quartiles of dietary B6 intake were 0–1.1 mg/day, 1.1–1.4 mg/day, 1.4–1.7 mg/day and >1.7 mg/day, respectively. Individuals with low household income had significantly lower dietary B6 intake compared to individuals with high household income (mean ± SD: 1.4 ± 0.42 vs. 1.5 ± 0.47, respectively; $p = 0.045$). Plasma PLP concentration and relative dietary B6 intake were positively but weakly correlated ($r = 0.17$; $p = 0.02$).

Dietary vitamin B6 intake derived mainly from meat and meat alternatives in this sample of young adult women of South Asian and European descent, as shown by multiple linear regression of dietary B6 intake (Table 3). There was no significant difference in the intake of meat and meat alternatives between women of South Asian and European descent (2.8 versus 3.0 servings; $p = 0.2$).

Table 3. Food sources of vitamin B6.

Variables	Adjusted change in dietary B6 intake, mg/day (95%CI)	Adjusted p value
Grains, serving	0.03 (0.01, 0.04)	<0.001
Fruits and Vegetables, serving	0.10 (0.08, 0.11)	<0.001
Dairy, serving	0.10 (0.07, 0.13)	<0.001
Meat and Alternatives, serving	0.19 (0.16, 0.22)	<0.001

Adjusted changes and p value were from multiple linear regression model controlled for intake of grains, fruits and vegetables, dairy, and meat and alternatives. Number of observation = 184, Model p value < 0.001, R^2: 0.79, Adjusted R^2: 0.79.

3.4. Multivariate Analyses

Relative dietary B6 intake, BMI, ethnicity and the use of supplemental B6 were significant predictors of plasma PLP concentration (Table 4). Relative dietary B6 intake and the use of supplemental B6 were positively associated with plasma PLP concentration; BMI and South Asian ethnicity were negatively associated with plasma PLP concentration. The model explained 32% (R^2) of the variance in plasma PLP concentration.

Table 4. Predictors of plasma PLP concentration from unadjusted and adjusted linear regression models.

Variables	Unadjusted % change in plasma PLP (95% CI) *	Unadjusted p value	Adjusted % change in plasma PLP (95% CI) *	Adjusted p value
Relative B6 intake				
Q2 (1.1–1.4 mg/day)	7.7 (–20.0, 45.0)	0.62	9.0 (–15.8, 41.2)	0.51
Q3 (1.4–1.7 mg/day)	27.5 (–5.3, 71.6)	0.11	23.1 (–4.4, 58.6)	0.11
Q4 (>1.7 mg/day)	35.6 (0.7, 82.4)	0.045	29.3 (0.3, 66.7)	0.048
BMI, kg/m^2	–3.7 (–6.3, –1.0)	0.007	–2.7 (–5.1, –0.2)	0.034
South Asian descent	–28.9 (–33.6, –24.0)	0.002	–21.1 (–35.7, –3.1)	0.024
Supplemental B-6 use	127.7 (115.6, 140.8)	<0.001	114.5 (75.6, 162.0)	<0.001

Unadjusted percentage changes and p value were from simple linear regression models. Adjusted percentage changes and p value were from multiple linear regression model controlled for relative dietary B-6 intake, South Asian ethnicity, BMI, and supplemental B-6 use. Number of observation = 184, Model p value <0.001, R^2: 0.32, Adjusted R^2: 0.29. * The percentage change in plasma PLP concentration was calculated by $(e^{\beta 1} - 1) \times 100\%$.

Women taking supplemental B6 are expected to have ~113% higher plasma PLP after adjusting for relative dietary B6 intake, BMI and ethnicity (compared to ~127% higher plasma PLP in the unadjusted model) (Table 4). South Asian descent was associated with 21% lower plasma PLP concentration compared to women of European descent ($p = 0.026$), after adjusting for relative dietary B6 intake, BMI and the use of supplemental B6.

4. Discussion

Since the vitamin B6 status of Canadian women was previously unknown, and the relationship between demographic, dietary, and lifestyle factors and plasma PLP had not been assessed, we conducted a study of B6 status in a convenience sample of 202 healthy young Canadian adult women. We identified a combined prevalence of B6 deficiency and suboptimal B6 status of 12.4%. We also found that body mass index, South Asian ethnicity, relative dietary B6 intake, and the use of supplemental B6 were significant predictors of plasma PLP.

As defined by the Institute of Medicine, a plasma PLP concentration of <20 nmol/L corresponds with B6 deficiency [21]. The prevalence of B6 deficiency (1.5%) in this sample was much lower than the 40% prevalence of B6 deficiency reported for women aged 21–44 years in the NHANES 2003–2004 [13]. This large discrepancy may partly be due to the high socioeconomic status of the women in our study compared with participants of the NHANES, a representative population-based survey in the US. Low socioeconomic status has been associated with low B6 status [15,17] and overall poorer nutritional intake [26]. Education and income status accounted for 6% of the variation in plasma PLP in the NHANES [15]. The discrepancy between our study and the NHANES may also be attributed to different analytical methods employed for quantification of plasma PLP. The enzymatic assay used for the NHANES 2003–2004 samples has been reported to underestimate plasma PLP concentrations to a degree that would result in a doubling of the prevalence of B6 deficiency compared to the HPLC method we employed [27]. In the recent Alberta Pregnancy Outcomes and Nutrition (APrON) cohort study, none of the 119 pregnant women in the first trimester and only one out of 528 (0.2%) second-trimester pregnant women was B6 deficient; the prevalence of suboptimal B6 status was not reported [28]. Like our study, the APrON cohort is comprised of women of high socioeconomic status and the lack of B6 deficiency observed is likely due to the high rate (>94%) of multivitamin supplement use throughout pregnancy [28].

Suboptimal B6 status has been associated with an increased risk of several chronic diseases, including cardiovascular disease [29], colorectal cancer [30], breast cancer [31] and ovarian cancer [32]. In our study, 11% of our subjects had suboptimal B6 status. A cross-sectional study in Boston reported 18% of suboptimal B6 status among Puerto Rican women aged 45–75 years (n = 1236) [17]. The lower education level and income of subjects in that study may explain the higher prevalence of suboptimal B6 status compared with our study. In light of the limited data on B6 status in Canadians [12,28] and our finding of a substantial rate of suboptimal status in a cohort of healthy women of high socioeconomic status, a representative, population-based study to determine B6 status of Canadians is timely and crucial. We predict a higher prevalence of B6 deficiency and suboptimal B6 status would be observed in a representative sample of Canadian women compared to our study.

The use of supplemental B6 was a strong predictor of plasma PLP concentration both before and after multivariate adjustment. This is consistent with large scale studies that reported higher plasma PLP concentrations and a lower prevalence of B6 deficiency in nutritional supplement users [13] and supplemental B6 users [14] compared with non-users. In this sample, 48% of women used nutritional supplements (i.e., any type of vitamin or mineral supplement) of whom 58% were retrospectively categorized as supplemental B6 users. The prevalence of nutritional supplement use in this sample (48%) was higher than the prevalence reported in the CCHS in 2004 [33] with 35% of Canadian women aged 19–30 years reporting nutritional supplement use.

Relative dietary B6 intake was not a strong predictor of plasma PLP concentration both before and after multivariate adjustment. The weak association may partially be due to the use of a semi-quantitative FFQ. The validation study of the FFQ reported an 11% underestimation of relative dietary B6 intake compared to the use of dietary recalls [24]. Although the FFQ was validated to assess micronutrient intakes in the Canadian population [24], it is possible that it was unable to record certain ethnic specific foods. Further, under-reporting appears to be a factor, as a 1566 kcal/day average daily energy intake is lower than would be anticipated. In the NHANES 2003–2004, a stronger association between total B6 intake (from food sources and supplements combined) and plasma PLP (r = 0.32, p < 0.001) was observed [13]. We are unable to report quantitative intake of B6 from supplements due to limitations of secondary analysis. The weaker association between plasma PLP and dietary B6 intake in this study compared to the NHANES data might be explained by our data reflecting dietary B6 from food alone and not supplemental B6.

Our study is the first to report that women of South Asian descent may have lower plasma PLP concentrations compared with women of European descent. The difference in B6 status between South Asian and European women was not related to the consumption of different food sources of B6; meat and meat alternatives were the main dietary B6 sources in these healthy adult women. The negative association between South Asian ethnicity and plasma PLP concentrations remained significant after adjustment for relative dietary B6 intake, BMI, and supplemental B6 use. Although the South Asian population was only 56, compared to the European population of 146 in this study, the sample size was sufficient to give over 80% of power with a small effect size of 0.2 and significance level of 0.05 in the multiple linear regression model. Ethnicity has been shown to correlate with nutritional biomarker levels of other micronutrients [34].

Body mass index was inversely associated with plasma PLP concentration after adjustment for relative dietary B6 intake, supplemental B6 use, and South Asian ethnicity. An inverse relationship of BMI and plasma PLP was also reported in the NHANES; every 25% increase in BMI was associated with a 13% decrease in plasma PLP [15]. The volumetric dilution of the blood was suggested as a potential underlying mechanism for the linkage between increasing body mass and decreasing concentrations of B6 as well as other B-vitamins [35]. In addition, plasma PLP concentration has been inversely associated with circulating concentration of C-reactive protein (CRP), a marker of systemic inflammation that is elevated in obesity [36,37].

Compared to other studies, we did not find OC use to be a significant predictor of B6 status. In recent literature, lower-dose OC use was associated with low B6 status [38]. In the NHANES 2003–2004, plasma PLP concentration was also significantly lower in OC users compared to non-users [13]. It was suggested that this may be due to the disruption of tryptophan metabolism by estrogen, independent of B6 status [39]. In our study, the effect of OC use on plasma PLP concentration was small and we had insufficient sample size to detect a statistically significant difference. We also lacked power to detect associations with other variables including physical activity and smoking.

The predictors of B6 status we assessed explained only 32% of the variability in plasma PLP. Our results might be confounded by unexplained biological factors or genetic modifiers. One recent study reported some variants in tissue nonspecific alkaline phosphatase gene influenced plasma PLP concentration, but the clinical implications of these variants were unclear [40].

Some weaknesses of this study include the recruitment of a convenience sample of relatively healthy women of high education and the lack of data on genetic variants. Over 71% of our study participants obtained a bachelor's degree or higher, where a comparatively lower proportion (35%) of women aged 25 to 64 in Metro Vancouver reported this high level of education, according to the National Household Survey [41]. We used plasma PLP as our single biomarker to assess B6 status since it is currently the only established biomarker with cut-offs to define B6 deficiency [21]. However, plasma PLP only reflects the circulating concentration of B6 and is influenced by several factors, such as inflammation, serum albumin and alkaline phosphatase concentrations [42]. The derivation of reference intervals for sensitive functional biomarkers, e.g., plasma cystathionine [43], is crucial for evaluation of intracellular B6 status.

5. Conclusions

We report a 12.4% combined prevalence of B6 deficiency and suboptimal B6 status in healthy young adult women in Metro Vancouver ($n = 202$). Periconceptional B6 adequacy is crucial for healthy pregnancy outcomes; and women with higher BMI and South Asian ethnicity might be more likely to have low B6 status. The lower prevalence of B6 deficiency and suboptimal B6 status in these women compared to reports from representative samples in other countries may be due to the high socioeconomic status of these women. Given the central roles of B6 in key biological functions and health, more research is warranted to determine B6 status in the general Canadian population.

Acknowledgments: The authors thank Bryna Shatenstein and Mira Jabbour (Centre de Recherche, Institut Universitaire de Gériatrie de Montréal) for analysis of the dietary data. This research was supported by funding from the "Food, Nutrition and Health Vitamin Research Fund", Faculty of Land and Food Systems, UBC. Y.L. acknowledges funding from the Canada Research Chairs program of the Canadian Institutes of Health Research. A.M.D. is supported by the Investigator Grant Award Program, Research Institute, British Columbia Children's Hospital.

Author Contributions: C.L.H. performed data analysis and wrote the initial draft of this study report. T.A.W.Q. and Y.L. designed and conducted the original study. A.M.D. commented on the study design and provided input to the manuscript. Y.L. had primary responsibility for the final content. All authors read and approved the final manuscript.

References

1. Stover, P.J.; Field, M.S. Vitamin B-6. *Adv. Nutr.* **2015**, *6*, 132–133. [CrossRef] [PubMed]
2. Lamers, Y.; Williamson, J.; Ralat, M.; Quinlivan, E.P.; Gilbert, L.R.; Keeling, C.; Stevens, R.D.; Newgard, C.B.; Ueland, P.M.; Meyer, K.; et al. Moderate dietary vitamin B-6 restriction raises plasma glycine and cystathionine concentrations while minimally affecting the rates of glycine turnover and glycine cleavage in healthy men and women. *J. Nutr.* **2009**, *139*, 452–60. [CrossRef] [PubMed]
3. Mann, J.; Truswell, A.S. The B vitamins. In *Essentials of Human Nutrition*, 4th ed.; Mann, T., Ed.; Oxford University Press: New York, NY, USA, 2012.
4. Ulvik, A.; Theofylaktopoulou, D.; Midttun, Ø.; Nygard, O.; Eussen, S.J.P.M.; Ueland, P.M. Substrate product ratios of enzymes in the kynurenine pathway measured in plasma as indicators of functional vitamin B-6 status. *Am. J. Clin. Nutr.* **2013**, *98*, 934–940. [CrossRef] [PubMed]
5. Dror, D.K.; Allen, L.H. Interventions with Vitamins B6, B12 and C in pregnancy. *Paediatr. Perinat. Epidemiol.* **2012**, *26*, 55–74. [CrossRef] [PubMed]
6. Wachstein, M.; Graffeo, L.W. Influence of vitamin B6 on the incidence of preeclampsia. *Obstet. Gynecol.* **1956**, *8*, 177–180. [PubMed]
7. Roepke, J.L.; Kirksey, A. Vitamin B6 nutriture during pregnancy and lactation. Vitamin B6 intake, levels of the vitamin in biological fluids, and condition of the infant at birth. *Am. J. Clin. Nutr.* **1969**, *32*, 2249–2256.
8. Schuster, K.; Bailey, L.B.; Mahan, C.S. Vitamin B6 status of low-income adolescent and adult pregnant women and the condition of their infants at birth. *Am. J. Clin. Nutr.* **1981**, *34*, 1731–1735. [PubMed]
9. Ronnenberg, A.G.; Goldman, M.B.; Chen, D.; Aitken, I.W.; Willett, W.C.; Selhub, J.; Xu, X. Preconception folate and vitamin B(6) status and clinical spontaneous abortion in Chinese women. *Obstet. Gynecol.* **2002**, *100*, 107–113. [CrossRef] [PubMed]
10. Ronnenberg, A.G.; Venners, S.A.; Xu, X.; Chen, C.; Wang, L.; Guang, W.; Huang, A.; Wang, X. Preconception B-vitamin and homocysteine status, conception, and early pregnancy loss. *Am. J. Epidemiol.* **2007**, *166*, 304–312. [CrossRef] [PubMed]
11. Sedgh, G.; Singh, S.; Hussain, R. Intended and unintended pregnancies worldwide in 2012 and recent trends. *Stud. Fam. Plann.* **2014**, *45*, 301–314. [CrossRef] [PubMed]
12. Health Canada. *Canadian Community Health Survey 2.2, Nutrition (2004). Nutrient Intakes from Food Provincial, Regional and National Summary Data Tables*; Health Canada: Ottawa, ON, Canada, 2009; Volume 2.
13. Morris, M.S.; Picciano, M.F.; Jacques, P.F.; Selhub, J. Plasma pyridoxal 5'-phosphate in the US population: The National Health and Nutrition Examination Survey, 2003–2004. *Am. J. Clin. Nutr.* **2008**, *87*, 1446–1454. [PubMed]
14. Deac, O.M.; Mills, J.L.; Shane, B.; Midttun, Ø.; Ueland, P.M.; Brosnan, J.T.; Brosnan, M.E.; Laird, E.; Gibney, E.R.; Fan, R.; et al. Tryptophan catabolism and vitamin B-6 status are affected by gender and lifestyle factors in healthy young adults. *J. Nutr.* **2015**, *145*, 701–707. [CrossRef] [PubMed]
15. Pfeiffer, C.M.; Sternberg, M.R.; Schleicher, R.L.; Rybak, M.E. Dietary supplement use and smoking are important correlates of biomarkers of water-soluble vitamin status after adjusting for sociodemographic and lifestyle variables in a representative sample of U.S. adults. *J. Nutr.* **2013**, *143*, 957S–965S. [CrossRef] [PubMed]
16. Ulvik, A.; Ebbing, M.; Hustad, S.; Midttun, Ø.; Nygård, O.; Vollset, S.E.; Bønaa, K.H.; Nordrehaug, J.E.; Nilsen, D.W.; Schirmer, H.; et al. Long- and short-term effects of tobacco smoking on circulating concentrations of B vitamins. *Clin. Chem.* **2010**, *56*, 755–763. [CrossRef] [PubMed]

17.   Ye, X.; Maras, J.E.; Bakun, P.J.; Tucker, K.L. Dietary intake of vitamin B-6, plasma pyridoxal 5′-phosphate, and homocysteine in Puerto Rican adults. *J. Am. Diet. Assoc.* **2010**, *110*, 1660–1668. [CrossRef] [PubMed]

18.   Quay, T.A.W.; Schroder, T.H.; Jeruszka-Bielak, M.; Li, W.; Devlin, A.M.; Barr, S.I.; Lamers, Y. High prevalence of suboptimal vitamin B12 status in young adult women of South Asian and European ethnicity. *Appl. Physiol. Nutr. Metab.* **2015**, *40*, 1279–1286. [CrossRef] [PubMed]

19.   Ubbink, J.B.; Serfontein, W.J.; de Villiers, L.S. Stability of pyridoxal-5-phosphate semicarbazone: applications in plasma vitamin B6 analysis and population surveys of vitamin B6 nutritional status. *J. Chromatogr.* **1985**, *342*, 277–284. [CrossRef]

20.   Leklem, J.E. Vitamin B-6: A status report. *J. Nutr.* **1990**, *120*, 1503–1507. [PubMed]

21.   Institute of Medicine (US) Standing Committee on the Scientific Evaluation of Dietary Reference Intakes and its Panel on Folate, Other B Vitamins, and Choline. *Dietary Reference Intakes for Thiamin, Riboflavin, Niacin, Vitamin B6, Folate, Vitamin B12, Pantothenic Acid, Biotin, and Choline*; National Academies Press: Washington, DC, USA, 1998.

22.   IPAQ Research Committee. Guidelines for Data Processing and Analysis of the International Physical Activity Questionnaire (IPAQ)—Short Form. Available online: https://docs.google.com/viewer?a=v& pid=sites&srcid=ZGVmYXVsdGRvbWFpbnx0aGVpcGFxfGd4OjhlMTcxZGJkZmMxYTg1NQ (accessed on 30 September 2011).

23.   Craig, C.L.; Marshall, A.L.; Sjöström, M.; Bauman, A.E.; Booth, M.L.; Ainsworth, B.E.; Pratt, M.; Ekelund, U.; Yngve, A.; Sallis, J.F.; et al. International physical activity questionnaire: 12-country reliability and validity. *Med. Sci. Sports Exerc.* **2003**, *35*, 1381–1395. [CrossRef] [PubMed]

24.   Shatenstein, B.; Nadon, S.; Godin, C.; Ferland, G. Development and validation of a food frequency questionnaire. *Can. J. Diet. Pract. Res.* **2005**, *66*, 67–75. [CrossRef] [PubMed]

25.   Shatenstein, B.; Xu, H.; Luo, Z.C.; Fraser, W. Relative Validity of a Food Frequency Questionnaire: For Pregnant Women. *Can. J. Diet. Pract. Res.* **2011**, *72*, 60–69. [CrossRef] [PubMed]

26.   Kirkpatrick, S.I.; Dodd, K.W.; Parsons, R.; Ng, C.; Garriguet, D.; Tarasuk, V. Household Food Insecurity Is a Stronger Marker of Adequacy of Nutrient Intakes among Canadian Compared to American Youth and Adults. *J. Nutr.* **2015**, *145*, 1596–1603. [CrossRef] [PubMed]

27.   National Center for Health Statistics. National Health and Nutrition Examination Survey (NHANES). Data Documentation, Codebook, and Frequencies. Laboratory Component. Vitamin B6. Survey Years: 2005–2006. Available online: http://wwwn.cdc.gov/nchs/nhanes/2005-2006/VIT_B6_D.htm (accessed on 8 July 2016).

28.   Fayyaz, F.; Wang, F.; Jacobs, R.L.; O'Connor, D.L.; Bell, R.C.; Field, C.J. Folate, vitamin B12, and vitamin B6 status of a group of high socioeconomic status women in the Alberta Pregnancy Outcomes and Nutrition (APrON) cohort. *Appl. Physiol. Nutr. Metab.* **2014**, *39*, 1402–1408. [CrossRef] [PubMed]

29.   Lotto, V.; Choi, S.W.; Friso, S. Vitamin B6: A challenging link between nutrition and inflammation in CVD. *Br. J. Nutr.* **2011**, *106*, 183–195. [CrossRef] [PubMed]

30.   Zhang, X.H.; Ma, J.; Smith-Warner, S.A.; Lee, J.E.; Giovannucci, E. Vitamin B6 and colorectal cancer: Current evidence and future directions. *World J. Gastroenterol.* **2013**, *19*, 1005–1010. [CrossRef] [PubMed]

31.   Wu, W.; Kang, S.; Zhang, D. Association of vitamin B6, vitamin B12 and methionine with risk of breast cancer: A dose-response meta-analysis. *Br. J. Cancer* **2013**, *109*, 1926–1944. [CrossRef] [PubMed]

32.   Harris, H.R.; Cramer, D.W.; Vitonis, A.F.; DePari, M.; Terry, K.L. Folate, vitamin B(6), vitamin B(12), methionine and alcohol intake in relation to ovarian cancer risk. *Int. J. Cancer* **2012**, *131*, E518–E529. [CrossRef] [PubMed]

33.   Guo, X.; Willows, N.; Kuhle, S.; Jhangri, G.; Veugelers, P.J. Use of vitamin and mineral supplements among Canadian adults. *Can. J. Public Health.* **2009**, *100*, 357–360. [PubMed]

34.   Kant, A.K.; Graubard, B.I. Ethnicity is an independent correlate of biomarkers of micronutrient intake and status in American adults. *J. Nutr.* **2007**, *137*, 2456–2463. [PubMed]

35.   Bird, J.K.; Ronnenberg, A.G.; Choi, S.W.; Du, F.; Mason, J.B.; Liu, Z. Obesity is associated with increased red blood cell folate despite lower dietary intakes and serum concentrations. *J. Nutr.* **2015**, *145*, 79–86. [CrossRef] [PubMed]

36.   Morris, M.S.; Sakakeeny, L.; Jacques, P.F.; Picciano, M.F.; Selhub, J. Vitamin B-6 intake is inversely related to, and the requirement is affected by, inflammation status. *J. Nutr.* **2010**, *140*, 103–110. [CrossRef] [PubMed]

37.   Kitahara, C.M.; Trabert, B.; Katki, H.A.; Chaturvedi, A.K.; Kemp, T.J.; Pinto, L.A.; Moore, S.C.; Purdue, M.P.; Wentzensen, N.; Hildesheim, A.; et al. Body mass index, physical activity, and serum markers of

inflammation, immunity, and insulin resistance. *Cancer Epidemiol. Biomarkers Prev.* **2014**, *23*, 2840–2849. [CrossRef] [PubMed]

38. Rios-Avila, L.; Coats, B.; Chi, Y.; Midttun, Ø.; Ueland, P.M.; Stacpoole, P.W.; Gregory, J.F. Metabolite profile analysis reveals association of vitamin B-6 with metabolites related to one-carbon metabolism and tryptophan catabolism but not with biomarkers of inflammation in oral contraceptive users and reveals the effects of oral contraceptives o. *J. Nutr.* **2015**, *145*, 87–95. [CrossRef] [PubMed]

39. Wilson, S.M.C.; Bivins, B.N.; Russell, K.A.; Bailey, L.B. Oral contraceptive use: Impact on folate, vitamin B6, and vitamin B12 status. *Nutr. Rev.* **2011**, *69*, 572–583. [CrossRef] [PubMed]

40. Carter, T.C.; Pangilinan, F.; Molloy, A.M.; Fan, R.; Wang, Y.; Shane, B.; Gibney, E.R.; Midttun, Ø.; Ueland, P.M.; Cropp, C.D.; et al. Common Variants at Putative Regulatory Sites of the Tissue Nonspecific Alkaline Phosphatase Gene Influence Circulating Pyridoxal 5′-Phosphate Concentration in Healthy Adults. *J. Nutr.* **2015**, *145*, 1386–1393. [CrossRef] [PubMed]

41. Statistics Canada. *Education in Canada: Attainment, Field of Study and Location of Study*; Health Canada: Ottawa, ON, Canada, 2014.

42. Ueland, P.M.; Ulvik, A.; Rios-Avila, L.; Midttun, Ø.; Gregory, J.F. Direct and Functional Biomarkers of Vitamin B6 Status. *Annu. Rev. Nutr.* **2015**, *35*, 33–70. [CrossRef] [PubMed]

43. Lamers, Y. Indicators and methods for folate, vitamin B-12, and vitamin B-6 status assessment in humans. *Curr. Opin. Clin. Nutr. Metab. Care* **2011**, *14*, 445–454. [CrossRef] [PubMed]

9

B-Vitamin Intake and Biomarker Status in Relation to Cognitive Decline in Healthy Older Adults in a 4-Year Follow-Up Study

Catherine F. Hughes [1,*], Mary Ward [1], Fergal Tracey [2], Leane Hoey [1], Anne M. Molloy [3], Kristina Pentieva [1] and Helene McNulty [1]

[1] Northern Ireland Centre for Food and Health, Ulster University, Cromore Road, Coleraine BT52 1SA, Northern Ireland, UK; mw.ward@ulster.ac.uk (M.W.); l.hoey@ulster.ac.uk (L.H.); k.pentieva@ulster.ac.uk (K.P.); h.mcnulty@ulster.ac.uk (H.M.)
[2] Causeway Hospital, Northern Health and Social Care Trust, Coleraine BT52 1HS, Northern Ireland, UK; Fergal.Tracey@northerntrust.hscni.net
[3] School of Medicine, Trinity College Dublin, Dublin 2, Ireland; AMOLLOY@tcd.ie
* Correspondence: h.mcnulty@ulster.ac.uk

Abstract: Advancing age can be associated with an increase in cognitive dysfunction, a spectrum of disability that ranges in severity from mild cognitive impairment to dementia. Folate and the other B-vitamins involved in one-carbon metabolism are associated with cognition in ageing but the evidence is not entirely clear. The hypothesis addressed in this study was that lower dietary intake or biomarker status of folate and/or the metabolically related B-vitamins would be associated with a greater than expected rate of cognitive decline over a 4-year follow-up period in healthy older adults. Participants (aged 60–88 years; n = 155) who had been previously screened for cognitive function were reassessed four years after initial investigation using the Mini-Mental State Examination (MMSE). At the 4-year follow-up assessment when participants were aged 73.4 ± 7.1 years, mean cognitive MMSE scores had declined from 29.1 ± 1.3 at baseline to 27.5 ± 2.4 (p < 0.001), but some 27% of participants showed a greater than expected rate of cognitive decline (i.e., decrease in MMSE > 0.56 points per year). Lower vitamin B6 status, as measured using pyridoxal-5-phosphate (PLP; <43 nmol/L) was associated with a 3.5 times higher risk of accelerated cognitive decline, after adjustment for age and baseline MMSE score (OR, 3.48; 95% CI, 1.58 to 7.63; p < 0.05). Correspondingly, lower dietary intake (0.9–1.4 mg/day) of vitamin B6 was also associated with a greater rate of cognitive decline (OR, 4.22; 95% CI, 1.28–13.90; p < 0.05). No significant relationships of dietary intake or biomarker status with cognitive decline were observed for the other B-vitamins. In conclusion, lower dietary and biomarker status of vitamin B6 at baseline predicted a greater than expected rate of cognitive decline over a 4-year period in healthy older adults. Vitamin B6 may be an important protective factor in helping maintain cognitive health in ageing.

Keywords: one-carbon metabolism; B-vitamin biomarkers; dietary intakes; vitamin B6; pyridoxal-5-phosphate (PLP); cognition; ageing

1. Introduction

Advancing age can be associated with an increase in cognitive dysfunction, a spectrum of disability that ranges in severity from normal age-related changes through mild cognitive impairment (MCI) to dementia; with the latter defined as a progressive decline in memory, thinking, language and judgment that is sufficient to impair activities of daily living [1]. An estimated 50% of those diagnosed with MCI will go onto develop dementia within 5 years of diagnosis [?] Globally, it is estimated that

48 million people are currently suffering from dementia and the figures are predicted to triple by 2050 [3]. Dementia is a leading cause of disability, dependency and decreased quality of life among older people [3] and presents many social, economic and health care challenges that will continue to increase with an ageing population. Therefore, the identification of strategies to prevent or delay the onset of dementia has become a major global public health priority.

A number of nutritional and lifestyle factors have emerged as potential modifiable risk factors for cognitive decline in ageing [4]. In particular, there is considerable epidemiological evidence to suggest that sub-optimal status of folate, the related B-vitamins, and/or elevated concentrations of the metabolite homocysteine, contribute to cognitive dysfunction [5–10] and to a greater rate of cognitive decline in ageing [11–14]. Elevated plasma homocysteine and lower folate have been most consistently associated with cognitive dysfunction in ageing [6,8]. There is also evidence to support a role for vitamin B12 [15,16] and to a lesser extent vitamin B6, although the latter has been far less extensively investigated [9,17]. There is also some evidence in the form of randomised controlled trials to show beneficial effects of B-vitamin supplementation on cognition in ageing [18–20]. A number of other trials have failed to detect significant benefits [21–23] with recent meta-analyses concluding that there was no beneficial effect of B-vitamin supplementation on cognition [24,25]. However, a number of these trials may have been too short in duration; conducted in healthy individuals, patients with severe dementia; or in those with optimal B-vitamin status and so unlikely to benefit from vitamin supplementation [26]. The strongest evidence to date of a causal relationship between B-vitamins and cognition comes from the Homocysteine and B-vitamin in Cognitive Impairment (VITACOG) study. This study showed that combined B-vitamin supplementation for two years had beneficial effects on cognitive performance in participants with MCI and elevated plasma homocysteine concentrations [20]. More importantly, it also demonstrated that B-vitamin supplementation reduced the rate of brain atrophy by 30% as measured using MRI [27]. A subsequent report from the VITACOG investigators reported that the atrophy occurred in grey matter areas of the brain which are particularly vulnerable to Alzheimer's disease [28].

The intervention doses administered in VITACOG were well in excess of recommended dietary intakes and therefore whilst the VITACOG papers provide powerful evidence of a role for folate, vitamin B12, and/or vitamin B6 in cognition, the relevance of these results to nutrition, and thus prevention of cognitive dysfunction in ageing is unclear. Furthermore, epidemiological research generally in this area has predominantly focused on plasma homocysteine, folate and vitamin B12; most studies have overlooked vitamin B6 and all have ignored the role of vitamin B2. Consequently, the influence of all the relevant B-vitamins involved in one-carbon metabolism on cognition is not fully understood. Therefore, the aim of this study was to investigate whether lower dietary intake or biomarker status of B-vitamins (folate, vitamin B12, vitamin B6 or riboflavin) at baseline was associated with a greater rate of cognitive decline over a 4-year follow-up period in healthy older adults.

2. Materials and Methods

2.1. Participant Recruitment and Study Design

Potential participants were identified from our records of a previous cross sectional study funded by the UK Food Standards Agency investigating B-vitamin dietary intakes and biomarker status in the healthy younger and older adults in Northern Ireland as previously described [29]. Healthy participants ($n = 662$; aged $\geq$18 years) were recruited to the original study and as part of the protocol, those aged $\geq$60 years completed a cognitive function test (Folstein's Mini Mental State Examination MMSE; [30], the purpose of the original assessment was to ensure that the ability of participants to accurately recall food intake was not compromised. The current study involved the re-examination (4 years after initial screening) of those aged $\geq$60 years ($n = 255$). The exclusion criteria for the original study were: those with vitamin B12 deficiency (serum vitamin B12 < 111 pmol/L); self-reported history of cardiovascular, gastrointestinal, hepatic, renal, or haematological disease; use of medications that interfere with B-vitamin metabolism; taking supplements containing B-vitamins; having visited a country with a mandatory fortification policy for a period ≥2 weeks in the previous 6 months; plasma creatinine concentrations >130 µmol/L (generally indicative of renal impairment); and a score of <25 on the MMSE (indicative of cognitive impairment). Ethical approval was granted by the University of Ulster Research Ethics Committee (UUREC; Ref UUREC/07/005) and all participants provided written informed consent.

2.2. Cognitive Assessment

Cognitive function was assessed at baseline and at follow-up (between 3.5 to 4 years from initial screening for each participant) using the MMSE [30], one of the most widely used cognitive screening tools in a clinical setting. It is a global test of cognitive function and assesses the domains of orientation, registration, attention and concentration, recall and language. Overall the maximum score achievable is 30, with a score <25 indicating a possibility of cognitive impairment and a score <20 dementia [30].

2.3. Dietary and Lifestyle Assessment

Dietary intake was assessed using a 4-day food diary (for 4 consecutive days, including Saturday and Sunday, to account for the known variation in day-to-day intake) in combination with a food frequency questionnaire. This combined dietary method as described previously has been validated at this centre for the assessment of the four relevant B-vitamins against each of their blood biomarkers [29]. The food frequency questionnaire requested participants to state the frequency of consumption for food groups or specific branded products fortified with B-vitamins (e.g., ready-to-eat breakfast cereals, bars, breads and margarines). Participants provided details on brand names of the products consumed so that the fortification profile of any new foods could be established. By combining the 2 dietary collection methods, we were able to estimate dietary intakes of the relevant B-vitamins from both natural food sources and from fortified foods. Each participant received oral and written instructions on how to complete the food diary and food-frequency questionnaire. Any queries or discrepancies between the 2 dietary records were discussed with the participant and were clarified within 1 week of collection to enhance the accuracy of information on usual food intakes. Food portion sizes were estimated by the participant by using household measures and were later quantified by using published food portion size data [31]. The food-composition database WEIGHED INTAKE SOFTWARE PACKAGE (WISP, version 3; Tinuviel Software, Anglesey, UK) was used to calculate mean daily energy and B-vitamin intakes. This database has been customised at our centre to enable natural food folate to be distinguished from folic acid added to foods by manufacturers, and this allows the estimation of dietary folate equivalents (DFE; [29]).

A health and lifestyle questionnaire was used to obtain information on medical history including depression, smoking, use of alcohol and medication, and educational attainment. Height (m) and weight (kg) were measured at baseline and body mass index (kg/m^2) was calculated.

2.4. Laboratory Analysis

All participants provided a fasting 30 mL blood sample at baseline. Sample preparation and fractionation were performed within 4 h of blood collection, and blood aliquots were stored at −80 °C until batch analysis. Plasma homocysteine was measured by fluorescence polarization immunoassay using the Abbot Imx analyser [32]. Red blood cell folate was measured by microbiological assay using *Lactobacillus casei* [33]. Vitamin B12 status was determined using a number of biomarkers; the direct measures were serum total vitamin B12 by microbiological assay using *Lactobacillus leichmanni* [34] and serum holoTC (the metabolically active fraction of vitamin B12) by microparticle enzyme immunoassay (AxSym Active-B12; Axis-Shield, Heidelberg, Germany); the functional biomarker serum methylmalonic acid (MMA) by gas chromatography mass spectrometry using methylchloroformate derivatization at University of Bergen, Norway. Plasma vitamin B6 (PLP) was measured by reversed phase, high performance liquid chromatography with fluorescence detection [35]. Riboflavin status was assessed using the erythrocyte glutathione reductase activation (EGRAC) where the ratio of FAD stimulated to unstimulated enzyme activity is calculated; higher EGRAC values indicate lower riboflavin status, and sub-optimal riboflavin status is generally recognised as a coefficient ≥ 1.3 [36]. The methylenetetrahydrofolate reductase (MTHFR) 677C$\rightarrow$T polymorphism was identified by polymerase chain reaction amplification followed by *HinF1* restriction digestion [37]. Plasma creatinine was measured using a standard spectrophotometric assay with use of a chemistry analyzer (Hitachi; Roche Diagnostics Corporation, Indianapolis, IN, USA). Additionally, pepsinogen I and pepsinogen II were measured as markers of gastric atrophy by enzyme-linked immunosorbent assay (Biohit, Helsinki, Finland); a ratio of pepsinogen I:II < 3 is indicative of atrophic gastritis. All samples were analysed blind and duplicated. Quality controls were provided by repeated analysis of pooled samples.

2.5. Statistical Analysis

All statistical analysis was performed using SPSS software (version 22; SPSS UK Ltd., Chersey, UK). Prior to analysis, tests for normality were conducted and data were log transformed where appropriate. Differences at baseline and follow-up were assessed using a paired t-test for continuous data and chi-squared test for categorical data. Correlations between dietary intakes and corresponding blood biomarkers were calculated using Pearson's correlation coefficient (r). Annual cognitive decline was calculated (baseline MMSE$-$follow-up MMSE)/(duration of follow-up) on an individual basis for each participant, accelerated cognitive decline was defined as a decrease in MMSE > 0.56 points per year [38]. Binary logistic regression analysis was used to assess health and lifestyle predictors of cognitive decline. The impact of B-vitamin dietary intake and blood biomarker status as predictors of cognitive decline was assessed using binary logistic regression after controlling for significant predictors of cognitive decline (age and baseline MMSE).

3. Results

Of the 662 healthy volunteers, 255 $\geq$ 60 years were identified as potential participants and of these 155 were available to participate in the follow-up assessment (Figure 1). Only those that participated at both timepoints are presented in this paper; those lost to follow-up were older and had significantly lower vitamin B12 status (Appendix A).

The characteristics of participants at initial screening are shown in Table 1. Participants had a mean age of 70 years, were predominantly female, well-educated and had a low rate of depression. The majority of participants were regular consumers of foods fortified with B-vitamins (75%). Dietary intakes compared favourably with current UK dietary recommendations [39] as reflected in good overall B-vitamin biomarker status. As a result of the exclusion criteria, no participant was deficient in vitamin B12, however some 3% were identified as deficient in folate and 11% deficient in vitamin B6. Gastric function was assessed by using pepsinogen I:II ratio, 12% had evidence of atrophic gastritis (pepsinogen I:II ratio < 3; data not shown).

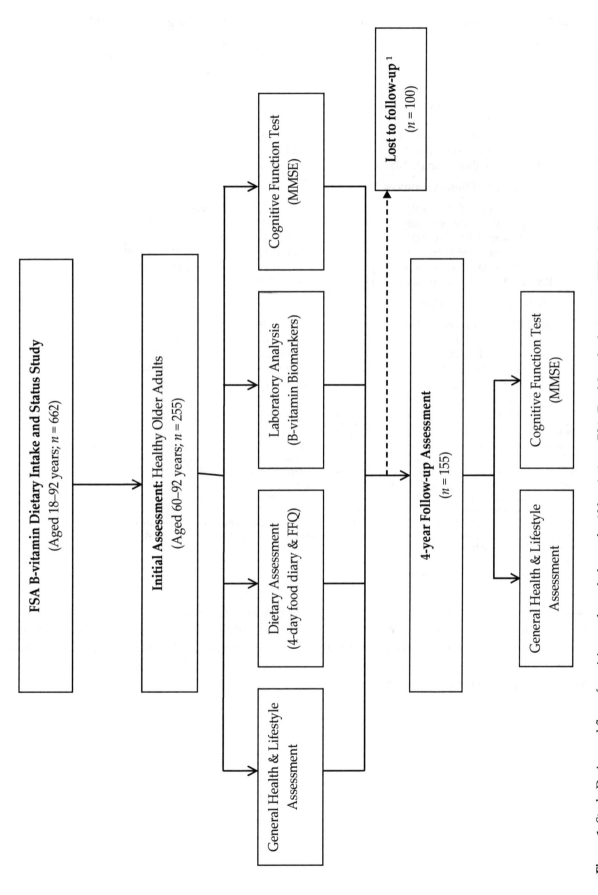

Figure 1. Study Design and flow of participants through the study. Abbreviations: FSA, Food Standards Agency; FFQ, Food Frequency Questionnaire; MMSE, Mini Mental State Examination; [1] Failed to meet inclusion criteria at follow-up assessment $n = 26$; declined to participate $n = 43$; deceased $n = 4$; non contactable $n = 21$; participation in other research $n = 6$.

Table 1. General characteristics of healthy older adults at initial investigation ($n = 155$).

	Participants	Reference Range
Age (years)	69.5 (7.3)	
Male n (%)	60 (39)	
BMI (kg/m^2)	27.5 (4.2)	20–25
Smokers n (%)	6 (4)	
3rd Level Education n (%)	48 (31)	
Depression n (%) *	11 (7)	
Cognitive Function (MMSE)	29.1 (1.3)	≤25
B-Vitamin Dietary Intakes †		
Energy (MJ/day)	7.621 (1.789)	9.71 (M); 7.96 (F)
Total Folate (µg/day)	303 (141)	200
Vitamin B12 (µg/day)	4.0 (2.4)	1.5
Vitamin B6 (mg/day)	2.3 (0.7)	1.4 (M); 1.2 (F)
Riboflavin (mg/day)	1.6 (0.4)	1.3 (M); 1.1 (F)
Fortified Food Consumer n (%) ‡	116 (75)	
B-Vitamin Biomarker Status §		
Red Blood Cell Folate (nmol/L)	954 (410)	340–2270
Serum total B12 (pmol/L)	282 (106)	111–740
Serum HoloTC (pmol/L)	50.8 (24.3)	40–200
Serum MMA (µmol/L)	0.24 (0.19	≤0.36
Vitamin B6 (Plasma PLP; nmol/L)	58.4 (25.8)	20–121
Riboflavin (EGRAC)	1.33 (0.14)	≤1.3
Plasma total homocysteine (µmol/L)	12.0 (3.7)	<10

Data presented as mean (SD) unless otherwise indicated. * History of depression was self-reported. † Reference ranges for dietary intakes based on reference nutrient intake values (RNIs) for 50+ years except for energy where the estimated energy requirements (EARs) for 65–74 years were used [39]; ‡ Consumers of fortified foods were defined as those who consumed foods fortified with B-vitamins at least once per week; § Reference ranges based on analytical laboratory where assay was performed. Abbreviations: BMI, body mass index; MMSE, mini mental state examination; HoloTC, Holotranscobalamin—functional indicator of metabolically active fraction of vitamin B12; MMA, methylmalonic acid—an indicator of vitamin B12 status, a higher MMA status indicates a lower vitamin B12 status; PLP, Pyridoxal-5-phosphate—a measure of vitamin B6 status; EGRAC, Erythrocyte glutathione reductase activation coefficient—a functional indicator of riboflavin status, a higher ratio indicates a lower riboflavin status

The relationship between dietary intakes and corresponding blood biomarker concentrations were examined for each B-vitamin of interest (Figure 2). Dietary intakes for total folate, vitamin B6 and riboflavin were each significantly correlated with the corresponding blood biomarker concentration. Of note, vitamin B12 intake was significantly correlated with serum holoTC but not serum total vitamin B12, the more typically measured biomarker ($r = 0.134$, $p = 0.104$; data not shown).

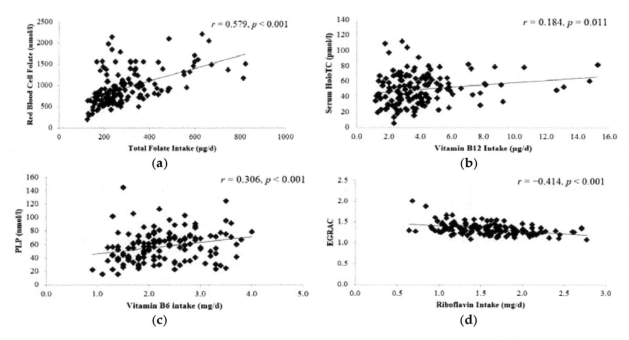

Figure 2. Relationship between dietary intake and biomarker status of B-vitamins at baseline (n = 148): (**a**) association between red blood cell folate and total folate intake; (**b**) association between holoTC and vitamin B12 intake; (**c**) association between pyridoxal-5-phosphate and vitamin B6 (**d**) association between EGRAC and riboflavin intake. Correlations were calculated using Pearson's correlation coefficients (r). $p < 0.05$ was considered significant. HoloTC, holo-transcobalamin; PLP, Pyridoxal-5-phosphate—a measure of vitamin B6 status; EGRAC: erythrocyte glutathione reductase activation coefficient, a functional indicator of riboflavin status. The change in cognitive function score, as measured using MMSE is shown in Table 2. Over the 4-year follow-up period, a significant decline in the mean MMSE by almost 2 points was observed; the scores for each component of the MMSE (i.e., orientation, attention, recall, total verbal and language) also declined significantly, with the exception of registration. Whilst all participants had a MMSE score within the normal range at baseline (i.e., according to the inclusion criteria), 12% had a score indicative of mild cognitive impairment (MMSE range 18–24) at the time of follow-up. Overall, the average decrease in MMSE score per year was 0.42 ± 0.56; but some participants 42 (27%) had a greater than expected rate of cognitive decline (i.e., decrease in MMSE score > 0.56 points per year; [38].

Table 2. Cognitive Characteristics of healthy older adults at initial examination and after 4-year follow-up (n = 155).

	Initial Assessment	Follow-Up Assessment	p-Value
Age	69.5 (7.2)	73.4 (7.1)	<0.001
Cognitive Function Score			
MMSE Total Score	29.1 (1.3)	27.5 (2.4)	<0.001
Orientation	9.9 (0.3)	9.8 (0.7)	0.014
Registration	3.0 (0.1)	3.0 (0.1)	0.565
Attention	4.7 (0.7)	4.4 (1.1)	0.004
Recall	2.7 (0.6)	1.8 (1.0)	<0.001
Total Verbal	20.3 (1.1)	19.0 (2.0)	<0.001
Language	8.8 (0.5)	8.5 (0.8)	<0.001
Impaired Cognition n (%) *	0 (0)	19 (12)	

Data presented as mean (standard deviation) unless otherwise indicated. * Impaired cognition defined as an MMSE score <25 [30]. Differences between the two time points were assessed using a paired t-test. $p \leq 0.05$ considered statistically significant. Abbreviations: MMSE, Mini mental state examination.

The influence of several lifestyle factors, B-vitamin dietary intake and B-vitamin biomarker status, as determinants of rate of cognitive decline are shown in Table 3. Of the general health and lifestyle factors examined only age and baseline MMSE score were predictive of cognitive decline. In addition, after adjustment for age and baseline MMSE score, no associations were observed between disease history (CVD, diabetes and gastrointestinal; data not shown) or medication use with the exception of use of analgesic medication ($p = 0.035$; data not shown). Vitamin B6 was found to be the only B-vitamin that was predictive of cognitive decline. After adjustment for age and baseline MMSE score, individuals with lower vitamin B6 biomarker status (PLP range $\leq$ 43.3 nmol/L; $p = 0.002$) or lower dietary B6 intakes (0.9–1.4 mg/day; $p = 0.018$) were at a 3.5–4 fold greater risk of cognitive decline. None of the other B vitamins or plasma homocysteine concentrations were associated with the risk of cognitive decline in this cohort.

Table 3. Lifestyle factors, B-vitamin dietary intake and B-vitamin biomarker status as predictors of cognitive decline in older adults.

	Range	Odds Ratio	95% CI	p-Value
Age		1.11	(1.05–1.16)	<0.001
Female Gender		0.69	(0.34–1.41)	0.310
BMI		1.04	(0.95–1.13)	0.410
Smoking		2.82	(0.55–14.56)	0.216
MTHFR TT genotype		1.82	(0.56–5.93)	0.318
Secondary level education		1.37	(0.62–3.03)	0.434
Depression		0.40	(0.08–2.18)	0.293
B-Vitamin Biomarker Status				
Low folate status (RBC Folate) *	(191–719 nmol/L)	1.81	(0.83–3.91)	0.134
Low vitamin B12 (serum total B12) *	(118–231 pmol/L)	1.14	(0.52–2.49)	0.750
Low vitamin B6 (PLP) *	(15.4–42.9 nmol/L)	3.49	(1.60–7.62)	0.002
Low riboflavin status (EGRAC) [†]	$\geq$1.3	1.01	(0.48–2.15)	0.972
High homocysteine	(12.6–25.4 µmol/L)	1.50	(0.58–3.85)	0.402
B-Vitamin Dietary Intake [‡]				
Low Folate intake	(124–166 µg/day)	2.55	(0.78–8.41)	0.123
Low vitamin B12 intake	(1.2–1.8 µg/day)	1.04	(0.29–3.78)	0.949
Low vitamin B6 intake	(0.9–1.4 mg/day)	4.08	(1.24–13.50)	0.021
Low riboflavin intake	0.6–1.0 mg/day)	0.41	(0.13–1.32)	0.136

Logistic regression was performed to determine predictors of cognitive decline (defined as a decrease in MMSE $\geq$ 0.56 points/year). The reference category for the lifestyle variables were as follows; sex, male gender; education, 3rd level; depression, no history; MTHFR 677 genotype, MTHFR 677 CC and CT genotype combined. * 'Low' B-vitamin status (with the exception of riboflavin) was defined as the bottom tertile of biomarkers; the reference category was the top two tertiles. [†] 'Low' riboflavin was defined by established cut-off values for EGRAC (low $\geq$1.3), the reference category was EGRAC < 1.3. [‡] 'Low' dietary intakes were identified by the bottom 10% of intake for each nutrient, the reference category was the remaining intake. Abbreviations: BMI, body mass index; MTHFR, methylenetetrahydrofolate; RCF, red cell folate; PLP, Pyridoxal-5-phosphate; EGRAC, Erythrocyte glutathione reductase activation coefficient.

4. Discussion

This study in healthy older adults, initially with normal cognitive performance, indicates that vitamin B6 is an important predictor of cognitive decline in ageing. Lower dietary intake and biomarker status of vitamin B6 were associated with a greater rate of cognitive decline over a subsequent 4 years follow-up period. No significant association of dietary intake or biomarker status with cognitive decline were observed for the other B-vitamins (folate, vitamin B12 and riboflavin). To our knowledge, this is the first longitudinal study to consider the impact of both dietary intake and biomarker status of all four relevant B-vitamins involved in one-carbon metabolism on cognitive health in ageing.

Whilst the influence of vitamin B6 on cognition has not been as fully investigated as folate and vitamin B12 a number of studies have reported observations consistent with the current study. Our results showed that participants with lower status of vitamin B6 (PLP; the measure of active vitamin B6) at baseline were 3.5 times more likely to have a greater rate of cognitive decline over a 4 years follow-up period. Furthermore, the association between vitamin B6 and cognitive decline was not confined to those with clinical deficiency, lower status included individuals in both the deficient (PLP < 30 nmol/L) and sufficient range (PLP 30–43 nmol/L) which would suggest that optimal vitamin B6 may be important for cognitive health in ageing. Consistent with the biomarker data, those with lower dietary intakes of vitamin B6 at baseline were 4 times more likely to have a greater rate of cognitive decline over the 4 years time period. Our results are in good agreement with findings from other studies, low vitamin B6 status (PLP < 46 nmol/L) and corresponding dietary intakes were previously associated with cognitive decline over a 3 years period in the Veteran Affairs Normative Ageing Study [40]. There is also evidence from several cross-sectional studies to support an association between low vitamin B6 and cognitive dysfunction [9,17,41,42] and Alzheimer's disease [43,44]. Furthermore, vitamin B6 status was associated with cognitive performance in high functioning older adults at baseline, though not with cognitive decline over the 7 years follow-up period in the MacArthur study of Successful Ageing [8]. Certain other studies have failed to detect any significant association between vitamin B6 and cognitive function, however, these studies have relied on dietary intake measures alone with no corresponding measurement of blood biomarker status [45–47]. Few RCTs have investigated the independent effect of vitamin B6 on cognitive function and only one very early study reported beneficial effects of vitamin B6 supplementation on memory [19]. Subsequent RCTs have investigated the effect of vitamin B6 in combination with folate and vitamin B12, with some studies reporting beneficial effects on cognitive function however the independent effect of vitamin B6 cannot be determined [18,20].

Whilst elevated plasma homocysteine, low folate and, to a lesser extent, vitamin B12 status have been frequently associated with cognitive decline [11–15,48] there was no evidence of significant associations for these biomarkers in the current study. A number of other studies have reported similar findings [49–52]. The findings in the current study may be explained to some degree by the fact that vitamin B6 seemed to be the limiting nutrient within the cohort. There was a greater incidence of deficiency of vitamin B6 (11% clinical deficiency) compared with folate (3%) or vitamin B12 (0%). Also, the lack of a significant association between cognitive decline and plasma homocysteine concentration is almost certainly is a reflection of the low prevalence of folate deficiency. Furthermore, the concept that the association between B-vitamin status and cognition is determined by the limiting nutrient within that population group is further supported by evidence from published RCTs. One trial of healthy older adults in New Zealand reported no benefit of combined B-vitamin supplementation on cognitive function [21], whereas another similar study from the Netherlands showed that supplementation with folic acid significantly improved cognitive performance [18]. A notable difference between these two studies was that baseline folate status tended to be far lower in the Dutch trial, suggesting that the cognitive benefit related to the correction of sub-optimal B-vitamin status whereas additional B-vitamins to an already optimal population may have no beneficial effect.

The mechanism linking vitamin B6 with cognitive health in this and other studies in ageing is not clear however, it is biologically plausible given the widespread functions of vitamin B6 within the brain and nervous system [53,54]. Vitamin B6 has a crucial role in the synthesis of a variety of neurotransmitters including dopamine and serotonin [55] and can act as a potent antioxidant [56,57]. In addition, higher vitamin B6 intakes have been associated with greater grey matter volume [58] and combined B-vitamin supplementation (including vitamin B6) has been shown to slow brain atrophy, an important feature cognitive dysfunction [27].

The current study has a number of strengths and limitations that merit comment. To our knowledge, this is the first longitudinal study to investigate the association between cognitive decline and all relevant B-vitamins along with their corresponding dietary intakes. The MMSE is the most widely used screening tools for cognitive dysfunction and although it has been criticised for lacking sensitivity, few previous studies have used it to measure cognitive change in a healthy older population. However, a meta-analysis reported a mean decline in MMSE of between 0.16 and 0.56 points per year in cognitively healthy people which compares favourably to the overall rate of decline observed in this study (mean 0.39 points per year) [38]. In addition, the rate of decline observed in this study was identical to that observed in the Rotterdam Study of community dwelling older adults free from cognitive impairment [59]. While the use of the MMSE may be perceived as a limiting factor in the current study, it could be argued that its use would only attenuate the associations observed and that the use of more sensitive tools would have, if anything, detected more subtle differences thus strengthening the results. Another well-recognised limitation of longitudinal studies of this kind is that individuals with the greatest decline in cognitive function are more likely to be lost to follow-up [60]. Indeed, in this study the non-participants were more likely to be older but any non-response bias would ultimately underestimate the associations between baseline B-vitamin status and cognitive decline and this could not have influenced the current findings.

5. Conclusions

In conclusion, vitamin B6 may be an important (often overlooked) protective factor in helping maintain cognitive health in ageing, especially in a folate and vitamin B12 replete population. Lower vitamin B6 status (as assessed by both dietary intake and biomarker status) at baseline predicted a greater than expected rate of cognitive decline over a 4-year period in healthy free living older adults. These findings are important because optimising vitamin B6 status in older people, through the use of fortified foods or supplements, may have a positive impact on cognition in ageing. Further research in this area in the form of well-designed randomised controlled trials targeted at populations with sub-optimal status are required in order to confirm a cause and effect relationship between B-vitamin status and cognitive health in ageing.

Acknowledgments: This research was part funded by a grant from the United Kingdom Food Standards Agency (Project No. N0505042) and Northern Ireland Department for Employment and Learning (DEL; PhD studentship Catherine F Hughes).

Author Contributions: H.M., M.W. and K.P. conceived and designed the experiments; L.H. and C.F.H. performed the experiments; C.F.H. analyzed the data; F.T. provided cognitive assessment training; C.F.H., H.M., M.W. and L.H. wrote the paper. Authorship must be limited to those who have contributed substantially to the work reported.

Abbreviations

MMSE	Mini-mental state examination
HoloTC	Holotranscobalamin—functional indicator of metabolically active fraction of vitamin B12
MMA	methymalonic acid—an indicator of vitamin B12 status, a higher MMA status indicates a lower vitamin B12 status
PLP	Pyridoxal-5-phosphate—a measure of vitamin B6 status
EGRAC	Erythrocyte glutathione reductase activation coefficient—a functional indicator of riboflavin status, a higher ratio indicates a lower riboflavin status

Appendix A

Table A1. A comparison of baseline characteristics between participants and non-participants (i.e., those lost to follow-up).

	Participants ($n = 155$)	Non-Participants ($n = 100$)	p-Value
General Characteristics			
Age (years)	69.5 (7.3)	72.2 (8.1)	0.007
Male n (%)	60 (39)	34 (34)	0.530
BMI (kg/m^2)	27.5 (4.2)	27.3 (3.5)	0.981
Smokers n (%)	6 (4)	5 (5)	
Cognitive Function Score			
MMSE Total Score	29.1 (1.3)	28.7 (1.4)	0.093
Orientation	9.9 (0.3)	9.8 (0.5)	0.140
Registration	3.0 (0.1)	3.0 (0.1)	0.273
Attention	4.7 (0.7)	4.6 (0.9)	0.243
Recall	2.7 (0.6)	2.6 (0.6)	0.825
Total Verbal	20.0 (1.1)	20.0 (1.2)	0.263
Language	8.8 (0.5)	8.6 (0.6)	0.094
B-vitamin Biomarker Status			
Red blood cell folate (nmol/L)	954 (410)	851 (359)	0.080
Serum total vitamin B12 (pmol/L)	282 (106)	257 (127)	0.013
Serum HoloTC (pmol/L)	50.8 (24.3)	47.1 (28.8)	0.381
Serum MMA (μmol/L)	0.24 (0.19)	0.36 (0.56)	0.035
Vitamin B6 (Plasma PLP; nmol/L)	58.4 (25.8)	54.3 (22.9)	0.314
Riboflavin (EGRAC)	1.33 (0.14)	1.34 (0.15)	0.387
Plasma total homocysteine (μmol/L)	12.0 (3.7)	13.1 (4.4)	0.117
Gastric Function			
Pepsinogen I (μg/L)	126.8 (70.8)	135.3 (78.2)	0.515
Pepsinogen Ratio^2	8.4 (6.7)	8.0 (6.6)	0.713

Values represented as mean (SD). Differences in baseline characteristics between those that participated in the 4-year follow-up and those that did not participate in the follow-up were compared using one-way ANCOVA with adjustment for age for continuous variables (on log transformed data were appropriate). Differences in categorical variables were assessed using Chi-squared analysis. $p < 0.05$ was significant.

References

1. McKhann, G.M.; Knopman, D.S.; Chertkow, H.; Hyman, B.T.; Jack, C.R., Jr.; Kawas, C.H.; Klunk, W.E.; Koroshetz, W.J.; Manly, J.J.; Mayeux, R.; et al. The diagnosis of dementia due to Alzheimer's disease: Recommendations from the national institute on Aging-Alzheimer's association workgroups on diagnostic guidelines for Alzheimer's disease. *Alzheimers Dement.* **2011**, *7*, 263–269. [CrossRef] [PubMed]
2. Gauthier, S.; Reisberg, B.; Zaudig, M.; Petersen, R.C.; Ritchie, K.; Broich, K.; Belleville, S.; Brodaty, H.; Bennett, D.; Chertkow, H.; et al. Mild cognitive impairment. *Lancet* **2006**, *367*, 1262–1270. [CrossRef]
3. Alzheimer's Disease International. *World Alzheimer Report 2015 the Global Impact of Dementia an Analysis of Prevalence, Incidence, Cost & Trends*; Alzheimer's Disease International (ADI): London, UK, 2015.
4. Morris, M.S. The role of B vitamins in preventing and treating cognitive impairment and decline. *Adv. Nutr.* **2012**, *3*, 801–812. [CrossRef] [PubMed]
5. Clarke, R.; Smith, A.; Jobst, K.A.; Refsum, H.; Sutton, L.; Ueland, P.M. Folate, vitamin B12, and serum total homocysteine levels in confirmed Alzheimer disease. *Arch. Neurol.* **1998**, *55*, 1449–1455. [CrossRef] [PubMed]
6. Doets, E.L.; Ueland, P.M.; Tell, G.S.; Vollset, S.E.; Nygård, O.K.; van't Veer, P.; de Groot, L.C.P.G.M.; Nurk, E.; Refsum, H.; Smith, A.D.; et al. Interactions between plasma concentrations of folate and markers of vitamin B12 status with cognitive performance in elderly people not exposed to folic acid fortification: The hordaland health study. *Br. J. Nutr.* **2014**, *111*, 1085–1095. [CrossRef] [PubMed]
7. Ford, A.H.; Flicker, L.; Singh, U.; Hirani, V.; Almeida, O.P. Homocysteine, depression and cognitive function in older adults. *J. Affect. Disord.* **2013**, *151*, 646–651. [CrossRef] [PubMed]

8.   Kado, D.M.; Karlamangla, A.S.; Huang, M.-H.; Troen, A.; Rowe, J.W.; Selhub, J.; Seeman, T.E. Homocysteine versus the vitamins folate, B6, and B12 as predictors of cognitive function and decline in older high-functioning adults: Macarthur studies of successful aging. *Am. J. Med.* **2005**, *118*, 161–167. [CrossRef] [PubMed]

9.   Moorthy, D.; Peter, I.; Scott, T.M.; Parnell, L.D.; Lai, C.-Q.; Crott, J.W.; Ordovás, J.M.; Selhub, J.; Griffith, J.; Rosenberg, I.H.; et al. Status of vitamins B-12 and B-6 but not of folate, homocysteine, and the methylenetetrahydrofolate reductase C677T polymorphism are associated with impaired cognition and depression in adults. *J. Nutr.* **2012**, *142*, 1554–1560. [CrossRef] [PubMed]

10. McCaddon, A.; Davies, G.; Hudson, P.; Tandy, S.; Cattell, H. Total serum homocysteine in senile dementia of Alzheimer type. *Int. J. Geriatr. Psychiatry* **1998**, *13*, 235–239. [CrossRef]

11. Blasko, I.; Hinterberger, M.; Kemmler, G.; Jungwirth, S.; Krampla, W.; Leitha, T.; Heinz Tragl, K.; Fischer, P. Conversion from mild cognitive impairment to dementia: Influence of folic acid and vitamin B12 use in the vita cohort. *J. Nutr. Health Aging* **2012**, *16*, 687–694. [CrossRef] [PubMed]

12. Haan, M.N.; Miller, J.W.; Aiello, A.E.; Whitmer, R.A.; Jagust, W.J.; Mungas, D.M.; Allen, L.H.; Green, R. Homocysteine, B vitamins, and the incidence of dementia and cognitive impairment: Results from the sacramento area latino study on aging. *Am. J. Clin. Nutr.* **2007**, *85*, 511–517. [PubMed]

13. Hooshmand, B.; Solomon, A.; Kareholt, I.; Rusanen, M.; Hanninen, T.; Leiviska, J.; Winblad, B.; Laatikainen, T.; Soininen, H.; Kivipelto, M. Associations between serum homocysteine, holotranscobalamin, folate and cognition in the elderly: A longitudinal study. *J. Intern. Med.* **2012**, *271*, 204–212. [CrossRef] [PubMed]

14. Zylberstein, D.E.; Lissner, L.; Björkelund, C.; Mehlig, K.; Thelle, D.S.; Gustafson, D.; Östling, S.; Waern, M.; Guo, X.; Skoog, I. Midlife homocysteine and late-life dementia in women. A prospective population study. *Neurobiol. Aging* **2011**, *32*, 380–386. [CrossRef] [PubMed]

15. Clarke, R.; Birks, J.; Nexo, E.; Ueland, P.M.; Schneede, J.; Scott, J.; Molloy, A.; Evans, J.G. Low vitamin B-12 status and risk of cognitive decline in older adults. *Am. J. Clin. Nutr.* **2007**, *86*, 1384–1391. [PubMed]

16. Morris, M.S.; Selhub, J.; Jacques, P.F. Vitamin B-12 and folate status in relation to decline in scores on the mini-mental state examination in the framingham heart study. *J. Am. Geriatr. Soc.* **2012**, *60*, 1457–1464. [CrossRef] [PubMed]

17. Riggs, K.M.; Spiro, A.; Tucker, K.; Rush, D. Relations of vitamin B-12, vitamin B-6, folate, and homocysteine to cognitive performance in the normative aging study. *Am. J. Clin. Nutr.* **1996**, *63*, 306–314. [PubMed]

18. Durga, J.; van Boxtel, M.P.J.; Schouten, E.G.; Kok, F.J.; Jolles, J.; Katan, M.B.; Verhoef, P. Effect of 3-year folic acid supplementation on cognitive function in older adults in the facit trial: A randomised, double blind, controlled trial. *Lancet* **2007**, *369*, 208–216. [CrossRef]

19. Deijen, J.B.; Beek, E.J.; Orlebeke, J.F.; Berg, H. Vitamin B-6 supplementation in elderly men: Effects on mood, memory, performance and mental effort. *Psychopharmacology* **1992**, *109*, 489–496. [CrossRef] [PubMed]

20. De Jager, C.A.; Oulhaj, A.; Jacoby, R.; Refsum, H.; Smith, A.D. Cognitive and clinical outcomes of homocysteine-lowering B-vitamin treatment in mild cognitive impairment: A randomized controlled trial. *Int. J. Geriatr. Psychiatry* **2012**, *27*, 592–600. [CrossRef] [PubMed]

21. McMahon, J.A.; Green, T.J.; Skeaff, C.M.; Knight, R.G.; Mann, J.I.; Williams, S.M. A controlled trial of homocysteine lowering and cognitive performance. *N. Engl. J. Med.* **2006**, *354*, 2764–2772. [CrossRef] [PubMed]

22. Ford, A.H.; Flicker, L.; Alfonso, H.; Thomas, J.; Clarnette, R.; Martins, R.; Almeida, O.P. Vitamins B12, B6, and folic acid for cognition in older men. *Neurology* **2010**, *75*, 1540–1547. [CrossRef] [PubMed]

23. Van der Zwaluw, N.L.; Dhonukshe-Rutten, R.A.M.; van Wijngaarden, J.P.; Brouwer-Brolsma, E.M.; van de Rest, O.; In 't Veld, P.H.; Enneman, A.W.; van Dijk, S.C.; Ham, A.C.; Swart, K.M.A.; et al. Results of 2-year vitamin B treatment on cognitive performance: Secondary data from an RCT. *Neurology* **2014**, *83*, 2158–2166. [CrossRef] [PubMed]

24. Wald, D.S.; Kasturiratne, A.; Simmonds, M. Effect of folic acid, with or without other B vitamins, on cognitive decline: Meta-analysis of randomized trials. *Am. J. Med.* **2010**, *123*, 522–527. [CrossRef] [PubMed]

25. Ford, A.H.; Almeida, O.P. Effect of homocysteine lowering treatment on cognitive function: A systematic review and meta-analysis of randomized controlled trials. *J. Alzheimers Dis.* **2012**, *29*, 133–149. [PubMed]

26. McGarel, C.; Pentieva, K.; Strain, J.J.; McNulty, H. Emerging roles for folate and related B-vitamins in brain health across the lifecycle. *Proc. Nutr. Soc.* **2015**, *74*, 46–55. [CrossRef] [PubMed]

27. Smith, A.D.; Smith, S.M.; de Jager, C.A.; Whitbread, P.; Johnston, C.; Agacinski, G.; Oulhaj, A.; Bradley, K.M.; Jacoby, R.; Refsum, H. Homocysteine-lowering by B vitamins slows the rate of accelerated brain atrophy in mild cognitive impairment: A randomized controlled trial. *PLoS ONE* **2010**, *5*, e12244. [CrossRef] [PubMed]

28. Douaud, G.; Refsum, H.; de Jager, C.A.; Jacoby, R.; Nichols, T.E.; Smith, S.M.; Smith, A.D. Preventing Alzheimer's disease-related gray matter atrophy by B-vitamin treatment. *Proc. Natl. Acad. Sci. USA* **2013**, *110*, 9523–9528. [CrossRef] [PubMed]

29. Hoey, L.; McNulty, H.; Askin, N.; Dunne, A.; Ward, M.; Pentieva, K.; Strain, J.; Molloy, A.M.; Flynn, C.A.; Scott, J.M. Effect of a voluntary food fortification policy on folate, related B vitamin status, and homocysteine in healthy adults. *Am. J. Clin. Nutr.* **2007**, *86*, 1405–1413. [PubMed]

30. Folstein, M.F.; Folstein, S.E.; McHugh, P.R. "Mini-mental state": A practical method for grading the cognitive state of patients for the clinician. *J. Psychiatr. Res.* **1975**, *12*, 189–198. [CrossRef]

31. Food Standards Agency. *Food Portion Sizes*, 3rd ed.Mills, A., Patel, S., Crawley, H., Eds.; Stationery Office Books: London, UK, 2002.

32. Leino, A. Fully automated measurement of total homocysteine in plasma and serum on the Abbott iMx analyzer. *Clin. Chem.* **1999**, *45*, 569–570. [PubMed]

33. Molloy, A.M.; Scott, J.M. Microbiological assay for serum, plasma, and red cell folate using cryopreserved, microtiter plate method. In *Methods in Enzymology*; Academic Press: Cambridge, MA, USA, 1997; Volume 281, pp. 43–53.

34. Kelleher, B.P.; Broin, S.D. Microbiological assay for vitamin B12 performed in 96-well microtitre plates. *J. Clin. Pathol.* **1991**, *44*, 592–595. [CrossRef] [PubMed]

35. Bates, C.J.; Pentieva, K.D.; Matthews, N.; Macdonald, A. A simple, sensitive and reproducible assay for pyridoxal 5′-phosphate and 4-pyridoxic acid in human plasma. *Clin. Chim. Acta* **1999**, *280*, 101–111. [CrossRef]

36. Powers, H.J.; Bates, C.J.; Prentice, A.M.; Lamb, W.H.; Jepson, M.; Bowman, H. The relative effectiveness of iron and iron with riboflavin in correcting a microcytic anaemia in men and children in rural Gambia. *Hum. Nutr. Clin. Nutr.* **1983**, *37*, 413–425. [PubMed]

37. Frosst, P.; Blom, H.J.; Milos, R.; Goyette, P.; Sheppard, C.A.; Matthews, R.G.; Boers, G.J.; den Heijer, M.; Kluijtmans, L.A.; van den Heuvel, L.P.; et al. A candidate genetic risk factor for vascular disease: A common mutation in methylenetetrahydrofolate reductase. *Nat. Genet.* **1995**, *10*, 111–113. [CrossRef] [PubMed]

38. Park, H.L.; O'Connell, J.E.; Thomson, R.G. A systematic review of cognitive decline in the general elderly population. *Int. J. Geriatr. Psychiatry* **2003**, *18*, 1121–1134. [CrossRef] [PubMed]

39. Britain, G. *Dietary Reference Values for Food Energy and Nutrients for the United Kingdom: Report of the Panel on Dietary Reference Values of the Committee on Medical Aspects of Food Policy*; Reports of Health and Social Subjects; Stationery Office Books: London, UK, 1991.

40. Tucker, K.L.; Qiao, N.; Scott, T.; Rosenberg, I.; Spiro, A. High homocysteine and low B vitamins predict cognitive decline in aging men: The veterans affairs normative aging study. *Am. J. Clin. Nutr.* **2005**, *82*, 627–635. [PubMed]

41. Bryan, J.; Calvaresi, E.; Hughes, D. Short-term folate, vitamin B-12 or vitamin B-6 supplementation slightly affects memory performance but not mood in women of various ages. *J. Nutr.* **2002**, *132*, 1345–1356. [PubMed]

42. Kim, H.; Kim, G.; Jang, W.; Kim, S.Y.; Chang, N. Association between intake of B vitamins and cognitive function in elderly Koreans with cognitive impairment. *Nutr. J.* **2014**, *13*, 118. [CrossRef] [PubMed]

43. Luchsinger, J.A.; Tang, M.; Miller, J.; Green, R.; Mayeux, R. Relation of higher folate intake to lower risk of Alzheimer disease in the elderly. *Arch. Neurol.* **2007**, *64*, 86–92. [CrossRef] [PubMed]

44. Miller, J.W.; Green, R.; Mungas, D.M.; Reed, B.R.; Jagust, W.J. Homocysteine, vitamin B6, and vascular disease in ad patients. *Neurology* **2002**, *58*, 1471–1475. [CrossRef] [PubMed]

45. Agnew-Blais, J.C.; Wassertheil-Smoller, S.; Kang, J.H.; Hogan, P.E.; Coker, L.H.; Snetselaar, L.G.; Smoller, J.W. Folate, vitamin B6 and vitamin B12 intake and mild cognitive impairment and probable dementia in the women's health initiative memory study. *J. Acad. Nutr. Diet.* **2015**, *115*, 231–241. [CrossRef] [PubMed]

46. Nelson, C.; Wengreen, H.J.; Munger, R.G.; Corcoran, C.D.; The Cache County Investigators. Dietary folate, vitamin B-12, vitamin B-6 and incident Alzheimer's disease: The cache county memory, health, and aging study. *J. Nutr. Health Aging* **2009**, *13*, 899–905. [CrossRef] [PubMed]

47. Vercambre, M.-N.; Boutron-Ruault, M.-C.; Ritchie, K.; Clavel-Chapelon, F.; Berr, C. Long-term association of food and nutrient intakes with cognitive and functional decline: A 13-year follow-up study of elderly french women. *Br. J. Nutr.* **2009**, *102*, 419–427. [CrossRef] [PubMed]

48. Seshadri, S.; Beiser, A.; Selhub, J.; Jacques, P.F.; Rosenberg, I.H.; D'Agostino, R.B.; Wilson, P.W.F.; Wolf, P.A. Plasma homocysteine as a risk factor for dementia and Alzheimer's disease. *N. Engl. J. Med.* **2002**, *346*, 476–483. [CrossRef] [PubMed]

49. Eussen, S.J.; de Groot, L.C.; Joosten, L.W.; Bloo, R.J.; Clarke, R.; Ueland, P.M.; Schneede, J.; Blom, H.J.; Hoefnagels, W.H.; van Staveren, W.A. Effect of oral vitamin B-12 with or without folic acid on cognitive function in older people with mild vitamin B-12 deficiency: A randomized, placebo-controlled trial. *Am. J. Clin. Nutr.* **2006**, *84*, 361–370. [PubMed]

50. Mooijaart, S.P.; Gussekloo, J.; Frölich, M.; Jolles, J.; Stott, D.J.; Westendorp, R.G.; de Craen, A.J. Homocysteine, vitamin B-12, and folic acid and the risk of cognitive decline in old age: The leiden 85-plus study. *Am. J. Clin. Nutr.* **2005**, *82*, 866–871. [PubMed]

51. Kalmijn, S.; Launer, L.J.; Lindemans, J.; Bots, M.L.; Hofman, A.; Breteler, M.M.B. Total homocysteine and cognitive decline in a community-based sample of elderly subjects: The rotterdam study. *Am. J. Epidemiol.* **1999**, *150*, 283–289. [CrossRef] [PubMed]

52. Ravaglia, G.; Forti, P.; Maioli, F.; Vettori, C.; Grossi, G.; Mario Bargossi, A.; Caldarera, M.; Franceschi, C.; Facchini, A.; Mariani, E.; et al. Elevated plasma homocysteine levels in centenarians are not associated with cognitive impairment. *Mech. Ageing Dev.* **2001**, *121*, 251–261. [CrossRef]

53. Guilarte, T.R. Vitamin B6 and cognitive development: Recent research findings from human and animal studies. *Nutr. Rev.* **1993**, *51*, 193–198. [CrossRef] [PubMed]

54. Wei, I.-L.; Huang, Y.-H.; Wang, G.-S. Vitamin B6 deficiency decreases the glucose utilization in cognitive brain structures of rats. *J. Nutr. Biochem.* **1999**, *10*, 525–531. [CrossRef]

55. Karlsson, I. Neurotransmitter changes in aging and dementia. *Nord. J. Psychiatry* **1993**, *47*, 41–44. [CrossRef]

56. Kannan, K.; Jain, S.K. Effect of vitamin B6 on oxygen radicals, mitochondrial membrane potential, and lipid peroxidation in H_2O_2-treated U937 monocytes. *Free Radic. Biol. Med.* **2004**, *36*, 423–428. [CrossRef] [PubMed]

57. Shen, J.; Lai, C.-Q.; Mattei, J.; Ordovas, J.M.; Tucker, K.L. Association of vitamin B-6 status with inflammation, oxidative stress, and chronic inflammatory conditions: The boston puerto rican health study. *Am. J. Clin. Nutr.* **2010**, *91*, 337–342. [CrossRef] [PubMed]

58. Erickson, K.I.; Suever, B.L.; Prakash, R.S.; Colcombe, S.J.; McAuley, E.; Kramer, A.F. Greater intake of vitamins B6 and B12 spares gray matter in healthy elderly: A voxel-based morphometry study. *Brain Res.* **2008**, *1199*, 20–26. [CrossRef] [PubMed]

59. Zhu, L.; Viitanen, M.; Guo, Z.; Winblad, B.; Fratiglioni, L. Blood pressure reduction, cardiovascular diseases, and cognitive decline in the mini-mental state examination in a community population of normal very old people: A three-year follow-up. *J. Clin. Epidemiol.* **1998**, *51*, 385–391. [CrossRef]

60. Lindeboom, J.; Weinstein, H. Neuropsychology of cognitive ageing, minimal cognitive impairment, Alzheimer's disease, and vascular cognitive impairment. *Eur. J. Pharmacol.* **2004**, *490*, 83–86. [CrossRef] [PubMed]

10

Excess Folic Acid Increases Lipid Storage, Weight Gain and Adipose Tissue Inflammation in High Fat Diet-Fed Rats

Karen B. Kelly [1]**, John P. Kennelly** [1]**, Marta Ordonez** [2]**, Randal Nelson** [1]**, Kelly Leonard** [1]**, Sally Stabler** [3]**, Antonio Gomez-Muñoz** [2]**, Catherine J. Field** [1] **and René L. Jacobs** [1,4,*]

[1]   Department of Agricultural, Food & Nutritional Science, University of Alberta, Edmonton, AB T6G2P5, Canada; kkelly1@ualberta.ca (K.B.K.); jkennell@ualberta.ca (J.P.K.); rn1@ualberta.ca (R.N.); kmd4@ualberta.ca (K.L.); cjfield@ualberta.ca (C.J.F.)

[2]   Department of Biochemistry and Molecular Biology, Faculty of Science and Technology, University of the Basque Country (UPV/EHU), Bilbao 48080, Spain; marta.ordonez87@gmail.com (M.O.); antonio.gomez@ehu.es (A.G.-M.)

[3]   Department of Medicine, University of Colorado School of Medicine, Aurora, CO 80206, USA; Sally.Stabler@ucdenver.edu

[4]   Department of Biochemistry, University of Alberta, Edmonton, AB T6G2R7, Canada

*   Correspondence: rjacobs@ualberta.ca

Abstract: Folic acid intake has increased to high levels in many countries, raising concerns about possible adverse effects, including disturbances to energy and lipid metabolism. Our aim was to investigate the effects of excess folic acid (EFA) intake compared to adequate folic acid (AFA) intake on metabolic health in a rodent model. We conducted these investigations in the setting of either a 15% energy low fat (LF) diet or 60% energy high fat (HF) diet. There was no difference in weight gain, fat mass, or glucose tolerance in EFA-fed rats compared to AFA-fed rats when they were fed a LF diet. However, rats fed EFA in combination with a HF diet had significantly greater weight gain and fat mass compared to rats fed AFA ($p < 0.05$). Gene expression analysis showed increased mRNA levels of peroxisome proliferator-activated receptor γ (PPARγ) and some of its target genes in adipose tissue of high fat-excess folic acid (HF-EFA) fed rats. Inflammation was increased in HF-EFA fed rats, associated with impaired glucose tolerance compared to high fat-adequate folic acid (HF-AFA) fed rats ($p < 0.05$). In addition, folic acid induced PPARγ expression and triglyceride accumulation in 3T3-L1 cells. Our results suggest that excess folic acid may exacerbate weight gain, fat accumulation, and inflammation caused by consumption of a HF diet.

Keywords: folic acid; obesity; metabolic syndrome; adipose tissue

---

1. Introduction

The metabolic syndrome, which encompasses excess abdominal adiposity, insulin resistance, dyslipidaemia, and hypertension, represents the largest public health challenge in developed countries [1]. The rise in metabolic syndrome prevalence in recent decades has been mirrored by changes in dietary patterns, reflecting increased nutrient availability [2]. Diets rich in fat and rapidly-digestible carbohydrates have increased total energy intake [2]. At the same time, fortification of staple foods and widespread supplement use has increased folic acid intake in many Western countries, placing importance on investigations into possible adverse effects [3].

Folates are a family of structurally-similar compounds involved in the transfer of one-carbon units for the production of nucleotides used in DNA synthesis; for the methylation of a variety of biological substrates; and for cell division [4]. These functions make folates especially important during the anabolic stages of foetal and childhood development [4]. Sources of natural folates (pteroylpolyglutamates) include green leafy vegetables, orange juice and legumes [4]. Folic acid (monoglutamate) is a synthetic member of the folate family commonly used in fortified foods and supplements due to its stability and low cost [4]. The current Recommended Daily Allowance (RDA) for folate is 400 μg Dietary Folate Equivalents (DFEs)/day for the general adult population [5]. While mandatory folic acid fortification of grains since 1998 has reduced the incidence of neural tube defects (NTDs) and other developmental disorders in Canada and the USA, population-wide intake of folic acid has increased to unprecedented levels, leading to concern that there may be adverse consequences [3,6,7]. Children and elderly populations are likely to have high folic acid intake because large proportions of their diet typically consist of cereals and bread [3]; while pregnant women are likely to have high intakes due to high supplement use [8]. High folic acid intake by women planning pregnancy is prevalent in many countries, including countries without mandatory folic acid fortification, due to worldwide recommendations for this population to consume 400 μg/day folic acid for the prevention of neural tube defects [9,10]. Human observational evidence has linked high folic acid intake to increased risk of colorectal and prostate cancer [11,12]; impaired immune function [13,14], and impaired cognition [15]. Further observational evidence has linked folate status to obesity, sparking investigations into the relationship between folic acid intake and lipid and energy metabolism [16,17].

Maternal excess folate [17,18] or methyl donor [19] intake during pregnancy in animal models causes weight gain or components of the metabolic syndrome in offspring. These effects may be more pronounced when offspring are fed a high fat diet [20,21]. In humans, high erythrocyte folate status during pregnancy was associated with increased fat mass of children at six years of age [22]. Folic acid appears to influence energy and lipid metabolism by modulating DNA methylation and gene expression patterns [17,18,23]. Diet-gene interactions remain important determinants of health throughout the lifespan [24], and so excess folic acid may continue to promote changes to energy and lipid metabolism in adulthood. However, the effects of excess folic acid intake on metabolic syndrome risk and adiposity in adulthood remains poorly understood.

The effects of excess dietary folic acid intake on the liver, an important site of both folate and lipid metabolism, have been investigated in rodent models [23,25]. Excess folic acid intake may promote changes to one carbon metabolic pathways and gene expression patterns, leading to liver injury [25]. There is evidence that the influence of methyl donors, including folic acid, on gene expression may be tissue-, site-, and gene-specific, and so investigations into the influence of excess folic acid on other tissues (e.g., adipose) are warranted [3].

The aim of our study was to investigate the effects of excess folic acid (EFA) intake compared to adequate folic acid (AFA) intake on metabolic health of rats. We hypothesized that consumption of a diet containing EFA would induce changes to lipid and glucose metabolism. High fat diets are commonly used to study weight gain and components of the metabolic syndrome in animal models. Therefore, we conducted our investigations in the setting of a 15% of energy low fat (LF) and a 60% of energy high fat (HF) diet. Our data suggest that EFA, in combination with a HF diet increases weight gain, adipose tissue mass and markers of inflammation compared to AFA, and that these effects are not seen in the setting of a LF diet. We conducted supporting experiments in vitro, the results of which suggest that folic acid can increase triglyceride accumulation in 3T3-L1 cells by inducing peroxisome proliferator-activated receptor γ (PPARγ).

2. Materials and Methods

2.1. Animals and Diets

All procedures were approved by the University of Alberta's Institutional Animal Care Committee (AUP00000175) in accordance with guidelines of the Canadian Council on Animal Care. All animals had free access to food and water and were housed on a 12-h light-dark cycle. The diet was supplied by Harlan Teklad, with basal diet formulations designed to AIN-93G specifications. In the first feeding trial, twelve eight-week old male Sprague–Dawley rats were fed a 15% of energy low fat diet with excess folic acid (7.5 mg/kg diet) or control levels of folic acid (0.75 mg/kg diet) (Table 1) [23]. In the second feeding trial, twelve rats were fed a 60% of energy high fat diet containing excess folic acid (7.5 mg/kg) or control levels of folic acid (0.75 mg/kg) (Table 1). Food intake and body weights were recorded three times weekly for the duration of the experiments. Food intake is reported as the average daily intake over the 12-week feeding period. During the eighth weeks of feeding, body composition was analyzed by magnetic resonance imaging (MRI). Animals were euthanized after 12 weeks on diet. Fasting blood was collected in ethylenediaminetetraacetic acid (EDTA)-coated vials by cardiac puncture and plasma was collected after centrifugation of blood at $3000 \times g$ for 10 min. Tissues were weighed and snap frozen in liquid nitrogen before being stored at -80 °C until analysis.

Table 1. Composition of diets (per kilogram diet).

Ingredients	LF-AFA	LF-EFA	HF-AFA	HF-EFA
Folic acid (mg)	0.75	7.5	0.75	7.5
L-cysteine (g)	3	3	4	4
Corn starch (g)	263.7	263.7	-	-
Sucrose (g)	209.7	209.7	106.3	106.3
Maltodextrin (g)	130	130	160	160
Soybean Oil (g)	60	60	30	30
Lard (g)	-	-	310	310
Cellulose (g)	50	50	20	20
Pectin (g)	50	50	50	50
Succinylsulphathiazole (g)	10	10	10	10
Vitamin-free casein (g)	195	195	265	265
Mineral Mix, AIN-93G (g)	35	35	48	48
Tertiary-Butylhydroquinone (mg)	12	12	3400	3400
Choline bitartrate (g)	2.5	2.5	3	3
Niacin (mg)	30	30	63	63
Calcium pantothenate (mg)	16	16	34	34
Pyridoxine HCl (μg)	7	7	15	15
Thiamin HCl (μg)	6	6	13	13
Riboflavin (mg)	6	6	13	13
Biotin (μg)	200	200	400	400
Vitamin B12 (μg)	25	25	40	40
DL-alpha tocopheryl acetate (500 IU/g) (mg)	150	150	315	315
Vitamin A palmitate (500,000 IU/g) (mg)	8	8	17	17
Cholecalciferol (500,000 IU/g) (mg)	2	2	4	4
Phylloquinone (μg)	800	800	1600	1600

2.2. Histological Analysis of Adipose and Liver Samples

Adipose tissue was collected, dehydrated, and embedded in paraffin. Cross-sections of tissue (5 μm) were prepared and stained with haematoxylin and eosin (H and E). Adipocyte size was estimated using ImageJ software, (the US National Institutes of Health, Bethesda, MD, USA).

2.3. Glucose Tolerance Tests

Eight weeks after initiation of the high fat diet (HFD) feeding trial, rats were fasted overnight before receiving 2 g/kg glucose by intraperitoneal (IP) injection. Blood samples were collected by tail vein bleeding at 15, 30, 60, 90, and 120 min.

2.4. Plasma Measurements

Plasma glucose and alanine aminotransferase (ALT) were measured using commercially available kits (WAKO Diagnostics (Mountain View, CA, USA) and Biotron (Diagnostic Inc., Hemet, CA, USA), respectively). Plasma insulin was measured by ELISA (ALPCO, Salem, NH, USA). Plasma levels of metabolites in the one carbon cycle, including folate, total homocysteine, methionine, cysteine, *N*,*N*-dimethylglycine, *N*-methylglycine, glycine, serine, cystathionine, α-aminobutyrate, were measured by capillary stable isotope dilution gas chromatography/mass spectrometry, as previously described [26]. Neutral lipids in plasma were quantified by gas-liquid chromatography as described previously [27], with tridecanoin as an internal standard.

2.5. Culture of 3T3L1 Adipocytes

3T3-L1 cells were cultured to confluence in Dulbecco's modified Eagle's medium (DMEM) supplemented with 10% (*v*/*v*) fetal bovine serum (FBS). At two days post-confluence (designated day 0), cells were induced to differentiate with DMEM supplemented with 10% (*v*/*v*) FBS, 1 μM dexamethasone, 0.5 mM isobutylmethylxanthine, 1 μg/mL insulin. Cells were incubated with 9 μM (standard level) or 20 μM (supplemented) folic acid. Differentiation media was refreshed daily. After 48 h, the media were replaced with DMEM supplemented with 10% FBS and 1 μg/mL insulin and the same level of folic acid that was used during differentiation. The cell media was refreshed every 24 following differentiation.

2.6. Analytical Procedures

Tissue levels of cytokines and chemokines were quantified using ELISA kits, according to manufacturer's instructions (Preprotech, Rocky Hill, NJ, USA or eBioscience, San Diego, CA, USA). To measure triglycerides in 3T3L1 adipocytes, cells were rinsed three times in sterile PBS then collected in 2 mL PBS by scraping. Cells were disrupted by vortexing, followed by sonication 3 × 15 s. Triglycerides were measured by colorimetric assay, according to the manufacturer's instructions (Sekisui Diagnostics, Lexington, MA, USA).

2.7. mRNA Quantification

mRNA was quantified as previously described [28]. Briefly, total RNA was isolated from tissue using Trizol reagent (Invitrogen, Carlsbad, CA, USA). RNA was then reverse transcribed using Superscript II (Invitrogen, Carlsbad, CA, USA). The Universal Probe Library (Roche Diagnostics, Indianapolis, IN, USA) was used to design primers and corresponding probes for each gene being evaluated. Quantitative PCR was run in triplicate on the Biomark system (Fluidigm, South San Francisco, CA, USA) for 40 cycles. Relative mRNA expression for each gene was calculated using the $\Delta\Delta$CT method, normalized to cyclophilin.

2.8. Statistical Analysis

Data are expressed as the means $\pm$ standard error of the mean (SEM). Data were analyzed using one-way ANOVA or Student's *t*-test where appropriate. All analyses were done using GraphPad Prism software version 6.00 for Windows (GraphPad Software, La Jolla, CA, USA). A *p*-value < 0.05 was taken as statistically significant.

3. Results

3.1. Excess Folic Acid Intake Does Not Influence Body Weight, Body Composition, or Glucose Tolerance on a Low Fat Diet

Rats were fed a LF diet with either AFA or EFA for 12 weeks. LF-AFA and LF-EFA fed rats had similar weight gain, fat mass and lean mass over the 12 weeks study period (Figure 1A–C). Glucose tolerance tests showed no difference in rate of glucose clearance between LF-AFA and LF-EFA fed rats (Figure 1D,E). Plasma ALT concentration, a marker of liver injury, was not different between groups (Figure 1F).

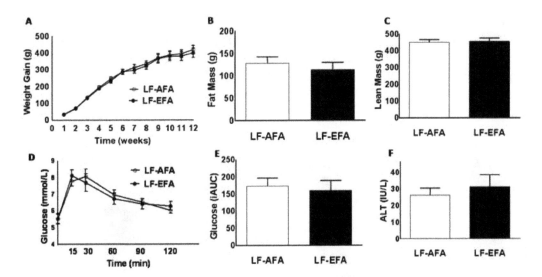

Figure 1. Excess folic acid intake does not influence body weight, body composition or glucose tolerance on a low fat diet (**A**); growth curves (**B**); fat mass (**C**); lean mass (**D**); glucose tolerance (**E**); area under the glucose curve, and (**F**) plasma ALT, of rats fed 15% LF diet with excess or adequate folic acid. Values are means ± SEM, * $p < 0.05$.

3.2. Excess Folic Acid Intake Increases Weight Gain, Fat Mass and Glucose Intolerance on a High Fat Diet

We next investigated the influence of AFA or EFA in rats challenged with a diet containing 60% kilocalories from fat for 12 weeks. Plasma homocysteine concentrations were significantly lower in HF-EFA fed rats (3.28 ± 0.17 compared to 2.650 ± 0.14 µM/L) at the end of the study period (Table 2). Plasma methionine and glycine concentrations were also lower in HF-EFA fed rats, while plasma folate concentration was similar between groups (Table 2). There was no significant difference in plasma concentrations of triglycerides, cholesterol, or cholesterol ester in rats fed HF-AFA or HF-EFA diets (Table 2).

Table 2. HF-EFA fed rats experience alterations in plasma one carbon metabolite profile, while plasma lipids remain unchanged, compared to HF-AFA fed rats.

	HF-AFA	HF-EFA
Plasma one carbon metabolites		
Folate (nmol/L)	41.56 ± 0.50	41.30 ± 0.72
Homocysteine (µM)	3.28 ± 0.17	2.650 ± 0.14 *
Methionine (µM)	69.73 ± 2.93	62.58 ± 1.01 *
Dimethylglycine (µM)	13.10 ± 0.98	15.68 ± 0.95
Methylglycine (µM)	7.19 ± 0.48	6.21 ± 0.31
Glycine (µM)	425.0 ± 21.6	345.5 ± 24.0 *
Serine (µM)	339.2 ± 11.2	364.5 ± 10.9
Cystathionine (nM)	914.7 ± 69.2	763.3 ± 37.2
Cysteine (nM)	311.3 ± 4.5	305.7 ± 9.7
α-aminobutyrate (µM)	27.68 ± 2.6	35.60 ± 4.0
Plasma lipids		
Triglyceride (µg/mL)	292.6 ± 43.26	211.8 ± 46.21
Cholesterol Ester (µg/mL)	72.92 ± 5.87	60.18 ± 7.97
Free Cholesterol (µg/mL)	134.4 ± 18.65	118.1 ± 15.41

Values are means ± SEM, * $p < 0.05$.

HF-EFA fed rats had 14% greater weight gain compared to HF-AFA fed controls after 12 weeks (Figure 2A). Estimated daily food intake was similar between groups (Figure 2B). Fat mass accounted for this difference in weight, with HF-EFA fed rats developing larger peri-renal fat pads (Figure 2C,D). There was no difference in lean body mass between HF-EFA and HF-AFA fed rats (Figure 2E). Fasting plasma glucose and insulin levels were similar between HF-EFA and HF-AFA fed rats (Figure 3A,B). However, IP glucose tolerance tests showed that HF-EFA fed rats had impaired glucose clearance compared to HF-AFA fed rats, as indicated by a significantly greater area under the glucose curve (Figure 3C,D). Therefore, EFA intake exacerbates weight gain, fat mass, and glucose intolerance in rats fed a HF diet.

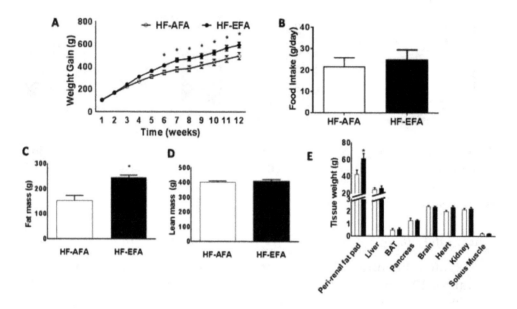

Figure 2. Excess folic acid intake increases weight gain and fat mass on a high fat diet. (**A**) Growth curves; (**B**) food intake; (**C**) fat mass; (**D**) lean mass; and (**E**) tissue weights. Values are means ± SEM, * $p < 0.05$.

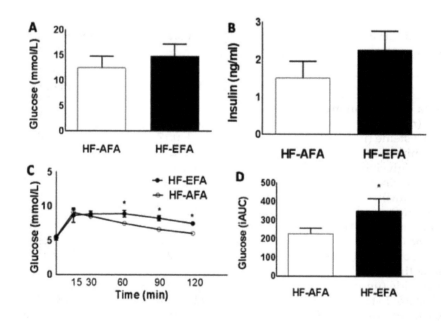

Figure 3. Excess folic acid intake impairs glucose tolerance on a high fat diet. (**A**) Fasting plasma glucose; (**B**) fasting plasma insulin; (**C**) blood glucose concentrations at different time points (15, 30, 60, 90, 120 min) after an intraperitoneal (IP) glucose injection; and (**D**) area under the glucose curve, for male rats fed 60% HF diet with excess or adequate folic acid. Values are means ± SEM, * $p < 0.05$.

3.3. Excess Folic Acid Increases Adipose Tissue Size and Mass By Inducing Lipogenic Genes in High Fat Diet-Fed Rats

Histologic examination of visceral adipose tissue after hematoxylin and eosin (H and E) staining showed increased adipocyte size in HF-EFA fed rats compared to HF-AFA fed controls (Figure 4). To further investigate this increased adiposity, we measured expression of key transcriptional regulators of lipid metabolism (Pparg, Srebf1, Srebf2, Nr1h2, Nr1h3), and lipogenic genes in adipose tissue. PPARγ regulates genes involved in lipid uptake and storage. Adipose tissue PPARγ mRNA was 2.5-fold higher in HF-EFA fed rats compared to HF-AFA fed controls (Figure 5A). Liver X receptor (LXR)-α and -β (encoded by Nr1h3 and Nr1h2) are nuclear transcription factors that have roles in adipose tissue lipid metabolism as well as inflammation [29]. LXR-α and -β mRNA levels were significantly higher in HF-EFA fed rats compared to HF-AFA fed rats (Figure 5A). Furthermore, there was increased mRNA levels of triglyceride synthetic genes (MGAT1, DGAT1 and DGAT2); genes involved in elongation (ELOV5 and ELOV6); and markers of adipogenesis (PLIN2) in adipose tissue of HF-EFA fed rats compared to HF-AFA fed rats (Figure 5B).

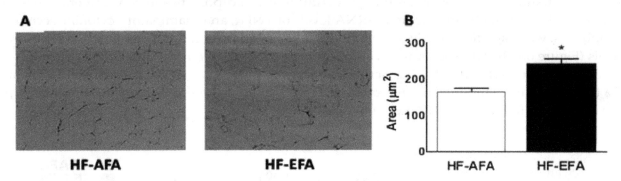

Figure 4. HF-EFA fed rats had larger adipocytes than HF-AFA fed rats. (**A**) Adipose tissue histology after H and E staining; (**B**) adipocyte size was quantified using ImageJ software. Values are means ± SEM, * $p < 0.05$.

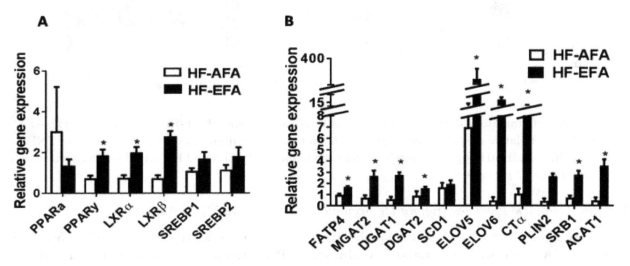

Figure 5. Gene expression analysis in adipose tissue of HF-EFA shows increased levels of lipogenic mediators. Relative mRNA levels of (**A**) transcription factors and (**B**) genes involved in lipid synthesis, storage and transport, in adipose tissue of HF-AFA and HF-EFA fed rats. Values are means ± SEM, * $p < 0.05$.

Increased adipocyte size and number increases demand for phosphatidylcholine (PC), which surrounds adipose tissue lipid droplets in a monolayer. Consistent with this increased demand, mRNA levels of the rate limiting enzyme in PC biosynthesis, cytidine triphosphate: phosphocholine cytidylyltransferase (CT) α, was increased in adipose tissue of HF-EFA fed rats compared to HF-AFA control rats (Figure 5B). Taken together, these observations indicate that EFA intake may induce lipogenic transcription factors and some of their dependent genes to promote adiposity in the setting of a HF diet.

3.4. Excess Folic Acid Increases Inflammation in White Adipose Tissue

White adipose tissue (WAT), in addition to its role in energy storage, secretes adipocytokines and chemokines which link increased fat mass to local and systemic insulin resistance [30]. In obesity, excess adipose tissue accumulation precedes immune cell infiltration and production of pro-inflammatory cytokines [30]. We measured adipose tissue protein levels of the chemokines monocyte chemoattractant protein-1 (MCP-1) and regulated on activation, normal T cell expressed and secreted (RANTES), and the cytokines tumor necrosis factor α(TNFα) and interleukin 10 (IL-10), as markers of inflammatory status. MCP-1 is a chemokine involved in monocyte and macrophage recruitment to adipose tissue [31]. Levels of MCP-1 were significantly higher in adipose tissue of HF-EFA fed rats (Figure 6B). Chronic low-grade inflammation after macrophage recruitment to adipose tissue can influence local and systemic insulin sensitivity. Protein and mRNA levels of TNFα, an inflammatory cytokine secreted by macrophages, were significantly higher in adipose tissue of HF-EFA fed rats compared to HF-AFA fed controls (Figure 6A,B). Adipose tissue levels of the cytokine IL-10 were not different between HF-AFA and HF-EFA fed rats (Figure 6B). Transcript levels of the inflammatory markers NADPH oxidase 1 (NOX1) and binding immunoglobulin protein (BiP) were found to be significantly increased in adipose tissue of HF-EFA fed rats after 12 weeks on diet (Figure 6A).

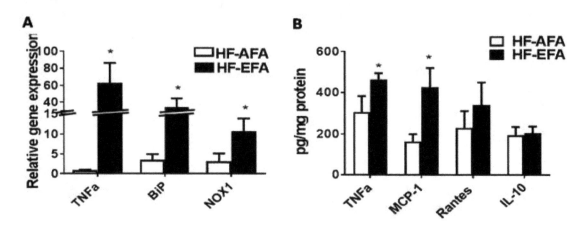

Figure 6. Inflammatory markers are increased in adipose tissue of HF-EFA compared to HF-AFA fed rats. (**A**) Relative mRNA levels of genes related to inflammation; and (**B**) protein levels of TNFα, MCP-1, Rantes, IL-10 in pg/mg protein, in adipose tissue of HF-EFA and HF-AFA fed rats. Values are means ± SEM, * $p < 0.05$.

3.5. Excess Folic Acid Promotes Triglyceride Accumulation in Mature 3T3L1 Adipocytes

We used 3T3-L1 cells to assess the lipogenic capacity of folic acid in vitro (Figure 7). We measured PPARγ mRNA expression as a marker of adipocyte differentiation in undifferentiated and mature 3T3-L1 cells cultured with 9 μM (normal) and 20 μM folic acid (excess). PPARγ was undetectable in undifferentiated 3T3-L1 cells. Treatment of differentiated adipocytes with 9 μM folic acid increased PPARγ expression and triglyceride (TG) accumulation compared to undifferentiated cells. High folic acid (20 μM) further promoted PPARγ expression and TG accumulation, indicating a dose-response to folic acid treatment in 3T3-L1 cells. These results support those found in adipose tissue of rats fed HF-EFA compared to HF-AFA diets.

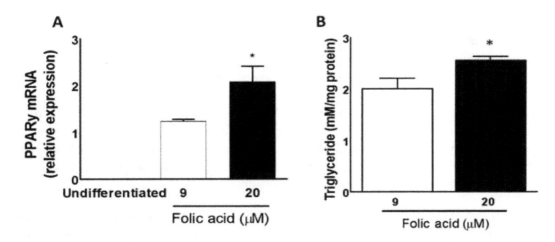

Figure 7. Folic acid increases PPARγ and triglyceride levels in a dose-dependent manner in cultured 3T3-L1 cells. (**A**) Relative PPARγ mRNA levels in cells cultured with 9 µM or 20 µM folic acid and (**B**) Triglyceride levels in cells after treatment with 9 µM compared to 20 µM folic acid. Values are means $\pm$ SEM, $^* p < 0.05$.

4. Discussion

Our results show that excess dietary folic acid exacerbates fat mass gain, adipose tissue inflammation, and systemic glucose intolerance in rats fed a HFD. These metabolic complications were not observed in rats fed a LF-EFA diet. Energy dense diets have long been implicated in fat mass gain and metabolic syndrome development [2]. Our results suggest that high dietary folic acid may aggravate these effects.

The body weight of rats in the HF-EFA group after 12 weeks was 14% higher than in rats in the HF-AFA group, with increased fat mass accounting for this difference in weight. Histological examination of adipose tissue revealed that HF-EFA fed rats had larger adipocytes. The capacity of folic acid or methyl-rich diets to promote weight gain has been reported previously in young rats fed 5 mg/kg folic acid [23], as well as in maternal rats fed a high fat diet enriched in methyl-containing vitamins [32]. Our data supports these findings and suggests that a high folic acid diet promotes fat gain.

Adipogenesis is a multistep process which is controlled by transcription factors that promote adipocyte development and adipose tissue expansion [33]. PPARγ is an important regulator of adipogenesis and is sensitive to nutrient composition of the diet [34]. Most pro-adipogenic factors appear to function by stimulating PPARγ [34]. Gene expression analysis showed that PPARγ mRNA levels were approximately three times higher in adipose tissue of HF-EFA fed rats compared to HF-AFA fed controls. Folic acid supplementation has previously been shown to decrease PPARγ promoter methylation in rat liver leading to an increase in PPARγ gene expression [35]. Other studies have reported that methylation status influences expression of key genes involved in lipid metabolism [23,36]. Therefore, it is conceivable that the increase in PPARγ expression observed in our study is related to changes to methylation status of adipose tissue PPARγ, induced by excess folic acid. Addition of folic acid to the medium stimulated PPARγ expression and increased TG storage in 3T3-L1 cells, which further supports the ability of folic acid to stimulate adipogenesis. The capacity of folic acid to stimulate PPARγ expression in adipose tissue has been previously reported [23]. LXRα and LXRβ, transcriptional regulators of lipid and glucose metabolism [29], mRNA levels were increased in HF-EFA compared to HF-AFA fed rats. These data suggest that the increased adiposity observed in HF-EFA fed rats is a result of increased induction of lipogenic transcription factors and their target genes in adipose tissue.

Excessive adiposity is associated with metabolic stress and inflammation which is induced when macrophages migrate to adipose tissue and secrete pro-inflammatory cytokines. HF-EFA fed rats had higher adipose tissue protein levels of MCP-1, a chemokine that recruits macrophages to obese adipose tissue [37]. Consistent with this observation, protein and mRNA levels of the pro-inflammatory cytokine TNFα were significantly elevated in adipose tissue of HF-EFA fed rats compared to HF-AFA fed controls. Elevated TNFα is linked to insulin resistance in humans and animals. Consistent with significantly increased TNFα protein and mRNA levels in adipose tissue, HF-EFA fed rats had impaired glucose tolerance compared to HF-AFA fed rats. Maternal EFA supplementation has previously been shown to impair glucose metabolism in HF diet fed offspring [20]. Our results support this cross-generational evidence and demonstrate a similar effect in a single-generational study of rats. Thus, our data suggest that the mechanism linking EFA intake to systemic glucose intolerance may be TNFα- mediated inflammation in adipose tissue.

Metabolic complications in adipose tissue generally precede similar complications in other tissues, such as the liver [38,39]. TNFα produced in adipose tissue may migrate into the circulation and exert pro-inflammatory effects on other tissues [38,39]. In addition, when adipose tissue has reached its capacity to store fatty acids there may be a 'spill-over' of fat to other tissues. This amplifies the importance of identifying and controlling factors that influence inflammation and glucose intolerance in adipose tissue as they can ultimately compromise systemic health. After observing increased triglyceride accumulation and inflammation in adipose tissue of HF-EFA fed rats, we examined hepatic neutral lipid accumulation and mRNA levels of inflammatory genes. No significant difference in triglyceride accumulation was observed, and mRNA levels of a select number of inflammatory genes were not increased in the HF-EFA fed groups (data not shown). It has been previously reported that while HFD-induced inflammation can occur relatively quickly in adipose tissue of murine models, hepatic inflammation can take up to 40 weeks to develop, suggesting that our 12 weeks study period may have been too short to observe effects of folic acid in the liver [39]. Twenty-four weeks of supplementary folic acid (20 mg/kg) was sufficient to alter lipid metabolism and cause liver injury in mildly MTHFR-deficient rats [25].

While there is increasing evidence that excess dietary folate intake may have adverse effects, it is important to acknowledge the necessity of adequate levels of folate for good health. The role of dietary folate in NTD prevention is widely acknowledged, but adequate folate is also essential for regulating lipid metabolism, especially in the liver where most methylation reactions occur [40]. Folate deficiency can lead to liver damage and steatosis, with impaired phosphatidylcholine (PC) synthesis and increased expression of lipogenic genes cited as possible mechanisms [40]. Folate is also essential for re-methylation of homocysteine to methionine, which can be used to synthesize protein, or recycled to S-adenosylmethionine (S-AdoMet), a key methyl donor [4]. Excessively high folic acid intake can increase levels of unmetabolized folic acid in circulation [13], and its transport into tissues [41]. Some of the adverse health effects linked to excessive folic acid intake have been attributed to unmetabolized folic acid. However, the molecular mechanisms involved in processing unmetabolized folic acid within different tissue and cell types, and the biological effects of this, is poorly understood. It is conceivable that the increased adiposity observed in our study is a result of altered gene methylation and expression patterns in adipose tissue by folic acid.

We decided to supplement the rat diet with 10 times the adequate level of folic acid. While this could be considered superphysiological, we have previously reported that a sub-set of pregnant Alberta women consume over 4 mg/day (10 times the RDA for the general population) of folic acid [8]. Rats reduce folic acid to tetrahydrofolate at a rate that far exceeds that seen in humans [42]. Therefore, the observation that 7.5 mg/kg folic acid induced fat mass gain and inflammation in rats despite their relatively high dihydrofolate reductase activity is striking. Interestingly, Burdge et al. reported that folic acid supplementation (5 mg/kg) induced weight gain in juvenile rats fed a high fat diet [23]. Nonenthless, the inter-species differences in capacity to handle high doses of folic acid need to be considered when drawing conclusions from animal studies and places importance on establishing the metabolic effects of excess folic acid in human populations.

5. Conclusions

Folic acid fortification has succeeded in reducing incidence of neural tube defects in North America. However, there is increasing evidence that high folic acid intake may have consequences. Our findings suggest that in adult males the dual insult of a high fat diet combined with excess folic acid may promote fat mass gain, adipose tissue inflammation and systemic glucose intolerance. Obesity and the metabolic syndrome represent major public burdens and the link between excess folic acid and metabolic complications warrants further investigation given the ubiquitous presence of folic acid in the human food chain.

Acknowledgments: This research was supported by grants to R.L.J. from the Canadian Institutes of Health Research and Canadian Foundation for Innovation and the Alberta Ministry for Advanced Education and Technology. R.L.J. is a new investigator of the Canadian Institutes of Health Research. K.B.K. was supported by an Alexander Graham Bell graduate scholarship from the Natural Sciences and Engineering Research Council of Canada. We thank Nicole Coursen for her excellent technical assistance.

Author Contributions: K.B.K. and R.L.J. conceived and designed the experiments; K.B.K., M.O., R.N., K.L., S.S. and C.J.F. performed the experiments; K.B.K., J.P.K. and R.L.J. analyzed the data; J.P.K. and K.B.K. wrote the first draft of the paper. All Authors reviewed and edited the manuscript.

References

1. James, P.T.; Rigby, N.; Leach, R.; Force, I.O.T. The obesity epidemic, metabolic syndrome and future prevention strategies. *Eur. J. Cardiovasc. Prev. Rehabil.* **2004**, *11*, 3–8. [CrossRef] [PubMed]

2. Cordain, L.; Eaton, S.B.; Sebastian, A.; Mann, N.; Lindeberg, S.; Watkins, B.A.; O'Keefe, J.H.; Brand-Miller, J. Origins and evolution of the Western diet: Health implications for the 21st century. *Am. J. Clin. Nutr.* **2005**, *81*, 341–354. [PubMed]

3. Smith, A.D.; Kim, Y.I.; Refsum, H. Is folic acid good for everyone? *Am. J. Clin. Nutr.* **2008**, *87*, 517–533. [PubMed]

4. Chan, Y.M.; Bailey, R.; O'Connor, D.L. Folate. *Adv. Nutr.* **2013**, *4*, 123–125. [CrossRef] [PubMed]

5. Institute of Medicine (U.S.) Standing Committee on the Scientific Evaluation of Dietary Reference Intakes; Institute of Medicine (U.S.) Panel on Folate Other B Vitamins and Choline; Institute of Medicine (U.S.) Subcommittee on Upper Reference Levels of Nutrients. *Dietary Reference Intakes for Thiamin, Riboflavin, Niacin, Vitamin B6, Folate, Vitamin B12, Pantothenic Acid, Biotin, and Choline*; National Academy Press: Washington, DC, USA, 1998; p. 564.

6. Pfeiffer, C.M.; Sternberg, M.R.; Fazili, Z.; Yetley, E.A.; Lacher, D.A.; Bailey, R.L.; Johnson, C.L. Unmetabolized folic acid is detected in nearly all serum samples from US children, adolescents, and adults. *J. Nutr.* **2015**, *145*, 520–531. [CrossRef] [PubMed]

7. Bailey, R.L.; Mills, J.L.; Yetley, E.A.; Gahche, J.J.; Pfeiffer, C.M.; Dwyer, J.T.; Dodd, K.W.; Sempos, C.T.; Betz, J.M.; Picciano, M.F. Serum unmetabolized folic acid in a nationally representative sample of adults ≥60 years in the United States, 2001–2002. *Food Nutr. Res.* **2012**, *56*. [CrossRef] [PubMed]

8. Fayyaz, F.; Wang, F.; Jacobs, R.L.; O'Connor, D.L.; Bell, R.C.; Field, C.J.; Team, A.S. Folate, vitamin B12, and vitamin B6 status of a group of high socioeconomic status women in the Alberta Pregnancy Outcomes and Nutrition (APrON) cohort. *Appl. Physiol. Nutr. Metab.* **2014**, *39*, 1402–1408. [CrossRef] [PubMed]

9. McNulty, B.; McNulty, H.; Marshall, B.; Ward, M.; Molloy, A.M.; Scott, J.M.; Dornan, J.; Pentieva, K. Impact of continuing folic acid after the first trimester of pregnancy: Findings of a randomized trial of Folic Acid Supplementation in the Second and Third Trimesters. *Am. J. Clin. Nutr.* **2013**, *98*, 92–98. [CrossRef] [PubMed]

10. Pentieva, K.; Selhub, J.; Paul, L.; Molloy, A.M.; McNulty, B.; Ward, M.; Marshall, B.; Dornan, J.; Reilly, R.; Parle-McDermott, A.; et al. Evidence from a Randomized Trial That Exposure to Supplemental Folic Acid at Recommended Levels during Pregnancy Does Not Lead to Increased Unmetabolized Folic Acid Concentrations in Maternal or Cord Blood. *J. Nutr.* **2016**, *146*, 494–500. [CrossRef] [PubMed]

11. Fife, J.; Raniga, S.; Hider, P.N.; Frizelle, F.A. Folic acid supplementation and colorectal cancer risk: A meta-analysis. *Colorectal Dis.* **2011**, *13*, 132–137. [CrossRef] [PubMed]

12. Hultdin, J.; Van Guelpen, B.; Bergh, A.; Hallmans, G.; Stattin, P. Plasma folate, vitamin B12, and homocysteine and prostate cancer risk: A prospective study. *Int. J. Cancer* **2005**, *113*, 819–824. [CrossRef] [PubMed]

13. Troen, A.M.; Mitchell, B.; Sorensen, B.; Wener, M.H.; Johnston, A.; Wood, B.; Selhub, J.; McTiernan, A.; Yasui, Y.; Oral, E.; et al. Unmetabolized folic acid in plasma is associated with reduced natural killer cell cytotoxicity among postmenopausal women. *J. Nutr.* **2006**, *136*, 189–194. [PubMed]

14. Sawaengsri, H.; Wang, J.; Reginaldo, C.; Steluti, J.; Wu, D.; Meydani, S.N.; Selhub, J.; Paul, L. High folic acid intake reduces natural killer cell cytotoxicity in aged mice. *J. Nutr. Biochem.* **2016**, *30*, 102–107. [CrossRef] [PubMed]

15. Morris, M.C.; Evans, D.A.; Bienias, J.L.; Tangney, C.C.; Hebert, L.E.; Scherr, P.A.; Schneider, J.A. Dietary folate and vitamin B12 intake and cognitive decline among community-dwelling older persons. *Arch. Neurol.* **2005**, *62*, 641–645. [CrossRef] [PubMed]

16. Bird, J.K.; Ronnenberg, A.G.; Choi, S.W.; Du, F.; Mason, J.B.; Liu, Z. Obesity is associated with increased red blood cell folate despite lower dietary intakes and serum concentrations. *J. Nutr.* **2015**, *145*, 79–86. [CrossRef] [PubMed]

17. Cho, C.E.; Sánchez-Hernández, D.; Reza-López, S.A.; Huot, P.S.; Kim, Y.I.; Anderson, G.H. High folate gestational and post-weaning diets alter hypothalamic feeding pathways by DNA methylation in Wistar rat offspring. *Epigenetics* **2013**, *8*, 710–719. [CrossRef] [PubMed]

18. Hoile, S.P.; Lillycrop, K.A.; Grenfell, L.R.; Hanson, M.A.; Burdge, G.C. Increasing the folic acid content of maternal or post-weaning diets induces differential changes in phosphoenolpyruvate carboxykinase mRNA expression and promoter methylation in rats. *Br. J. Nutr.* **2012**, *108*, 852–857. [CrossRef] [PubMed]

19. Szeto, I.M.; Aziz, A.; Das, P.J.; Taha, A.Y.; Okubo, N.; Reza-Lopez, S.; Giacca, A.; Anderson, G.H. High multivitamin intake by Wistar rats during pregnancy results in increased food intake and components of the metabolic syndrome in male offspring. *Am. J. Physiol. Regul. Integr. Comp. Physiol.* **2008**, *295*, R575–R582. [CrossRef] [PubMed]

20. Huang, Y.; He, Y.; Sun, X.; Li, Y.; Sun, C. Maternal high folic acid supplement promotes glucose intolerance and insulin resistance in male mouse offspring fed a high-fat diet. *Int. J. Mol. Sci.* **2014**, *15*, 6298–6313. [CrossRef] [PubMed]

21. Szeto, I.M.; Das, P.J.; Aziz, A.; Anderson, G.H. Multivitamin supplementation of Wistar rats during pregnancy accelerates the development of obesity in offspring fed an obesogenic diet. *Int. J. Obes. (Lond.)* **2009**, *33*, 364–372. [CrossRef] [PubMed]

22. Yajnik, C.S.; Deshpande, S.S.; Jackson, A.A.; Refsum, H.; Rao, S.; Fisher, D.J.; Bhat, D.S.; Naik, S.S.; Coyaji, K.J.; Joglekar, C.V.; et al. Vitamin B12 and folate concentrations during pregnancy and insulin resistance in the offspring: The Pune Maternal Nutrition Study. *Diabetologia* **2008**, *51*, 29–38. [CrossRef] [PubMed]

23. Burdge, G.C.; Lillycrop, K.A.; Phillips, E.S.; Slater-Jefferies, J.L.; Jackson, A.A.; Hanson, M.A. Folic acid supplementation during the juvenile-pubertal period in rats modifies the phenotype and epigenotype induced by prenatal nutrition. *J. Nutr.* **2009**, *139*, 1054–1060. [CrossRef] [PubMed]

24. McKay, J.A.; Mathers, J.C. Diet induced epigenetic changes and their implications for health. *Acta Physiol. (Oxf.)* **2011**, *202*, 103–118. [CrossRef] [PubMed]

25. Christensen, K.E.; Mikael, L.G.; Leung, K.Y.; Lévesque, N.; Deng, L.; Wu, Q.; Malysheva, O.V.; Best, A.; Caudill, M.A.; Greene, N.D.; et al. High folic acid consumption leads to pseudo-MTHFR deficiency, altered lipid metabolism, and liver injury in mice. *Am. J. Clin. Nutr.* **2015**, *101*, 646–658. [CrossRef] [PubMed]

26. Stabler, S.P.; Allen, R.H. Quantification of serum and urinary S-adenosylmethionine and S-adenosylhomocysteine by stable-isotope-dilution liquid chromatography-mass spectrometry. *Clin. Chem.* **2004**, *50*, 365–372. [CrossRef] [PubMed]

27. Myher, J.J.; Kuksis, A. Determination of plasma total lipid profiles by capillary gas-liquid chromatography. *J. Biochem. Biophys. Methods* **1984**, *10*, 13–23. [CrossRef]

28. Da Silva, R.P.; Kelly, K.B.; Leonard, K.A.; Jacobs, R.L. Creatine reduces hepatic TG accumulation in hepatocytes by stimulating fatty acid oxidation. *Biochim. Biophys. Acta* **2014**, *1841*, 1639–1646. [CrossRef] [PubMed]

29. Korf, H.; Vander Beken, S.; Romano, M.; Steffensen, K.R.; Stijlemans, B.; Gustafsson, J.A.; Grooten, J.; Huygen, K. Liver X receptors contribute to the protective immune response against Mycobacterium tuberculosis in mice. *J. Clin. Investig.* **2009**, *119*, 1626–1637. [CrossRef] [PubMed]

30. Waki, H.; Tontonoz, P. Endocrine functions of adipose tissue. *Annu. Rev. Pathol.* **2007**, *2*, 31–56. [CrossRef] [PubMed]

31. Suganami, T.; Ogawa, Y. Adipose tissue macrophages: Their role in adipose tissue remodeling. *J. Leukoc. Biol.* **2010**, *88*, 33–39. [CrossRef] [PubMed]

32. Pannia, E.; Cho, C.E.; Kubant, R.; Sánchez-Hernández, D.; Huot, P.S.; Chatterjee, D.; Fleming, A.; Anderson, G.H. A high multivitamin diet fed to Wistar rat dams during pregnancy increases maternal weight gain later in life and alters homeostatic, hedonic and peripheral regulatory systems of energy balance. *Behav. Brain Res.* **2015**, *278*, 1–11. [CrossRef] [PubMed]

33. Ali, A.T.; Hochfeld, W.E.; Myburgh, R.; Pepper, M.S. Adipocyte and adipogenesis. *Eur. J. Cell Biol.* **2013**, *92*, 229–236. [CrossRef] [PubMed]

34. Symonds, M.E. *Adipose Tissue Biology*; Springer: New York, NY, USA, 2012; p. 413.

35. Sie, K.K.; Li, J.; Ly, A.; Sohn, K.J.; Croxford, R.; Kim, Y.I. Effect of maternal and postweaning folic acid supplementation on global and gene-specific DNA methylation in the liver of the rat offspring. *Mol. Nutr. Food Res.* **2013**, *57*, 677–685. [CrossRef] [PubMed]

36. Ehara, T.; Kamei, Y.; Takahashi, M.; Yuan, X.; Kanai, S.; Tamura, E.; Tanaka, M.; Yamazaki, T.; Miura, S.; Ezaki, O.; et al. Role of DNA methylation in the regulation of lipogenic glycerol-3-phosphate acyltransferase 1 gene expression in the mouse neonatal liver. *Diabetes* **2012**, *61*, 2442–2450. [CrossRef] [PubMed]

37. Weisberg, S.P.; Hunter, D.; Huber, R.; Lemieux, J.; Slaymaker, S.; Vaddi, K.; Charo, I.; Leibel, R.L.; Ferrante, A.W. CCR2 modulates inflammatory and metabolic effects of high-fat feeding. *J. Clin. Investig.* **2006**, *116*, 115–124. [CrossRef] [PubMed]

38. Moschen, A.R.; Molnar, C.; Geiger, S.; Graziadei, I.; Ebenbichler, C.F.; Weiss, H.; Kaser, S.; Kaser, A.; Tilg, H. Anti-inflammatory effects of excessive weight loss: Potent suppression of adipose interleukin 6 and tumour necrosis factor alpha expression. *Gut* **2010**, *59*, 1259–1264. [CrossRef] [PubMed]

39. Van der Heijden, R.A.; Sheedfar, F.; Morrison, M.C.; Hommelberg, P.P.; Kor, D.; Kloosterhuis, N.J.; Gruben, N.; Youssef, S.A.; de Bruin, A.; Hofker, M.H.; et al. High-fat diet induced obesity primes inflammation in adipose tissue prior to liver in C57BL/6j mice. *Aging* **2015**, *7*, 256–268. [CrossRef] [PubMed]

40. Da Silva, R.P.; Kelly, K.B.; Al Rajabi, A.; Jacobs, R.L. Novel insights on interactions between folate and lipid metabolism. *Biofactors* **2014**, *40*, 277–283. [CrossRef] [PubMed]

41. Qiu, A.; Jansen, M.; Sakaris, A.; Min, S.H.; Chattopadhyay, S.; Tsai, E.; Sandoval, C.; Zhao, R.; Akabas, M.H.; Goldman, I.D. Identification of an intestinal folate transporter and the molecular basis for hereditary folate malabsorption. *Cell* **2006**, *127*, 917–928. [CrossRef] [PubMed]

42. Bailey, S.W.; Ayling, J.E. The extremely slow and variable activity of dihydrofolate reductase in human liver and its implications for high folic acid intake. *Proc. Natl. Acad. Sci. USA* **2009**, *106*, 15424–15429. [CrossRef] [PubMed]

11

Pyridoxine (Vitamin B6) and the Glutathione Peroxidase System: A Link between One-Carbon Metabolism and Antioxidation

Danyel Bueno Dalto [1,2] and Jean-Jacques Matte [1,*]

[1]   Sherbrooke Research Centre, Agriculture and Agri-Food Canada, Sherbrooke, QC J1M 0C8, Canada; danyel.buenodalto@agr.gc.ca
[2]   Department of Biology, Université de Sherbrooke, Sherbrooke, QC J1K 2R1, Canada
*   Correspondence: jacques.matte@agr.gc.ca

Abstract: Vitamin B_6 (B_6) has a central role in the metabolism of amino acids, which includes important interactions with endogenous redox reactions through its effects on the glutathione peroxidase (GPX) system. In fact, B_6-dependent enzymes catalyse most reactions of the transsulfuration pathway, driving homocysteine to cysteine and further into GPX proteins. Considering that mammals metabolize sulfur- and seleno-amino acids similarly, B_6 plays an important role in the fate of sulfur-homocysteine and its seleno counterpart between transsulfuration and one-carbon metabolism, especially under oxidative stress conditions. This is particularly important in reproduction because ovarian metabolism may generate an excess of reactive oxygen species (ROS) during the peri-estrus period, which may impair ovulatory functions and early embryo development. Later in gestation, placentation raises embryo oxygen tension and may induce a higher expression of ROS markers and eventually embryo losses. Interestingly, the metabolic accumulation of ROS up-regulates the flow of one-carbon units to transsulfuration and down-regulates remethylation. However, in embryos, the transsulfuration pathway is not functional, making the understanding of the interplay between these two pathways particularly crucial. In this review, the importance of the maternal metabolic status of B_6 for the flow of one-carbon units towards both maternal and embryonic GPX systems is discussed. Additionally, B_6 effects on GPX activity and gene expression in dams, as well as embryo development, are presented in a pig model under different oxidative stress conditions.

Keywords: glutathione peroxidase; one-carbon; pig; pyridoxine; remethylation; transsulfuration

1. Introduction

Among various metabolic pathways present in the organism, the metabolism of sulfur- (S) methionine and its seleno- (Se) analogous (Se-methionine) are particularly important because they not only contribute to protein mass but also produce (Se) homocysteine, a key metabolite connecting two fundamental metabolic functions, the one-carbon metabolism and the antioxidative system.

The transfer of one-carbon groups, represented by methyl (–CH3), methylene (–CH2–), formyl (–CHO), formimino (–CHNH), and methenyl (–CH=), is involved in the remethylation of (Se) homocysteine to (Se) methionine, as well as related pathways such as the folate cycle and the choline oxidation pathway [1]. Additionally, during the demethylation of (Se) methionine to (Se) homocysteine, the universal bioactive methyl donor S-adenosylmethionine (SAM) is synthesized and donates its methyl group to a large number of methyl acceptors catalyzed by methyltransferases [1,2] with profound impacts on DNA synthesis, protection and repair, cellular metabolism, and cell proliferation and, consequently, with direct effects on embryo/fetal growth [3,4].

During redox challenges, however, the high level of reactive oxygen species (ROS) induces a negative feedback on methionine synthase (MTR) [5] and betaine-homocysteine S-methyltransferase (BHMT) [6], which are enzymes that catalyze the regeneration of methionine from homocysteine [7]. Concomitantly, a positive feedback on cystathionine β-synthase (CBS), the first enzyme of the transsulfuration pathway, increases the flow of carbon towards transsulfuration reactions [8].

The transsulfuration of homocysteine, catalyzed by two vitamin B_6- (B_6) dependent reactions, consumes one-carbon units and is a major source of cysteine, contributing with about 50% of the cysteine used for glutathione (GSH) synthesis [8], the major redox buffer in mammalian cells. Se-homocysteine follows these same B_6-dependent steps of the transsulfuration pathway but syntheses Se-cysteine (SeCys). Due to the action of the B_6-dependent and Se-specific enzyme selenocysteine lyase (SCLY), SeCys loses its organic part and releases selenide. Selenide is also formed after dietary selenite (mineral Se) supplementation [9]. Considering the high cytotoxicity of selenide, it has to be immediately metabolized through either methylation reactions consuming SAM or phosphorylation to merge Se into an organic moiety in a B_6-dependent reaction (Figure 1). After another B_6-dependent reaction, phosphorylated Se is incorporated into tRNA Se-cysteinyl with further translation into Se-proteins such as Se-dependent glutathione peroxidases (SeGPX), the enzyme responsible for the oxidation of GSH during the important detoxification of ROS [10].

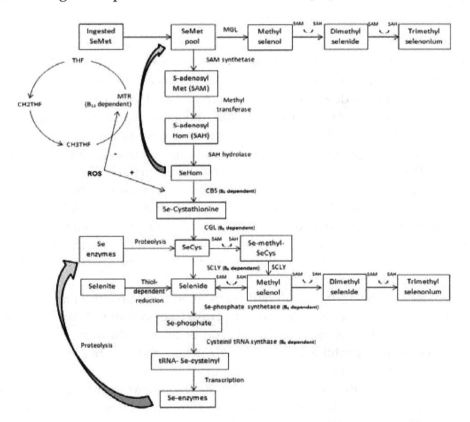

Figure 1. Transmethylation and transsulfuration pathways of selenium (similar for sulfur counterparts) in adults. Selenomethionine (SeMet) is methylated to methyl selenol by methionine γ lyase (MGL) or demethylated to selenohomocysteine (SeHom). SeHom may follow remethylation back to SeMet or transsulfuration to form selenocysteine (SeCys). The substrate-specific enzyme selenocysteine lyase (SCLY), which represents the landmark between sulfur and selenium metabolisms, catalyses the synthesis of selenide from SeCys. Selenide may also be formed from dietary selenite after thiol-dependent reactions. Selenide may be methylated and excreted or phosphorylated and its selenium (Se) incorporated into tRNA Se-cysteinyl with further translation to Se-enzymes. THF = tetrahydrofolate; CH2THF = 5,10-methylene-THF; CH3THF = 5-methyl-THF; MTR = methionine synthase; CBS = cystathionine β synthase; CGL = cystathionine γ lyase; ROS = reactive oxygen species.

Although the transmethylation of (Se) methionine is not dependent on B_6 [11], the direct impact of this vitamin on the transsulfuration of (Se) homocysteine to (Se) cysteine and the intrinsic relation between these two metabolic pathways make the B_6 status of an individual important not only for the antioxidant system but for the one-carbon pool as well. Considering that the transsulfuration of homocysteine to the synthesis of GSH requires two B_6-dependent reactions, whereas Se-homocysteine requires five B_6-dependent reactions to synthesize SeGPX, the impact of B_6 is expected to be more evident for Se metabolism. Additionally, the dissimilar metabolisms between organic and mineral Se, including different mechanisms of regulation for the synthesis of selenoprotein, indicate possible different fates for the one-carbon metabolism.

All the above concepts are even more fundamental in developing embryos because of the singular transfer of Se to pre-implantation embryos [12], the redox alterations brought by the placentation process [13], and the incomplete transsulfuration pathway [14].

The present review discusses the impact of B_6 on the equilibrium between the synthesis and the consumption of one-carbon units under different oxidative stress conditions, focusing not only sulfur-related metabolism but also Se metabolism and the differences between Se sources both in adults and embryos at 5- and 30-days of gestation using a pig model.

2. Vitamin B_6 Metabolism

Vitamers and Their Metabolism

Vitamin B_6 is a general description of six interconvertible metabolites, pyridoxine (alcohol), pyridoxamine (amine), pyridoxal (aldehyde), and their respective phosphates. Its main metabolic form differs between plant (pyridoxine) and animal (pyridoxal and/or pyridoxamine) sources, but, independently of origin, they are mainly found in the phosphorylated state or bound to proteins [15].

The enteric absorption of the phosphorylated protein-bound B_6 vitamers, mostly at jejunum and ileum, is dependent on their dephosphorylation by membrane-bound alkaline phosphatases present in the intestinal mucosa [16]. All three dephosphorylated vitamers are absorbed by passive diffusion, and, within the enterocytes, these metabolites are re-phosphorylated, generating a metabolic trapping of the vitamin with further oxidation to pyridoxal-5-phosphate (P-5-P), its metabolically active form [17]. This latter metabolite must be dephosphorylated at the intestinal serosal surface before its release into the portal circulation. Dephosphorylated forms of B_6 are readily taken up by membranes, whereas the phosphorylated analogs are not; therefore, phosphorylation may be considered a mechanism for the intracellular retention of this vitamin [15].

Pyridoxal released into the portal circulation is absorbed in the liver by passive diffusion, followed by re-phosphorylation within the cells. In order to cross liver cell membranes, P-5-P is hydrolyzed to pyridoxal and released into the general circulation bound to albumin and/or hemoglobin [18]. Any P-5-P that is not bound to proteins is readily hydrolyzed and the free pyridoxal remaining in the liver is oxidized to 4-pyridoxic acid and excreted.

Considering that no specific tissular storage of B_6 is present in the organism, both short- and long-term whole body pools of B_6 (about 12 h and 1 month, respectively) are present as P-5-P bound to enzymes/proteins [15]. Blood plasma is the major source of extrahepatic B_6, which occurs mainly as P-5-P bound to albumin [16]. Circulatory P-5-P must be hydrolyzed (by extracellular alkaline phosphatases) to pyridoxal that can cross cell membranes and then is trapped intracellularly by phosphorylation. Pyridoxal-5-P is over six times more concentrated in erythrocytes than in plasma possibly because the Schiff base with hemoglobin is stronger than the one with albumin, driving the uptake of the vitamin to erythrocytes; however, its storage in these cells is saturable [16,19].

3. Vitamin B_6 Metabolic Functions

In addition to the role of B_6 as a cofactor for the degradation of stored carbohydrates [20] and its function as a protective agent against ROS generated in vitro [21], P-5-P was shown to interact with steroid hormone-receptors, affecting their genes expression [22]. Pyridoxal-5-P also acts as a cofactor in the biosynthesis of many neurotransmitters such as dopamine, epinephrine, gamma-aminobutyric acid, histamine, norepinephrine, and serotonin, as well as the neuromodulator serine [17]. However, the most recognized role of P-5-P is the catalysis of many important steps in the metabolism of amino acids, such as transamination, racemization, decarboxylation, and α,β-elimination reactions [23,24]. The various reactions of P-5-P in the metabolism of amino acids depend on its ability to stabilize amino acid carbanions. In the absence of a substrate, P-5-P forms an internal aldimine (Schiff base) with the lysyl residue (ε-amino group) of the enzyme. Once a substrate amino acid displaces its lysyl residue (α-amino group), P-5-P transfers the aldimine linkage from the ε-amino group to the α-amino group.

4. Transmethylation vs. Transsulfuration

4.1. Transmethylation and the One-Carbon Metabolism

Methylation is an essential metabolic function that controls the addition of –CH3 groups to a variety of organic compounds in every cell of the body. Transmethylation represents metabolic reactions in which –CH3 groups are transferred from one compound to another, comprising both demethylation and remethylation reactions. The methionine cycle contains good examples of transmethylation reactions, in which methionine is demethylated to homocysteine, S-adenosylmethionine acts as a methyl donor, with a further possible remethylation to methionine with either 5-methyl tetrahydrofolate or betaine as the methyl donor.

During the methionine cycle, the –CH3 group of methionine, which contains a sulfur atom, is activated by adenosine triphosphate (ATP) through the addition of adenosine to its sulfur. This reaction, which is catalyzed by methionine adenosyltransferase (MAT), forms S-adenosylmethionine (SAM) [25], which is an important donor of –CH3 groups to nucleic acids, proteins, and neurotransmitters.

Upon transfer of its –CH3 group, SAM is rapidly converted to S-adenosylhomocysteine (SAH) that, by removal of the adenosine molecule catalyzed by SAH hydrolase (SAHH), is immediately hydrolyzed to homocysteine [26]. Homocysteine can then follow two major pathways; transsulfuration (see next sub-item) or remethylation (Figure 1). Two remethylation pathways regenerate methionine; one is independent of cobalamin (Cbl) but depends on betaine as the one-carbon donor, and the other is Cbl-dependent and requires folate (5-methyltetrahydrofolate) as the one-carbon donor [27].

Folate has two carbon-carbon double bonds that yield dihydrofolate (DHF) and tetrahydrofolate (THF) after saturation of its first and second carbon, respectively, by hydrogen. Folates serve as donors of single carbons in their reduced (5-methyl-THF; CH3THF), intermediate (5,10-methylene-THF; CH2THF), and oxidized (10-formyl-THF; CHOTHF) states [28]. Although not clearly shown in the literature [11,29,30], B_6 status may influence the flux –CH3 groups through remethylation because 5,10-methylene-THF is formed by the methylene group of the side-chain of serine (after its conversion into glycine) along with THF in a reaction catalyzed by the B_6-dependent enzyme serine hydroxylmethyltransferase. Although THF and serine, respectively, are the most important metabolic carrier and source of one-carbon groups, they do not promote the most energetically favorable reactions. The interaction of methionine with ATP produces SAM that easily donates its –CH3 group; SAM is considered the most important one-carbon donor [3]. Folate and SAM transfer of single carbons, which are volatile and bind easily to other molecules, generates the one-carbon metabolism. The one-carbon metabolism creates interplay between amino acid and nucleotide metabolisms, playing a fundamental role in DNA synthesis, repair, and replication [3]. The one-carbon donor 5-methyl-THF is used to convert homocysteine into methionine. The overall reaction transforms 5-methyl-THF into THF while transferring a –CH3 group to homocysteine to form methionine [4].

Methionine synthase (MTR), a vitamin B_{12} (Cbl)-dependent enzyme, catalyzes the final step in the regeneration of methionine from homocysteine [7]. The complex Cbl(I)MTR binds the –CH3 group of 5-methyl-THF to form methylCbl(III)MTR, activating the enzyme. The activated –CH3 group is transferred from methylCbl(III)MTR (regenerating Cbl(I)MTR) to homocysteine synthesizing methionine, which is released from the enzyme [31]. Under folate and/or vitamin B_{12} deficiency, MTR reactions are severely impaired.

4.2. Transsulfuration and the GPX System

As described above, after its synthesis from SAH, homocysteine can follow the remethylation or the transsulfuration pathway (Figure 1). Transsulfuration is a metabolic pathway involving the conversion of homocysteine into cysteine through the intermediate metabolite cystathionine. Briefly, in a reaction catalyzed by cystathionine β-synthase (CBS; B_6-dependent enzyme), a β-replacement of the thiol group of homocysteine by the acetyl or succinyl group of homoserine forms cystathionine [32]. By acting at the homocysteine junction, CBS represents a critical step, regulating both the maintenance of the methionine pool and the synthesis of cysteine. Therefore, this enzyme would be expected to be strictly regulated. In fact, CBS is allosterically regulated by SAM, in which low SAM concentrations direct homocysteine into remethylation, whereas at high SAM concentrations, transsulfuration is favored [33]. Following cystathionine formation, the B_6-dependent enzyme cystathionine γ-lyase (CGL) cleaves the molecule by γ-elimination of its homocysteine portion. This reaction leaves an unstable amino acid that binds to water molecules to form cysteine, α-ketobutyrate, and ammonia [34]. By the action of gamma-glutamylcysteine synthetase (GCL), cysteine and glutamate synthesize gamma-glutamylcysteine, a rate-limiting step in GSH synthesis [35]. Further, glycine binds to the C-terminal of gamma-glutamylcysteine via the enzyme GSH synthetase to form GSH.

Therefore, the transsulfuration pathway is a straight connection between homocysteine and GSH, the major redox buffer in mammalian cells. Consequently, it is expected that enzymes related to this metabolism display sensitivity to redox changes. Indeed, studies on purified mammalian MTR and CBS have revealed the reciprocal sensitivity of these two major homocysteine-utilizing enzymes to oxidative conditions [5,36]. In mammals, CBS contains a heme cofactor that functions as a redox sensor, increasing CBS activity and consequently transsulfuration under oxidizing conditions [36]. In contrast, under these same conditions, remethylation is depressed because MTR activity is reduced, most likely due to the lability of the reactive cofactor intermediate Cbl(I) [5]. Additionally, the betaine-related enzyme BHMT was also shown to be inhibited by oxidizing agents [6]. Considering that mammals metabolize seleno-amino acids in the same way as their sulfur counterparts [37], recent studies by this laboratory on the effects of selenium (Se) sources and levels combined or not with B_6 provided indirect support to this effect of ROS. Dalto et al. [38] reported that, under the oxidative stress of ovulation, the gene expression of GPX1, 3, and 4 in the livers (Table 1) and kidneys (Table 2) of Se-supplemented animals were higher than in the control Se-unsupplemented group, and animals supplemented with organic Se plus B_6 had the highest gene expression of GPX1 and selenocysteine lyase (SCLY), indicating that the transsulfuration pathway was stimulated. In contrast, Dalto et al. [39] observed, under basal oxidative stress conditions, no differential expression for the same genes (Tables 1 and 2).

Table 1. Real-time mRNA abundance of liver glutathione peroxidase (GPX) and selenocysteine-lyase (SCLY) genes in gilts three days after the fourth estrus and at day 30 of gestation, according to selenium and vitamin B_6 treatments.

	Day 3 Post-Estrus [a]					30 Days Gestation [b]				
	CONT	MSe $B_6$0 [c]	MSe $B_6$10 [c]	OSe $B_6$0 [c]	OSe $B_6$10 [c]	CONT	MSe $B_6$0 [c]	MSe $B_6$10 [c]	OSe $B_6$0 [c]	OSe $B_6$10 [c]
GPX1	0.44	1.02	1.09	0.77	1.57	1.15	1.19	1.37	1.27	1.15
GPX3	0.43	1.02	1.22	0.67	1.17	0.77	1.03	0.87	0.96	0.93
GPX4	0.59	1.00	1.08	0.66	1.19	1.05	1.05	1.19	1.07	0.98
SCLY	0.72	0.82	0.84	0.89	1.45	0.82	0.92	0.84	0.71	0.82

Adapted from Dalto et al. [38,39]. Standard error means for day three post estrus and 30 days gestation respectively equal 0.06 and 0.17 for GPX1, 0.05 and 0.12 for GPX3, 0.05 and 0.10 for GPX4, and 0.07 and 0.12 for SCLY. [a] For all treatments, GPX1, GPX3, GPX4, and SCLY were higher expressed than in the control diet ($p < 0.01$); Among all treatments, OSeB$_6$10 presented the highest gene expression for GPX1 and SCLY ($p < 0.01$); [b] No statistical difference ($p \geq 0.22$); [c] CONT = basal diet; MSe = inorganic selenium; OSe = organic selenium.

Table 2. Real-time mRNA abundance of kidney glutathione peroxidase (GPX) and selenocysteine-lyase (SCLY) genes in gilts three days after the fourth estrus and at day 30 of gestation, according to selenium and vitamin B_6 treatments.

	Day 3 Post-Estrus [a]					30 Days Gestation [b]				
	CONT [c]	MSe $B_6$0 [c]	MSe $B_6$10 [c]	OSe $B_6$0 [c]	OSe $B_6$10 [c]	CONT [c]	MSe $B_6$0 [c]	MSe $B_6$10 [c]	OSe $B_6$0 [c]	OSe $B_6$10 [c]
GPX1	0.72	1.16	1.25	1.19	1.83	0.97	1.11	0.95	1.03	1.14
GPX3	0.73	1.14	1.33	1.41	1.75	1.09	1.17	1.09	1.11	1.03
GPX4	1.06	1.12	1.18	1.18	1.47	1.10	1.22	1.12	1.18	1.17
SCLY	1.20	1.18	1.20	1.48	2.05	1.28	1.15	1.17	1.07	1.25

Adapted from Dalto et al. [38,39]. Standard error means for day three post estrus and 30 days gestation respectively equal 0.14 and 0.10 for GPX1, 0.10 and 0.09 for GPX3, 0.14 and 0.07 for GPX4, and 0.15 and 0.14 for SCLY. [a] For all treatments, GPX1 and GPX3 were higher ($p < 0.01$) expressed than control diet ($p < 0.01$); Among all treatments, OSe$B_6$10 presented the highest gene expression for GPX1 and SCLY ($p < 0.05$); Only for GPX3, OSe was higher than MSe ($p < 0.01$) and $B_6$10 was higher than $B_6$0 ($p < 0.01$); [b] No statistical difference ($p \geq 0.18$); [c] CONT = basal diet; MSe = inorganic selenium; OSe = organic selenium.

5. The Role of B_6

Differential Effects on Organic and Mineral Se Metabolisms in Gilts

Selenium is an essential trace element derived from inorganic (MSe) or organic (OSe) sources. Both forms are involved in the activation of SeGPX. The metabolism of Se-methionine, the natural organic source present in food, is interchangeable with a sulfur-methionine metabolism [37], and, therefore, the influence of B_6 on the one-carbon metabolism by the regulation between remethylation and transsulfuration is predictable. Although less evident, selenide, which is the metabolized form of selenite (commonly used dietary MSe) and a key intermediate for the utilization and/or excretion of both OSe and MSe [40,41], may represent another regulatory step influencing one-carbon metabolism. In this sense, two important B_6-dependent reactions direct selenide to be incorporated into Se-enzymes in preference to its excretion through the use of one-carbon groups in methylation reactions.

For Se-methionine, it is converted to Se-homocysteine through the action of SAM synthetase and SAHH, supplying the one-carbon system with –CH3 groups (Figure 1). As discussed above for sulfur-homocysteine, Se-homocysteine may be remethylated to Se-methionine or transsulfurated to Se-cystathionine, depending on the influence of SAM levels and ROS feedback on CBS. In this context, the SAM levels may promote equilibrium between remethylation and transsulfuration depending on dietary OSe levels, whereas the positive feedback of ROS on CBS (and the negative feedback of MTR) favors the transsulfuration pathway independently of dietary Se levels. Se-methionine may also be transaminated to methylselenol and then transformed to selenide via methyltransferases [42] or methylated to excretory forms. However, considering the importance of this amino acid in protein synthesis and the vital consequences of transmethylation, the partition of its pool to transamination and methylation may have a secondary relevance.

After SeCys synthesis from Se-cystathionine via Se-cystathionine gamma lyase (CGL; B_6-dependent enzyme), this amino acid can be incorporated into proteins or metabolized by the B_6-dependent enzyme SeCys lyase (SCLY) to alanine and selenide [43]. Considering that SCLY is substrate specific, this step is the landmark between sulfur and Se metabolisms and settles their fates in relation to the metabolism of glutathione. It has to be stated that the greater volume of sulfur, rather than SeCys, molecules available in the organism makes the impact of B_6 important not only for the enzyme SeGPX but also for its substrate (glutathione) as well.

Dietary selenite is non-enzymatically reduced via thiol-dependent reactions to selenide [44]. This direct reduction of selenite, short-cutting the transsulfuration pathway and with no regulatory mechanism, allows the accumulation of toxic levels of selenide. To avoid toxicity, selenide from both OSe (synthesized from SeCys) and MSe may follow two pathways: synthesis of Se-proteins or methylation (excretion). By the action of Se-phosphate synthetase 2 (B_6-dependent enzyme), selenide is converted into Se-phosphate [45]. This last molecule acts as a Se donor in the exchange of the phosphate moiety of serine-tRNA for Se, generating the SeCys-specific tRNA(Ser)Sec, in a B_6-dependent reaction [46]. This special tRNA, which contains the SeCys-insertion sequence (SECIS) along with a SeCys-tRNA-specific elongation factor (eEFSEC) and a specific SECIS binding protein (SECISBP2), is essential for SeCys incorporation into Se-proteins [47]. Remaining selenide must be successively methylated using –CH3 groups from SAM to generate the monomethylated intermediate methylselenol and multimethylated excretory metabolites (dimethylselenide and trimethylselenonium) [48].

Although the metabolism of OSe also generates selenide, the balance between SeCys incorporation into protein and its degradation by the saturable enzyme SCLY prevents the accumulation of excessive selenide. It is known that methylation and demethylation reactions between selenide and methylselenol promote equilibrium between the two molecules [41,42,49]; however, considering that low levels of dietary selenite supplementation provoke toxicity, whereas dietary Se-methionine is tolerated up to extreme high levels [50], one can assume that the utilisation of dietary selenite will direct the metabolism to consume greater amounts of one-carbon groups for the methylation of selenide than dietary Se-methionine. In contrast, OSe metabolism may not only preserve –CH3 molecules through the controlled synthesis of selenide, but also acts generating these one-carbon groups via demethylation/remethylation reactions between Se-methionine and Se-homocysteine. In this context, the regulatory steps (SAM levels, ROS feedback on CBS and MTR, and controlled synthesis of selenide from SCLY) in this metabolic pathway may promote a balance between the synthesis of one-carbon molecules and Se-proteins with possible beneficial effects to the organism.

Recent studies on Se and B_6 metabolisms by this laboratory, using the peri-estrus period as a model for oxidative stress in gilts [38,39,51], provided peculiar information about the control of this metabolic pathway. Although those studies did not specifically address the homeostasis of –CH3 groups, based on the above information this review makes some indirect inferences about the one-carbon metabolism from responses reported in relation to the transsulfuration pathway.

According to Dalto et al. [38,39], B_6 supplementation (10 mg/kg) does not affect the deposition of blood or tissue Se on a long-term basis (3 to 5 estrus), as well as blood Se levels during the peri-estrus period (oxidative stress condition) for both MSe and OSe. For MSe it is not surprising because, independently of the physiological state, absorbed selenite is quickly transformed into selenide and then converted into functional Se-proteins or methylated instead of being actively stored [9]. Consequently, the impact of MSe on the pool of one-carbon molecules for the methylation of selenide would be mainly related to the level of selenite supplementation rather than to B_6 availability.

For OSe supplemented animals however, the explanation is not so straightforward. Under basal oxidative stress conditions, the absence of positive feedback of ROS on CBS suggests that the remethylation of Se-homocysteine would be the preferential pathway, whereas the high SAM levels would stimulate CBS to transsulfurate Se-homocysteine. However, according to Bekaert et al. [52], in humans, high doses of daily supplementation with selenium yeast (a source of OSe) over six months did not affect the homocysteine concentrations in plasma. Also, considering that CBS is a B_6-dependent enzyme, its activity would direct more Se to SeGPX synthesis under B_6 supplementation. Davis [53] and Lima [54] reported that CBS is slightly affected by marginal vitamin B_6 status, whereas CGL is more sensitive, but neither of them affected cysteine synthesis. Although under marginal B_6 levels, these studies indicate that the B_6 status may not be a determining factor of the transsulfuration pathway flux, which is possibly mainly controlled by ROS and SAM levels. In fact, Dalto et al. [39] reported no effect of B_6 on either blood SeGPX activity or GPX and SCLY gene expression in gilts at 30-days of gestation (Tables 1 and 2), a conditions shown to be of low oxidative stress in this species. These results suggest that under basal oxidative stress conditions, in animals supplemented with Se and B_6, neither remethylation nor transsulfuration but Se deposition into proteins is the major route for this mineral.

In contrast, as also described above, Dalto et al. [38] reported that, under the oxidative stress of the peri-estrus period (3-days after estrus), GPX's and SCLY genes were highly expressed in OSe + B_6 supplemented animals in the liver and kidneys, in agreement with the positive feedback of ROS on CBS, increasing the ratio of transsulfuration. Interestingly, however, these same authors did not find any B_6 effect on SeGPX activity in the liver and kidneys (day 3 after estus) or whole blood (day − 4 to day + 3 of the peri-estrus period). In this regard, Lubos et al. [55] reported that GPX can be regulated by transcriptional, post-transcriptional, translational, or post-translational factors, and changes in gene transcription may not be reflected on GPX protein or its related enzymatic activity.

6. Embryo Metabolism

6.1. 5-Days Porcine Embryos

Using microarray technology to evaluate the global gene expression in 5-days porcine embryos, Dalto et al. [56] provided unique and interesting information on Se and B_6 metabolisms and, consequently, on the distinct interplay between remethylation and transsulfuration during early porcine embryo development.

The first aspect to be considered in 5-days embryos is the transfer of Se from dam to embryos. Dalto et al. [56] showed that Se was undetectable in the uterine flushing, indicating that this is a negligible source of this mineral for the pre-implantation embryo. Nevertheless, embryos from OSe supplemented dams are richer in Se than those from MSe supplemented dams. It was hypothesized that the most probable source is the pre-ovulatory oocyte that might be affected by the systemic maternal blood Se concentration through follicular fluid, considering that OSe is known to be more common deposited in tissues than is MSe [39,51,57,58]. In fact, Dalto et al. [56] observed that maternal supplementation with OSe plus B_6 stimulated 28.8 times more genes than MSe plus B_6 (six and 173 genes for MSe and OSe, respectively). These findings suggest that embryos coming from OSe supplemented dams have greater Se-methionine reserves and, therefore, are more suitable to go through demethylation steps to Se-homocysteine than are embryos from MSe supplemented dams.

A crucial aspect when studying the remethylation/transsulfuration pathway in embryos, fetuses, and newborns is the absence of CGL activity, in spite of its mRNA expression [10,14] (Figure 2). This relevant finding implies that, from conception to neonatal age, individuals are not able to convert Se-methionine into SeCys via the transsulfuration pathway. Therefore, Se-methionine would be directly incorporated into protein, methylated to methylselenol (with further methylation to excretory forms or demethylation to selenide), or demethylated to Se-homocysteine (generating the –CH3 donor SAM) and thereafter remethylated to Se-methionine via folate-dependent reactions, supplying the one-carbon metabolism. Dalto et al. [56] evaluated the expression of genes exclusively related to each source of Se (common genes between sources were excluded from the analysis) in 5-days embryos from gilts supplemented with OSe or MSe combined with B_6 and did not find differentially expressed genes related to the demethylation or remethylation of Se-methionine, whereas several genes related to general elongation factors and biological processes related to translation and mitotic cell cycle were stimulated by OSe. Those authors concluded that, in 5-days porcine embryos, Se-methionine preferentially follows protein deposition. However, recent results from this laboratory (data not yet published), using the database generated by Dalto et al. [56], evaluated global gene expression in 5-days embryos (common genes between sources of Se were not excluded from the analysis), showing that OSe, but not MSe, may affect DNA methylation and epigenetic events in 5-days embryos through the higher generation of –CH3 groups (stimulation of methyltransferases and SAM carrier genes). Therefore, although Se-methionine may be preferentially incorporated into protein, the magnitude of the demethylation and remethylation reactions that compose the one-carbon metabolism cannot be disregarded.

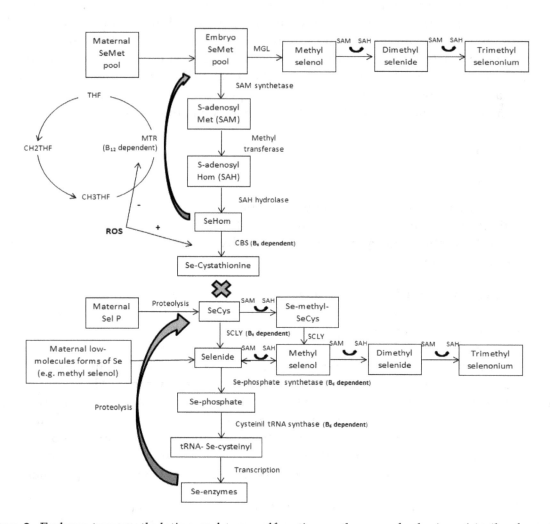

Figure 2. Embryo transmethylation and transsulfuration pathways of selenium (similar for sulfur counterparts) and possible maternal selenium transfer routes. Maternal selenomethionine (SeMet) is transferred to the embryo and may be methylated to methyl selenol by methionine γ lyase (MGL) or demethylated to selenohomocysteine (SeHom). SeHom may follow remethylation back to SeMet or transsulfuration to form selenocystathionine because the enzyme cystathionine γ lyase (CGL) that catalyzes the synthesis of selenocysteine (SeCys) from selenocystathionine is inactive in embryos. Pre-formed SeCys may be available after maternal selenoprotein P proteolysis in the placenta. Through the actions of selenocysteine lyase (SCLY), selenide is formed. Selenide may be methylated and excreted or phosphorylated and its selenium (Se) incorporated into tRNA Se-cysteinyl with further translation to Se-enzymes. THF = tetrahydrofolate; CH2THF = 5,10-methylene-THF; CH3THF = 5-methyl-THF; MTR = methionine synthase; CBS = cystathionine β synthase; ROS = reactive oxygen species.

Although the transsulfuration pathway is not complete in embryos, many genes involved in Se-enzymes synthesis were found in Dalto et al. [56] suggesting that 5-days embryos are potentially capable of synthesizing these enzymes. If so, the most probable sources of Se to the embryo are SeCys, methylselenol, and/or Se-proteins (after proteolysis in the embryo) coming from the pre-ovulatory oocyte. Furthermore, SeGPX synthesis would possibly not be under the feedback control by ROS but limited by the B_6-dependent enzyme SCLY, which controls the synthesis of selenide and, consequently, the consumption of one-carbon molecules for its methylation (Figure 2). Considering the importance of these one-carbon molecules for DNA processing and genetic stability, these routes of maternal Se transfer to early embryos may be considered a mechanism of defense to protect the pool of –CH3.

6.2. 30-Days Porcine Embryos

Similarly to 5-days embryos, the enzyme CGL is absent in 30-days embryos and, consequently, the above aspects related to remethylation/transsulfuration are expected to be analogous. However, at 30 days of gestation the presence of the placenta may change the dynamic of the interaction between these metabolic pathways.

One of the main features brought about by the presence of the placenta is the rise in the oxygen tension in the embryo, increasing the production of ROS. These levels are, in fact, higher in early gestation than thereafter [13], possibly because of the more immature embryonic antioxidant system. This suggests that, under oxidative stress conditions, the feedback of ROS stimulates CBS, directing Se-homocysteine to transsulfuration, whereas it would affect remethylation by reducing MTR activity. According to Kalhan [2], alterations to the metabolism of one-carbon may be the main cause of impaired fetal growth. Additionally, because the transsulfuration pathway is interrupted at Se-cystathionine, large amounts of this metabolite could possibly accumulate with negative effects in embryos from OSe supplemented dams. In this sense, under these conditions, B_6 supplementation levels might be carefully considered due to its effect on CBS activity. Evidences of this negative effect of B_6 on embryo development were observed in a study by Dalto et al. [39], in which maternal supplementation with 12.4 mg/kg of feed of B_6, with either MSe or OSe at 0.6 mg/kg of feed, increased the within-litter Se content variation and the within-litter weight variation, compared to animals receiving 2.4 mg/kg of B_6. Under similar experimental conditions and pig genetic lines, Fortier et al. [51] fed gilts with different sources of Se (MSe or OSe at 0.5 mg/kg of feed) but a fixed amount of B_6 at 3 mg/kg and observed improved within-litter Se content variation, embryo weight and length, and protein and DNA content, with no detrimental effect on the within-litter weight variation, compared to the control diet at similar levels of B_6 but 0.2 mg/kg of feed of Se.

As mentioned above, OSe increases body Se concentration more than MSe due to its deposition in proteins following the methionine metabolism, and B_6 does not interfere with Se deposition in the tissues of adult individuals [38,39]. Also in 30-days porcine embryos, Fortier et al. [51] and Dalto et al. [39] showed that, independently of B_6 status, gilts supplemented with OSe produced embryos with higher Se concentrations than gilts supplemented with MSe. Considering that the transsulfuration pathways is not complete at this stage of development, this higher load of Se-methionine in OSe embryos is not utilized in the synthesis of selenoenzymes but rather will be deposited in proteins and/or transmethylated, producing one-carbon groups. However, it has to be stated that even MSe supplemented gilts supply their embryos with OSe, not as Se-methionine but as SeCys, after selenoprotein P catabolism in the placenta [12]. In spite of the low activity of SCLY in vivo [59], one can assume that the majority of SeCys would be metabolized through SCLY because its concentration in tissues is enough to metabolize all SeCys available and the K_M (Michaelis constant) value of the enzyme is greater than the tissue levels of the substrate. However, Fortier et al. [51] and Dalto et al. [39] reported no effect of maternal Se levels (control vs. Se-supplemented gilts) and sources (OSe vs. MSe) on SeGPX activity in 30-days porcine embryos, indicating that at this stage of development the enzyme flux is not primarily substrate driven. Therefore, it is reasonable to hypothesize that embryo SeCys, from the catabolism of selenoprotein P in the placenta, follows primarily protein deposition and secondarily catabolism by SCLY, which is not controlled by the feedback of ROS, for the synthesis of selenide and further selenoenzymes. This mechanism would protect the embryo from wasting one-carbon groups for the methylation and elimination of excess selenide.

7. Conclusions

Both sulfur and Se methionine are important metabolic suppliers of one-carbon molecules through transmethylation reactions. The equilibrium between transmethylation and transsulfuration pathways, majorly regulated by redox conditions on CBS and MTR, influences the flow of –CH3 molecules between the one-carbon and antioxidation metabolisms.

Vitamin B_6 is important for the interplay between the synthesis (transmethylation) and the utilization (transsulfuration) of one-carbon groups by acting in most of their regulatory enzymes. However, its effects on the GPX system depend on other parameters such as the oxidative stress conditions and metabolic maturity.

Finally, whereas MSe may act by wasting one-carbon molecules to methylate the excess of selenide produced, OSe not only preserves one-carbon groups (due to the control of SCLY) but also promotes equilibrium between transsulfuration and transmethylation via the control of B_6-dependent CBS by SAM and ROS.

Author Contributions: Both authors equally contributed to the writing of the manuscript, revision of its content and approval of the final version submitted for publication.

References

1.   Joseph, J.; Loscalzo, J. Methoxistasis: Integrating the roles of homocysteine and folic acid in cardiovascular pathobiology. *Nutrients* **2013**, *5*, 3235–3256. [CrossRef] [PubMed]

2.   Kalhan, S.C. One carbon metabolism in pregnancy: Impact on maternal, fetal and neonatal health. *Mol. Cell. Endocrinol.* **2016**, *435*, 48–60. [CrossRef] [PubMed]

3.   Selhub, J. Homocysteine metabolism. *Annu. Rev. Nutr.* **1999**, *19*, 217–246. [CrossRef] [PubMed]

4.   Berg, J.M.; Tymoczko, J.L.; Stryer, L. *Biochemistry*, 5th ed.; W.H. Freeman and Company: New York, NY, USA, 2002; pp. 571–572, 674–678, 686, 694, 698–700, 704, 771–772.

5.   Chen, Z.; Chakraborty, S.; Banerjee, R. Demonstration that mammalian methionine synthases are predominantly cobalamin-loaded. *J. Biol. Chem.* **1995**, *270*, 19246–19249. [PubMed]

6.   Castro, C.; Millian, N.S.; Garrow, T.A. Liver betaine-homocysteine S-methyltransferase activity undergoes a redox switch at the active site zinc. *Arch. Biochem. Biophys.* **2008**, *472*, 26–33. [CrossRef] [PubMed]

7.   Li, Y.N.; Gulati, S.; Baker, P.J.; Brody, L.C.; Banerjee, R.; Kruger, W.D. Cloning, mapping and RNA analysis of the human methionine synthase gene. *Hum. Mol. Genet.* **1996**, *5*, 1851–1858. [CrossRef] [PubMed]

8.   Mosharov, E.; Cranford, M.R.; Banerjee, R. The quantitatively important relationship between homocysteine metabolism and glutathione synthesis by the transsulfuration pathway and its regulation by redox changes. *Biochemistry* **2000**, *39*, 13005–13011. [CrossRef] [PubMed]

9.   Windisch, W. Interaction of chemical species with biological regulation of the metabolism of essential trace elements. *Anal. Bioanal. Chem.* **2002**, *372*, 421–425. [CrossRef] [PubMed]

10.   Gardiner, C.S.; Reed, D.J. Glutathione redox cycle-driven recovery of reduced glutathione after oxidation by tertiary-butyl hydroperoxide in preimplantation mouse embryos. *Arch. Biochem. Biophys.* **1995**, *321*, 6–12. [CrossRef]

11.   Davis, S.; Scheer, J.; Quinlivan, E.; Coats, B.; Stacpoole, P.; Gregory, J. Dietary vitamin B_6 restriction does not alter rates of homocysteine remethylation or synthesis in healthy young women and men. *Am. J. Clin. Nutr.* **2005**, *81*, 648–655. [PubMed]

12.   Burk, R.F.; Olson, G.E.; Hill, K.E.; Winfrey, V.P.; Motley, A.K.; Kurokawa, S. Maternal-fetal transfer of selenium in the mouse. *FASEB J.* **2013**, *27*, 3249–3256. [CrossRef] [PubMed]

13.   Jauniaux, E.; Watson, A.L.; Hempstock, J.; Bao, Y.P.; Skepper, J.N.; Burton, G.J. Onset of maternal arterial blood flow and placental oxidative stress. A possible factor in human early pregnancy failure. *Am. J. Pathol.* **2000**, *157*, 2111–2122. [CrossRef]

14.   Levonen, A.L.; Lapatto, R.; Saksela, M.; Raivio, K.O. Human cystathionine gamma-lyase: Developmental and in vitro expression of two isoforms. *Biochem. J.* **2000**, *347*, 291–295. [CrossRef] [PubMed]

15.   Bender, D.A. *Nutritional Biochemistry of the Vitamins*, 2nd ed.; Cambridge University Press: Cambridge, UK, 2003.

16.   Combs, G.F., Jr. *The Vitamins*, 4th ed.; Academic Press: San Diego, CA, USA, 2012.

17.   Combs, G.F. *The Vitamins: Fundamental Aspects in Nutrition and Health*; Elsevier: San Diego, CA, USA, 2008.

18.   Berdanier, C.D. Water-Soluble Vitamins. In *Advanced Nutrition-Micronutrients*; Berdanier, C.D., Ed.; CRC Press: New York, NY, USA, 1998.

19. Matte, J.J.; Girard, C.L.; Sève, B. Effects of long-term parenteral administration of vitamin B_6 on B_6 status and some aspects of the glucose and protein metabolism of early-weaned piglets. *Br. J. Nutr.* **2001**, *85*, 11–21. [CrossRef] [PubMed]

20. Helmreich, E.J. How pyridoxal 5'-phosphate could function in glycogen phosphorylase catalysis. *Biofactors* **1992**, *3*, 159–172. [PubMed]

21. Bilski, P.; Li, M.Y.; Ehrenshaft, M.; Daub, M.E.; Chignell, C.F. Vitamin B_6 (pyridoxine) and its derivatives are efficient singlet oxygen quenchers and potential fungal antioxidants. *Photochem. Photobiol.* **2000**, *71*, 129–134. [CrossRef]

22. Oka, T. Modulation of gene expression by vitamin B6. *Nutr. Res. Rev.* **2001**, *14*, 257–265. [CrossRef] [PubMed]

23. Drewke, C.; Leistner, E. Biosynthesis of vitamin B_6 and structurally related derivatives. *Vitam. Horm.* **2001**, *61*, 121–155. [PubMed]

24. Mittenhuber, G. Phylogenetic analyses and comparative genomics of vitamin B_6 (pyridoxine) and pyridoxal phosphate biosynthesis pathways. *J. Mol. Microbiol. Biotechnol.* **2001**, *3*, 1–20. [PubMed]

25. Mudd, S.H.; Cantoni, G.L. Activation of methionine for transmethylation. III. The methionine-activating enzyme of Bakers' yeast. *J. Biol. Chem.* **1958**, *231*, 481–492. [PubMed]

26. Ulrey, C.L.; Liu, L.; Andrews, L.G.; Tollefsbol, T.O. The impact of metabolism on DNA methylation. *Hum. Mol. Genet.* **2005**, *14*. [CrossRef] [PubMed]

27. Födinger, M.; Hörl, W.; Sunder-Plassmann, G. Molecular biology of 5,10-methylenetetrahydrofolate reductase. *J. Nephrol.* **2000**, *13*, 20–33. [PubMed]

28. Tibbetts, A.S.; Appling, D.R. Compartmentalization of mammalian folate-mediated one-carbon metabolism. *Annu. Rev. Nutr.* **2010**, *30*, 57–81. [CrossRef] [PubMed]

29. Martinez, M.; Cuskelly, G.J.; Williamson, J.; Toth, J.P.; Gregory, J.F. Vitamin B_6 deficiency in rats reduces hepatic serine hydroxymethyltransferase and cystathionine beta-synthase activities and rates of in vivo protein turnover, homocysteine remethylation and transsulfuration. *J. Nutr.* **2000**, *130*, 1115–1123. [PubMed]

30. Perry, C.; Yu, S.; Chen, J.; Matharu, K.; Stover, P. Effect of vitamin B_6 availability on serine hydroxymethyltransferase in MCF-7 cells. *Arch. Biochem. Biophys.* **2007**, *462*, 21–27. [CrossRef] [PubMed]

31. Matthews, R.G.; Smith, A.E.; Zhou, Z.S.; Taurog, R.E.; Bandarian, V.; Evans, J.C.; Ludwig, M. Cobalamin-dependent and cobalamin-independent methionine synthases: Are there two solutions to the same chemical problem? *Helv. Chim. Acta* **2003**, *86*, 3939–3954. [CrossRef]

32. Aitken, S.M.; Lodha, P.H.; Morneau, D.J.K. The enzymes of the transsulfuration pathways: Active-site characterizations. *Biochim. Biophys. Acta Proteins Proteom.* **2011**, *1814*, 1511–1517. [CrossRef] [PubMed]

33. Ereno-Orbea, J.; Majtan, T.; Oyenarte, I.; Kraus, J.P.; Martinez-Cruz, L.A. Structural insight into the molecular mechanism of allosteric activation of human cystathionine beta-synthase by *S*-adenosylmethionine. *Proc. Natl. Acad. Sci. USA* **2014**, *111*, E3845–E3852. [CrossRef] [PubMed]

34. Flavin, M.; Slaughter, C. Cystathionine cleavage enzymes of neurospora. *J. Biol. Chem.* **1964**, *239*, 2212–2219. [PubMed]

35. Franklin, C.C.; Backos, D.S.; Mohar, I.; White, C.C.; Forman, H.J.; Kavanagh, T.J. Structure, function, and post-translational regulation of the catalytic and modifier subunits of glutamate cysteine ligase. *Mol. Aspects Med.* **2009**, *30*, 86–98. [CrossRef] [PubMed]

36. Taoka, S.; Ohja, S.; Shan, X.; Kruger, W.D.; Banerjee, R. Evidence for heme-mediated redox regulation of human cystathionine β-synthase activity. *J. Biol. Chem.* **1998**, *273*, 25179–25184. [CrossRef] [PubMed]

37. Schrauzer, G.N. The nutritional significance, metabolism and toxicology of selenomethionine. *Adv. Food Nutr. Res.* **2003**, *47*, 73–112. [PubMed]

38. Dalto, D.B.; Roy, M.; Audet, I.; Palin, M.-F.; Guay, F.; Lapointe, J.; Matte, J.J. Interaction between vitamin B_6 and source of selenium on the response of the selenium-dependent glutathione peroxidase system to oxidative stress induced by oestrus in pubertal pig. *J. Trace Elem. Med. Biol.* **2015**, *32*, 21–29. [CrossRef] [PubMed]

39. Dalto, D.B.; Audet, I.; Lapointe, J.; Matte, J.J. The importance of pyridoxine for the impact of the dietary selenium sources on redox balance, embryo development, and reproductive performance in gilts. *J. Trace Elem. Med. Biol.* **2016**, *34*, 79–89. [CrossRef] [PubMed]

40. Birringer, M.; Pilawa, S.; Flohe, L. Trends in selenium biochemistry. *Nat. Prod. Rep.* **2002**, *19*, 693–718. [CrossRef] [PubMed]

41. Suzuki, K.T.; Doi, C.; Suzuki, N. Metabolism of ^{76}Se-methylselenocysteine compared with that of ^{77}Se-selenomethionine and ^{82}Se-selenite. *Toxicol. Appl. Pharmacol.* **2006**, *217*, 185–195. [CrossRef] [PubMed]

42. Suzuki, K.T.; Kurasaki, K.; Suzuki, N. Selenocysteine β-lyase and methylselenol demethylase in the metabolism of Se-methylated selenocompounds into selenide. *Biochim. Biophys. Acta* **2007**, *1770*, 1053–1061. [CrossRef] [PubMed]

43. Esaki, N.; Nakamura, T.; Tanaka, H.; Soda, K. Selenocysteine lyase, a novel enzyme that specifically acts on selenocysteine. Mammalian distribution and purification and properties of pig liver enzyme. *J. Biol. Chem.* **1982**, *257*, 4386–4391. [PubMed]

44. Foster, L.H.; Sumar, S. Selenium in health and disease: A review. *Crit. Rev. Food Sci. Nutr.* **1997**, *37*, 211–228. [CrossRef] [PubMed]

45. Xu, X.-M.; Carlson, B.A.; Mix, H.; Zhang, Y.; Saira, K.; Glass, R.S.; Berry, M.J.; Gladyshev, V.N.; Hatfield, D.L. Biosynthesis of selenocysteine on its tRNA in eukaryotes. *PLoS Biol.* **2007**, *5*, 96–105. [CrossRef] [PubMed]

46. Sunde, R.A.; Thompson, B.M.; Palm, M.D.; Weiss, S.L.; Thompson, K.M.; Evenson, J.K. Selenium regulation of selenium-dependent glutathione peroxidases in animals and transfected CHO cells. *Biomed. Environ. Sci.* **1997**, *10*, 346–355. [PubMed]

47. Johansson, L.; Gafvelin, G.; Arnér, E.S.J. Selenocysteine in proteins—Properties and biotechnological use. *Biochim. Biophys. Acta Gen. Subj.* **2005**, *1726*, 1–13. [CrossRef] [PubMed]

48. Hsieh, S.H.; Ganther, H.E. Biosynthesis of dimethyl selenide from sodium selenite in rat liver and kidney cell-free systems. *Biochim. Biophys. Acta Gen. Subj.* **1977**, *497*, 205–217. [CrossRef]

49. Ganther, H.E. Enzymic synthesis of dimethyl selenide from sodium selenite in mouse liver extracts. *Biochemistry* **1966**, *5*, 1089–1098. [CrossRef] [PubMed]

50. Kim, Y.Y.; Mahan, D.C. Comparative effects of high dietary levels of organic and inorganic selenium on selenium toxicity of growing-finishing pigs. *J. Anim. Sci.* **2001**, *79*, 942–948. [CrossRef] [PubMed]

51. Fortier, M.-E.; Audet, I.; Giguère, A.; Laforest, J.-P.; Bilodeau, J.-F.; Quesnel, H.; Matte, J.J. Effect of dietary organic and inorganic selenium on antioxidant status, embryo development, and reproductive performance in hyperovulatory first-parity gilts. *J. Anim. Sci.* **2012**, *90*, 231–240. [CrossRef] [PubMed]

52. Bekaert, B.; Cooper, M.L.; Green, F.R.; McNulty, H.; Pentieva, K.; Scott, J.M.; Molloy, A.M.; Rayman, M.P. Effect of selenium status and supplementation with high-selenium yeast on plasma homocysteine and B vitamin concentrations in the UK elderly. *Mol. Nutr. Food Res.* **2008**, *52*, 1324–1333. [CrossRef] [PubMed]

53. Davis, S.R.; Quinlivan, E.P.; Stacpoole, P.W.; Gregory, J.F., 3rd. Plasma glutathione and cystathionine concentrations are elevated but cysteine flux is unchanged by dietary vitamin B-6 restriction in young men and women. *J. Nutr.* **2006**, *136*, 373–378. [PubMed]

54. Lima, C.P.; Davis, S.R.; Mackey, A.D.; Scheer, J.B.; Williamson, J.; Gregory, J.F., 3rd. Vitamin B-6 deficiency suppresses the hepatic transsulfuration pathway but increases glutathione concentration in rats fed AIN-76A or AIN-93G diets. *J. Nutr.* **2006**, *136*, 2141–2147. [PubMed]

55. Lubos, E.; Loscalzo, J.; Handy, D.E. Glutathione peroxidase-1 in health and disease: From molecular mechanisms to therapeutic opportunities. *Antioxid. Redox Signal.* **2011**, *5*, 1957–1997. [CrossRef] [PubMed]

56. Dalto, D.B.; Tsoi, S.; Audet, I.; Dyck, M.K.; Foxcroft, G.R.; Matte, J.J. Gene expression of porcine blastocysts from gilts fed organic or inorganic selenium and pyridoxine. *Reproduction* **2015**, *149*, 31–42. [CrossRef] [PubMed]

57. Svoboda, M.; Ficek, R.; Drabek, J. Efficacy of selenium from Se-enriched yeast on selenium transfer from sows to piglets. *Acta Vet. Brno* **2008**, *77*, 515–521. [CrossRef]

58. Ma, Y.L.; Lindemann, M.D.; Pierce, J.L.; Unrine, J.M.; Cromwell, G.L. Effect of inorganic or organic selenium supplementation on reproductive performance and tissue trace mineral concentrations in gravid first-parity gilts, fetuses, and nursing piglets. *J. Anim. Sci.* **2014**, *92*, 5540–5550. [CrossRef] [PubMed]

59. Soda, K.; Oikawa, T.; Esaki, N. Vitamin B$_6$ enzymes participating in selenium amino acid metabolism. *BioFactors* **1999**, *10*, 257–262. [CrossRef] [PubMed]

12

Intakes of Folate and Vitamin B12 and Biomarkers of Status in the Very Old: The Newcastle 85+ Study

Nuno Mendonça [1,2,3,*], John C. Mathers [2,3,4], Ashley J. Adamson [2,3,5], Carmen Martin-Ruiz [2], Chris J. Seal [1,3], Carol Jagger [2,5] and Tom R. Hill [1,2,3]

[1]   School of Agriculture Food and Rural Development, Newcastle University, Newcastle upon Tyne NE1 7RU, UK; Chris.seal@newcastle.ac.uk (C.J.S.); Tom.hill@newcastle.ac.uk (T.R.H.)
[2]   Newcastle University Institute for Ageing, Newcastle University, Newcastle upon Tyne NE2 4AX, UK; john.mathers@newcastle.ac.uk (J.C.M.); Ashley.Adamson@newcastle.ac.uk (A.J.A.); Carmen.martin-ruiz@newcastle.ac.uk (C.M.-R.); carol.jagger@newcastle.ac.uk (C.J.)
[3]   Human Nutrition Research Centre, Newcastle University, Newcastle upon Tyne NE2 4HH, UK
[4]   Institute of Cellular Medicine, Newcastle upon Tyne NE2 4HH, UK
[5]   Institute of Health and Society, Newcastle University, Newcastle upon Tyne NE2 5PL, UK
*   Correspondence: n.m.p.mendonca@newcastle.ac.uk

Abstract: Very old adults are at increased risk of folate and vitamin B12 deficiencies due to reduced food intake and gastrointestinal absorption. The main aim was to determine the association between folate and vitamin B12 intake from total diets and food groups, and status. Folate or vitamin B12 intakes (2×24 h multiple pass recalls) and red blood cell (RBC) folate or plasma vitamin B12 (chemiluminescence immunoassays) concentrations were available at baseline for 731 participants aged 85 from the Newcastle 85+ Study (North-East England). Generalized additive and binary logistic models estimated the associations between folate and vitamin B12 intakes from total diets and food groups, and RBC folate and plasma B12. Folate intake from total diets and cereal and cereal products was strongly associated with RBC folate ($p < 0.001$). Total vitamin B12 intake was weakly associated with plasma vitamin B12 ($p = 0.054$) but those with higher intakes from total diets or meat and meat products were less likely to have deficient status. Women homozygous for the *FUT2* G allele had higher concentrations of plasma vitamin B12. Cereals and cereal products are a very important source of folate in the very old. Higher intakes of folate and vitamin B12 lower the risk of "inadequate" status.

Keywords: 'aged 80 and over'; Newcastle 85+ Study; red blood cell folate; vitamin B12; *FUT2*; *MTHFR*; food groups

---

1. Introduction

B vitamins, specifically folate and vitamin B12, are essential for one-carbon transfer reactions which include amino acid interconversions, RNA and DNA synthesis and methylation of cell macromolecules [1]. Older adults are at increased risk of B vitamin deficiencies due to decreased food intake and increased malabsorption. Low folate and vitamin B12 status have been associated with adverse health outcomes, including cognitive impairment [2–4], stroke [5,6], fractures [7,8] and cancer in older adults [9]. A review of micronutrient deficiencies in community-dwelling older adults (aged 65 and over) living in western countries reported that 29% and 16% of men and, 30% and 19% of women had intakes below the Nordic Nutrition Recommendations (NNR) estimated average requirement (EAR) for folate (200 μg/day) and vitamin B12 (1.4 μg/day), respectively [10]. The current UK National Diet and Nutrition Survey (NDNS) rolling programme estimated that 1% of older adults (aged 65 and over) were below the UK lower reference nutrient intake (LRNI) for folate (100 μg/day) and vitamin B12 (1.0 µg/day) but that 7.3% of men and 10.8% of women had red blood cell folate (RBC) concentrations below 340 nmol/L and 5.9% of men and women had serum vitamin B12 concentrations below 150 pmol/L [11]. The complexity of the dose–response relationships between intake and status is influenced by limitations in dietary assessment, food composition data, choice of biomarkers, genotypic variation, bioavailability and complex metabolic pathways. About 10%–30% of older adults have atrophic gastritis (caused by *Helicobacter pylori* infection, long-term use of proton pump inhibitors, H_2 receptor antagonists and biguanides) which leads to hypochlorhydria [12]. This has a detrimental effect onacid–pepsin digestion and favours small bowel bacterial growth resulting in impaired vitamin B12 absorption [13]. In addition, those with autoimmune atrophic gastritis produce antibodies against the intrinsic factor which can lead to pernicious anemia [13]. Therefore, older adults may have adequate vitamin B12 intake but inadequate vitamin B12 plasma concentration. In addition, several single nucleotide polymorphisms (SNP) modulate folate and vitamin B12 status. For example, homozygosity of the T allele (forward orientation) (rs1801133) of the *MTHFR* gene (which encodes methylenetetrahydrofolate reductase) is associated with low folate status [14].

There is conflicting evidence about relationships between folate and vitamin B12 intake and, folate and vitamin B12 status, respectively, in older adults. Some studies report a significant association between folate and vitamin B12 intake and status in older adults [2,15–19] while others do not [20–22]. Differences in folate and vitamin B12 bioavailability from total diets and specific food sources may provide a partial explanation for the observed discrepancies. Folate bioavailability from foods is substantially lower than that from supplements or from foods fortified with folic acid with estimated bioavailability of 50% and 85%, respectively [23]. If intrinsic factor (IF) secretion is intact, approximately 40% of vitamin B12 is absorbed [24].

In light of the concerns about dietary inadequacy, it is imperative to assess folate and vitamin B12 status in older people, particularly the very old (85 years and older). The aims were to determine (i) the prevalence of "inadequate" folate and vitamin B12 intake and status in the Newcastle 85+ Study; (ii) the associations between the top contributing dietary sources of folate and vitamin B12, and status; and (iii) whether high dietary intakes of both vitamins are associated with a reduced risk of "inadequate" status.

2. Material and Methods

2.1. Newcastle 85+ Study

The Newcastle 85+ Study is a longitudinal population-based study of health trajectories and outcomes in the very old which approached all people turning 85 in 2006 (born in 1921) who were registered with participating general practices within Newcastle upon Tyne or North Tyneside primary care trusts (North East England). Details of the study have been reported elsewhere [25–27]. All procedures involving human subjects were approved by the Newcastle and North Tyneside local research ethics committee (06/Q0905/2). Written informed consent was obtained from all participants, and when unable to do so, consent was obtained from a carer or a relative. The recruited cohort was socio-demographically representative of the general UK population [25]. At baseline (2006/2007), multidimensional health assessment, complete general practice (GP) medical records data and complete dietary intake data (without protocol violation) were available for 793 participants [28].

2.2. Dietary Assessment and Food Groups

Dietary intake was collected at baseline using two 24 h Multiple Pass Recalls (24 h-MPR) on two non-consecutive occasions in the participant's usual residence by a trained research nurse and energy, folate and vitamin B12 intakes were estimated using the McCance and Widdowson's Food Composition tables 6th edition [29]. Individual foods were coded and allocated to 15 first level food groups that consisted of: cereals and cereal products, milk and milk products, eggs and egg dishes, oils and fat spreads, meat and meat products, fish and fish dishes, vegetables, potatoes, savoury snacks, nuts and seeds, fruit, sugar, preserves and confectionery, non-alcoholic beverages, alcoholic beverages and miscellaneous (soups, sauces and remaining foods that did not belong in other food groups) [28]. The top three food group contributors to folate or vitamin B12 intakes (accounted for >50% of total intake) were included in the analysis. These food groups were also widely consumed by this population and, therefore, a possible target for public health policies/fortification. Information on supplement use was limited to type and brand and, therefore, this was only used as a dichotomous covariate (yes/no) [30].

2.3. Nutritional Biomarkers and Single Nucleotide Polymorphisms

Blood samples were taken after an overnight fast at baseline. Forty mL of blood was drawn from the antecubital vein between 7:00 a.m. and 10:30 a.m., placed on ethylenediamine tetraacetic acid (EDTA) tubes and 95% of the samples were taken to the laboratory within 1 h [31]. Red blood cell folate (RBC folate) and plasma vitamin B12 concentrations were determined by chemiluminescence (Microparticle Immunoassay on an Abbott ARCHITECT analyser) and data were available for 731 and 732 participants, respectively. RBC folate was stabilized with ascorbic acid and adjusted for hematocrit. Whole blood DNA was extracted by means of a QiaGEN Amp Maxi DNA Purification Kit. As part of the EU Longevity Genetics Consortium, genome-wide association studies (GWAS) were performed on 765 participants from the Newcastle 85+ Study using Illumina Omni genotyping arrays. Data were obtained from 710 individuals and after quality control, 642 individuals were retained for the final analysis [32]. The single nucleotide polymorphisms (SNP) in the MTHFR (rs1801133, chromosome 1, position 11796321), FUT2 (rs492602, chromosome 19, position 48703160), MTR (rs1805087, chromosome 1, position 236885200) and TCN1 (rs526934, chromosome 11, position 59866020) genes were chosen as candidate modifiers of RBC folate and plasma vitamin B12 concentrations. All SNPs were assessed for deviation from the Hardy–Weinberg equilibrium.

2.4. Statistical Analysis

Normality was assessed graphically with the aid of Q-Q plots and histograms. Linearity and homoscedasticity assumptions were tested with residuals versus predicted values plots. Normally distributed continuous values are presented as means and standard deviations (SD), and non-Gaussian distributed variables as medians and interquartile ranges (IQR). Categorical data are presented as percentages (with corresponding sample size). Sex differences were assessed with the Chi-squared test (χ^2) for categorical variables and by independent t-test, and Mann–Whitney U test for parametric and non-parametric continuous data, respectively. Differences between RBC folate and plasma vitamin B12 concentrations according to MTHFR (rs1801133), MTR (rs1805087), TCN1 (rs526934) and FUT2 (rs492602) genotype were assessed using Kruskal–Wallis tests followed by Dunn–Bonferoni tests if the null hypothesis was rejected.

The semi-parametric generalized additive models (gam) were investigated in R version 3.0.1 (R foundation for statistical computing) using the package "gam" to plot the relationship between vitamin intakes (thin plate regression splines for smoothing) and corresponding biomarkers. The generated reference value of zero in the y-axis corresponds to the RBC folate/ plasma vitamin B12 concentrations for the mean intake of folate and vitamin B12, respectively. The odds ratio (OR) (and 95% confidence intervals (CI)) of RBC folate concentrations <600 nmol/L and plasma B12 <148 pmol/L according to quartiles of folate and vitamin B12 intake from total diets and top contributing food groups were computed using binary logistic regression. The commonly used cut-off to define folate deficiency of RBC folate <340 nmol/L [23] could not be used for these models due to the low percentage of deficiency among study participants. Gam and binary logistic regression models were adjusted for sex, energy intake, folic acid or vitamin B12 containing supplement use, folate/vitamin B12 intake from other food groups, MTHFR or FUT2 genotype. The vitamin B12 models were additionally adjusted for H_2 receptor antagonists, biguanides and proton pump inhibitor (PPI) use.

$p < 0.05$ was considered statistically significant. Apart from the gam models, all statistical analyses were conducted using the IBM statistical tool SPSS v22 (IBM, New York, NY, USA).

3. Results

3.1. Folate and Vitamin B12 Intake and Status "Inadequacies"

Although 43% of participants ($n = 335$) consumed one or more supplements on a regular basis [30], only 4.8% were users of folic acid and vitamin B12 as part of multivitamin supplements (Table 1). A low percentage of participants (3.1%) had folate intakes below the UK LRNI (100 µg/day) [33] or had RBC folate concentrations below the classic cut-off for deficiency of 340 nmol/L (3.6%) [23]. Folate intake and status were "inadequate" in only five participants. Cereals and cereal products, vegetables and fruit and fruit juice were the top food group contributors to folate intake, explaining almost 60% of total folate intake. Vitamin B12 intakes were below the UK LRNI (1 µg/day) [33] in 9.2% ($n = 67$) of the population while 17.1% ($n = 125$) were below 148 pmol/L of plasma vitamin B12 [24] (110 of these 125 had also total homocysteine concentrations >15 µmol/L). In addition, 17 participants had "inadequate" intakes and also deficient plasma concentrations of vitamin B12. There were twice as many women with vitamin B12 intakes below the UK LRNI than men (5.0% vs. 12.4%, $p < 0.001$) but not based on plasma vitamin B12 concentrations <148 pmol/L (17.4% vs. 16.9%, $p = 0.238$). Eighty-six percent ($n = 628$) of the participants had plasma vitamin B12 concentration <400 pmol/L, a concentration that has been associated with high total homocysteine and methylmalonic acid concentrations [34,35]. Intake of the top three food groups (meat, fish and dairy) explained more than 80% of total vitamin B12 intake.

Table 1. Population characteristics, folate and vitamin B12 intakes and biomarkers of one carbon metabolism in the Newcastle 85+ Study.

	All	Men	Women	p-Value [1]
Sex (%) (n)	732	39 (287)	61 (445)	-
BMI (kg/m^2) (mean ± SD)	24.4 ± 4.3	24.7 ± 3.9	24.3 ± 4.6	0.244 [2]
Smokers (%) (n)	5.6 (41)	4.2 (12)	6.5 (29)	0.183
Alcohol Drinkers (%) (n)	72 (364)	84 (192)	62 (172)	<0.001
Total Energy Intakes (MJ/day)	6.78 (5.62–8.31)	8.01 (6.65–9.59)	6.26 (5.17–7.38)	<0.001
Folate and vitamin B12 supplement use (%) (n)	4.8 (35)	3.8 (11)	5.4 (24)	0.334
H$_2$ antagonists, PPI and biguanides use (%) (n)	26.8 (196)	27.2 (78)	26.5 (118)	0.844
Total Homocysteine (µmol/L)	16.7 (13.5–21.4)	18.0 (14.5–21.9)	16.1 (13.1–21.0)	0.001
>15 µmol/L (%) (n)	63.1 (471)	70.3 (206)	58.5 (265)	0.001
Folate				
Intake (µg/day)	209 (157–265)	246 (185–296)	189 (144–242)	<0.001
<100 µg/day (%) (n)	3.1 (23)	0.7 (2)	4.7 (21)	0.002
Top food group contributors	Cereals (32%), Vegetables (16%), Fruit (9%)	Cereals (32%), Vegetables (15%), Fruit (8%)	Cereals (31%), Vegetables (17%), Fruit (10%)	-
Red Blood Cell Folate (nmol/L)	863 (451–1287)	868 (596–1282)	854 (614–1287)	0.728
<340 nmol/L (%) (n)	3.6 (26)	2.1 (6)	4.5 (20)	0.103
Vitamin B12				
Intake (µg/day)	2.9 (1.9–4.4)	3.5 (2.2–5.2)	2.5 (1.6–3.9)	<0.001
<1.0 µg/day (%) (n)	9.2 (67)	4.5 (13)	12.1 (54)	<0.001
Top food group contributors	Meat (53%), Fish (17%), Milk (13%)	Meat (59%), Fish (16%), Milk (10%)	Meat (48%), Fish (19%), Milk (15%)	-
Plasma Vitamin B12 (pmol/L)	232 (170–324)	228 (166–309)	238 (174–337)	0.238
<148 pmol/L (%) (n)	17.1 (125)	17.4 (50)	16.9 (75)	0.841

BMI, body mass index; Cereals, Cereals and cereal products; Fruit, Fruit and fruit juice; Meat, Meat and meat products; Fish, Fish and fish dishes; Milk, Milk and milk products; PPI, proton pump inhibitors. Values are medians and IQR unless otherwise stated. [1] No sex difference by Chi-squared test (χ^2) for categorical or Mann–Whitney test for non-parametric continuous variables; [2] Independent t-test.

3.2. Folate, Vitamin B12 Status and Genotype

RBC folate and plasma vitamin B12 concentrations according to *FUT2*, *MTHFR*, *MTR* and *TCN1* and genotypes are shown in Table 2. Individuals with the *MTHFR* (rs1801133) AG or GA genotype [minor allele frequency (MAF) = 0.33 in the Newcastle 85+ Study vs. 0.32 for the A allele from the 1000 Genomes Project British population phase 3 [36]] had higher RBC folate concentrations than those homozygous for G (p = 0.024). Participants with the *FUT2* (rs492602) GG genotype had higher concentrations of plasma vitamin B12 than other *FUT2* genotypes (p < 0.001) (MAF = 0.45 in the Newcastle 85+ Study vs. 0.48 for the G allele in residents of England and Scotland [36]). The association between *FUT2* genotype and plasma vitamin B12 concentrations was significant in women (p < 0.001) but not in men (p = 0.140).

Table 2. Plasma vitamin B12 and RBC folate concentrations by *FUT2*, *MTHFR*, *MTR*, and *TCN1* genotypes in the Newcastle 85+ Study.

	RBC Folate (nmol/L)	p-Value [1]	Plasma Vitamin B12 (pmol/L)	p-Value [1]
FUT2 (rs492602)		0.531		<0.001
AA (n = 128)	894 (629–1349		216 (146–281)	Ref.
A/G (n = 308)	917 (603–1322)		221 (163–309)	0.413
GG (n = 187)	835 (595–1206)		277 (209–381)	<0.001
MTHFR (rs1801133)		0.028		0.244
GG (n = 276)	871 (614–1275)	Ref.	234 (168–331)	
A/G (n = 279)	845 (584–1263)	1.000	230 (164–312)	
AA (n = 67)	1010 (693–1626)	0.060	249 (193–339)	
MTR (rs1805087)		0.547		0.277
AA (n = 419)	881 (613–1278)		240 (173–337)	
A/G (n = 178)	845 (596–1332)		226 (162–297)	
GG (n = 26)	1053 (580–1593)		247 (162–310)	
TCN1 (rs526934)		0.065		0.298
AA (n = 331)	877 (606–1317)		237 (178–336)	
A/G (n = 247)	845 (595–1223)		231 (160–325)	
GG (n = 45)	1074 (630–1439)		222 (182–273)	

RBC folate, Red blood cell folate; *FUT2*, Fucosyltrasnferase 2; *MTHFR*, Methylenetetrahydrofolate reductase; *MTR*, Methionine synthase; *TCN1*, Transcobalamin 1. Ref., Reference used for post hoc comparisons.
[1] Kruskal–Wallis test followed by Dunn–Bonferroni post-hoc test if the null hypothesis was rejected.

3.3. Association between Folate Intake and Status

The associations between folate intake from all food sources, from cereals and cereal products, from fruit and fruit juice and from vegetables, and RBC folate concentrations are shown in Figure 1 (gam model adjusted for sex, energy intake, *MTHFR* genotype, folate intake from the two other food groups and folic acid supplement use). Total folate intakes were associated with RBC folate (p < 0.001). The steepest part of the dose–response curve appeared to be for folate intakes of 50–200 µg per day but RBC folate concentrations continued to increase with increasing folate intake up to ≈500 µg per day. Folate intake from cereals and cereal products, and from fruit and fruit juice were also associated with RBC folate concentrations (p < 0.001 and p = 0.014, respectively) (Figure 1).

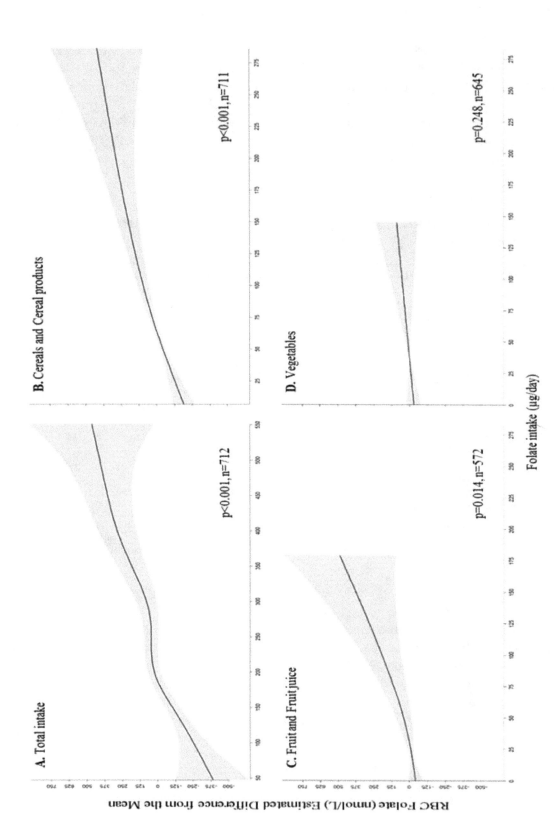

Figure 1. Estimated difference from the mean (and 95% CI) of RBC folate concentration according to folate intake from A. all dietary sources, B. from cereals and cereal products, C. from fruit and fruit juice and D. from vegetables. Generalized additive model (gam) adjusted for sex, energy intake, *MTHFR* genotype, folic acid supplement use and folate intake from the two other food sources. The highest 2.5th percentiles of RBC folate concentrations are not included. Three participants with a folate intake above 150 µg only from vegetables were not included. One participant with a folate intake of 327 µg only from fruit and fruit juice was excluded. *p* values are from the corresponding gam model.

3.4. Risk of Low Folate Status by Folate Intake

Table 3 shows the odds ratio (OR) (and 95% CI) of low RBC folate (<600 nmol/L) according to total, cereals and cereal products, vegetables and, fruit and fruit juice folate intake quartiles. Individuals in the highest quartile of total folate intake (>264 μg/day) were less likely to have RBC folate concentrations <600 nmol/L than those in the lowest quartile (<157 μg/day) in the unadjusted model (OR: 0.58, 95% CI: 0.36, 0.94) and adjusted model (OR: 0.43, 95% CI: 0.23, 0.82). Individuals in higher quartiles of folate intake from cereals and cereal products and from vegetables were also less likely to have low RBC folate concentrations (<600 nmol/L) than those in quartile 1. The same was not true for folate intake from fruit and fruit juice in any model.

Table 3. Odds ratio (95% CI) of low RBC folate concentration according to quartiles of total folate intake and intakes from cereals and cereal products, from vegetables and from fruit and fruit juice in the Newcastle 85+ Study.

Folate Intake	Model 1 (Unadjusted)		Model 2 (Adjusted)	
Total (μg/day)	<600 nmol/L (n = 170)	p	<600 nmol/L (n = 170)	p
<157	1.00 (ref.)	-	1.00 (ref.)	-
157–208	0.64 (0.40, 1.04)	0.071	0.65 (0.38, 1.09)	0.103
209–264	0.72 (0.45, 1.15)	0.173	0.58 (0.34, 1.02)	0.057
>264	0.58 (0.36, 0.94)	0.028	0.43 (0.23, 0.82)	0.010
Cereals and Cereal products (μg/day)	<600 nmol/L (n = 170)	p	<600 nmol/L (n = 170)	p
<36	1.00 (ref.)	-	1.00 (ref.)	-
36–59	0.96 (0.61, 1.49)	0.840	0.84 (0.51, 1.38)	0.493
59–92	0.40 (0.24, 0.66)	<0.001	0.32 (0.18, 0.57)	<0.001
>92	0.41 (0.25, 0.68)	0.001	0.33 (0.18, 0.61)	<0.001
Vegetables (μg/day)	<600 nmol/L (n = 154)	p	<600 nmol/L (n = 154)	p
<15	1.00 (ref.)	-	1.00 (ref.)	-
15–30	0.72 (0.43, 1.21)	0.212	0.49 (0.25, 0.95)	0.035
30–51	0.86 (0.52, 1.41)	0.550	0.59 (0.32, 1.08)	0.089
>51	0.79 (0.48, 1.30)	0.357	0.52 (0.28, 0.99)	0.045
Fruit and Fruit Juice (μg/day)	<600 nmol/L (n = 127)	p	<600 nmol/L (n = 127)	p
<7.3	1.00 (ref.)	-	1.00 (ref.)	-
7.3–16	0.90 (0.53, 1.52)	0.682	1.01 (0.56, 1.83)	0.979
16–34	0.61 (0.35, 1.07)	0.086	0.67 (0.36, 1.25)	0.213
>34	0.76 (0.44, 1.31)	0.329	0.79 (0.43, 1.44)	0.437

RBC folate, Red blood cell folate; p, p-value. Low folate status was defined as RBC folate concentration <600 nmol/L. Binary logistic regression model. Model 1 is unadjusted and Model 2 is adjusted for sex, energy intake, folate intake from the other two food sources (except for total folate), *MTHFR* genotype and folic acid-containing supplement use.

3.5. Association between Vitamin B12 Intake and Status

Total vitamin B12 intake was weakly associated with plasma vitamin B12 concentrations while adjusting for sex, energy intake, vitamin B12 intake from the other two food groups, *FUT2* genotype, vitamin B12 supplement use and H_2 antagonists, biguanides or PPI use (p = 0.054) (Figure 2). Plasma vitamin B12 concentration appeared to decrease when vitamin B12 intake exceeded 10 μg/day but the CI were very wide thereafter. Vitamin B12 intake from meat and meat products, milk and milk products and fish and fish dishes were not associated with plasma vitamin B12 concentration.

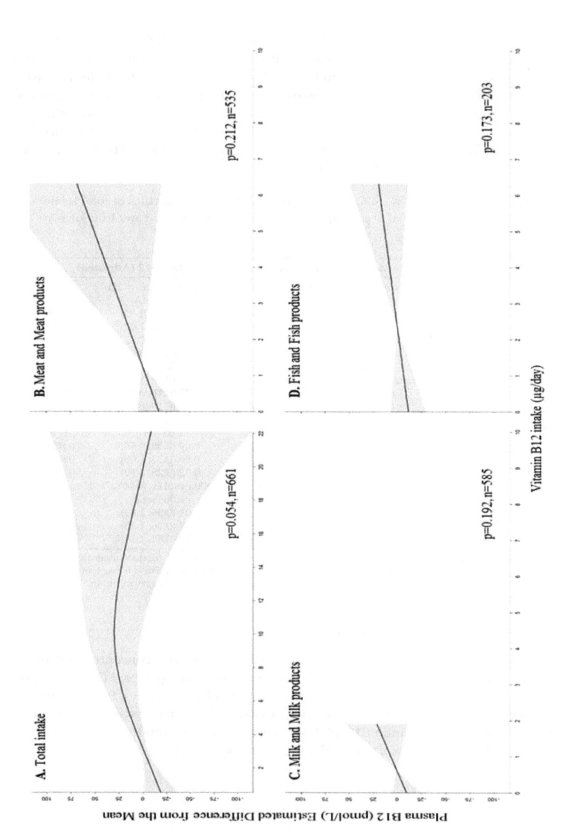

Figure 2. Estimated difference from the mean (and 95% CI) of plasma B12 concentrations according to vitamin B12 intake from A. all dietary sources, B. from meat and meat products, C. from milk and milk products and D. from fish and fish products. Generalized additive model (gam) adjusted for sex, energy intake, *FUT2* genotype, H_2 antagonists, proton pump inhibitors or biguanides use, vitamin B12 supplement use and vitamin B12 intakes from the other two food sources. The lowest and highest 2.5th percentiles of vitamin B12 intakes and plasma vitamin B12 concentrations are not included except for meat and meat products where the highest 5th percentile was excluded. *p* values are from the corresponding gam model.

3.6. Risk of Deficient Vitamin B12 Status by Vitamin B12 Intake

Participants with total vitamin B12 intake above the median (2.88 µg/day) were half as likely to be deficient for plasma B12 as those with the lowest intake (<1.87 µg/day) in the adjusted model (Table 4). Individuals in quartile 4 of vitamin B12 intake from meat and meat products (>2.10 µg/day) were also half as likely to be deficient for plasma vitamin B12 as those in quartile 1 in the unadjusted (OR: 0.55, 95% CI: 0.31–0.98) and adjusted models (OR: 0.41, 95% CI: 0.20–0.81). The same trend was present for milk and milk products but this did not reach statistical significance ($p = 0.054$).

Table 4. Odds ratio (95% CI) of plasma vitamin B12 deficiency according to quartiles of intake of total vitamin B12 and intakes from meat and meat products, from fish and fish products, and from milk and milk products in the Newcastle 85+ Study.

Vitamin B12 Intake	Model 1 (Unadjusted)	p	Model 2 (Adjusted)	p
Total (µg/day)	<148 pmol/L ($n = 125$)	p	<148 pmol/L ($n = 125$)	p
<1.87	1.00 (ref.)	-	1.00 (ref.)	-
1.87–2.88	0.70 (0.42, 1.18)	0.180	0.57 (0.32, 1.01)	0.056
2.88–4.40	0.60 (0.35, 1.02)	0.057	0.50 (0.28, 0.92)	0.026
>4.40	0.53 (0.31, 0.92)	0.024	0.40 (0.21, 0.76)	0.005
Meat and Meat products (µg/day)	<148 pmol/L ($n = 118$)	p	<148 pmol/L ($n = 118$)	p
<0.35	1.00 (ref.)	-	1.00 (ref.)	-
0.35–1.03	0.72 (0.42, 1.24)	0.236	0.69 (0.38, 1.25)	0.220
1.03–2.10	0.84 (0.50, 1.44)	0.533	0.78 (0.43, 1.42)	0.422
>2.10	0.55 (0.31, 0.98)	0.043	0.41 (0.20, 0.81)	0.010
Fish and Fish products (µg/day)	<148 pmol/L ($n = 43$)	p	<148 pmol/L ($n = 43$)	p
<0.46	1.00 (ref.)	-	1.00 (ref.)	-
0.46–1.06	0.61 (0.23, 1.65)	0.331	0.66 (0.23, 1.91)	0.444
1.06–2.45	0.86 (0.34, 2.15)	0.743	0.66 (0.23, 1.86)	0.427
>2.45	1.00 (0.41, 2.42)	0.992	0.70 (0.25, 1.97)	0.503
Milk and Milk products (µg/day)	<148 pmol/L ($n = 102$)	p	<148 pmol/L ($n = 102$)	p
<0.27	1.00 (ref.)	-	1.00 (ref.)	-
0.27–0.53	0.84 (0.47, 1.52)	0.562	0.88 (0.46, 1.71)	0.711
0.53–0.88	1.12 (0.64, 1.96)	0.698	1.28 (0.70, 2.37)	0.425
>0.88	0.58 (0.31, 1.08)	0.086	0.49 (0.24, 1.01)	0.054

p, p-value. Binary logistic regression model. Deficient plasma vitamin B12 concentration was defined as <148 pmol/L. Model 1 is unadjusted and Model 2 is adjusted for sex, energy intake, *FUT2* genotype, vitamin B12 intake from the other two food sources (except total vitamin B12 intake), vitamin B12 containing supplement use, H_2 antagonists, biguanides and proton pump inhibitors use.

4. Discussion

This study found that, in the very old, folate intakes from all food sources and from cereals and cereal products were significantly associated with RBC folate. Individuals with higher total folate intake or intake from cereals and cereal products were less likely to have low concentrations of RBC folate. The association between vitamin B12 intakes and plasma vitamin B12 was weak. Individuals with vitamin B12 intakes from all food sources and from meat and meat products were also less likely to be deficient for plasma vitamin B12. In addition, higher concentrations of RBC folate were found in participants with the *MTHFR* (rs1801133) AA genotype compared with those with A/G or GG genotypes. Women homozygous for the *FUT2* (rs492602) G allele also had higher concentrations of plasma vitamin B12 than those with other *FUT2* genotypes.

4.1. Folate and Vitamin B12 Intake and Status "Inadequacies"

In the Newcastle 85+ Study there was a relatively low prevalence of "inadequate" folate intake (3.1%) and status (3.6%). The NDNS rolling programme estimated that 1% of older adults (aged 65 and over) were below the UK LRNI for folate but that 7.3% of men and 10.8% of women had RBC folate concentrations <340 nmol/L. In the Newcastle 85+ Study, plasma vitamin B12 deficiency (<148 pmol/L) was present in 17.1% of participants and 9.2% were below the UK LRNI (1 µg/day) for vitamin B12 intake whilst the NDNS estimated that 1% were below the LRNI for vitamin B12 but

5.9% had serum vitamin B12 concentrations <150 pmol/L [11]. Age, dietary assessment method (4-day weighted diet record vs. 2 × 24 h-MPR) and other methodological differences are likely explanations for these observed discrepancies. Specifically, the novel method used to assess RBC folate in the NDNS (whole blood folate by a microbiological assay, serum total folate by LC-MS/MS and hematocrit) is likely to give higher estimates of folate "inadequacy" than the one used in this study. The NDNS used a similar method to the Newcastle 85+ Study to assess plasma vitamin B12 (competitive immunoassay with direct chemiluminescence (ADVIA Centaur B12 assay)).

In the post-fortification period in the US, less than 1% of older adults had deficient folate status (RBC folate <340 nmol/L) [37]. In the National Health and Nutrition Examination Survey (NHANES) 2003–2006, it was estimated that 9% of men and 24% of women >70 years old were below the North American EAR for folate (320 DFE/day [38,39]). In the same NHANES edition, 19% of older adults had plasma vitamin B12 concentrations below 221 pmol/L [40]. Moreover, less than 1% of men and 6% of women >70 years were below the EAR for vitamin B12 (2 μg/day) [39]. Almost 30% (n = 235) of the Newcastle 85+ Study participants were below the same EAR for vitamin B12 intake.

4.2. Association between Folate Intake and Status

Folate intake from total diets and from cereals and cereal products but not from vegetables or fruit and fruit juice were associated with RBC folate concentrations in the very old. Vegetables and fruit and fruit juice contributed to 16% and 9%, respectively to folate intake and the relatively lower contribution might explain the lack of associations. Further, folate bioavailability is dependent on the food matrix, stability of labile folates, presence of vitamin C and folate-binding proteins and folate pool sizes [23,41,42]. Nonetheless, there is a consensus that folic acid is better absorbed than dietary folate. Evidence also shows that that folic acid intake is a stronger predictor of RBC folate concentration than total folate intake [43]. The US Institute of Medicine estimated that the absorption efficiency of folic acid in supplements or fortified food was 85% taken with food or 100% from supplements taken on an empty stomach [23], whilst dietary folate absorption efficiency was 50% [23,42]. Breakfast cereals (grouped under cereals and cereal products in this study) have frequently been the target of voluntary fortification in the UK and elsewhere which might explain the stronger association between folate intake from cereals and cereal products and RBC folate concentrations. Cereals and cereal products were also the top contributors to folate intake (32%), suggesting that this is an important source of folate/folic acid in this population group. On the other hand, the incomplete release of dietary folate from plant foods cellular structures may explain a weaker association between folate from vegetables and fruit, and RBC folate.

4.3. Association between Vitamin B12 Intake and Status

Total vitamin B12 was weakly associated with plasma B12 in the very old (p = 0.054) and seemed to saturate at intakes ≈10 μg. The relatively weak association might be due to the low vitamin B12 intakes in relation to the large liver stores (1 μg/g of liver) so that intakes only slowly influence plasma concentrations [24]. Further, vitamin B12 absorption is complex. Bound to protein in food, vitamin B12 has to be released by pepsin and hydrochloric acid in the stomach. The ensuing free form of vitamin B12 binds to haptocorrin, forming a B12-haptocorrin complex. This complex is later broken down in the small intestine by pancreatic proteases which enable vitamin B12 to bind to the glycoprotein IF, be recognized (by cubilin) and absorbed by endocytosis in the enterocytes of the distal ileum. These steps present a problem to older adults as 10%–30% have atrophic gastritis and therefore, reduced gastric acid secretion which is essential to vitamin B12 release from food proteins [12]. The bioavailability of vitamin B12 in any form or dose is estimated to be 40% in healthy adults with intact IF secretion [24]. Meat and meat products, milk and milk products and, fish and fish products were the top sources of vitamin B12 in the Newcastle 85+ Study [30]. However, unlike some findings [44,45], but in agreement with others [46], vitamin B12 intake from meat and meat products was not associated significantly with plasma vitamin B12. Meat and meat products, especially liver (beef liver can reach to as much as 83 µg per 100 g [29]) and ruminant meat have very high concentrations of vitamin B12 and it is reported that ileal receptors saturate with intakes of 1.5–2.5 µg of vitamin B12 per meal [47]. Only 50% and 5% of vitamin B12 are absorbed with intakes of ~1 and 25 µg, respectively [24]. Others have found that vitamin B12 from dairy products is very bioavailable [48] but also that vitamin B12 in yogurt and cheese is not as bioavailable as that in milk in older individuals [46]. This could explain why vitamin B12 intake from dairy products (that includes yogurt and cheese) was not associated with plasma B12 in this study.

4.4. MTHFR and RBC Folate, and FUT2 and Plasma Vitamin B12

Interestingly, and in contrast to most previous findings [49], participants heterozygous for the A allele of the *MTHFR* gene had higher concentrations of RBC folate than those homozygous for the G allele. This was not a reflection of higher folate or folic acid containing supplements intake. Similar to previous findings [14,49,50], women with the *FUT2* GG genotype had higher concentrations of plasma vitamin B12. *FUT2* encodes galactoside 2-alpha-L-fucosyltransferase 2 (EC: 2.4.1.69) which is involved in the regulation of the H antigen and is a precursor of the ABO (H) antigens [50]. *FUT2* variants (from the allele A) are proposed to be protective against *Helicobacter pylori* infection or to increase IF production [14]. Both proposed explanations would explain the higher plasma vitamin B12 concentrations in those homozygous for the G allele.

4.5. Strengths and Weaknesses

The Newcastle 85+ Study is a unique cohort owing to the age group, the large number of participants and the extensive multidimensional health data. The study was socio-demographically representative of the UK but the lack of ethnic diversity warrants caution when generalizing the findings to a non-white population. The rapid processing of blood samples after venepuncture is another strength of this study.

As dietary intake assessment consisted of a 24 h-MPR applied on two non-consecutive days, the possibility of unusually high or low vitamin B12/folate intakes cannot be excluded. For practical reasons, 24 h-MPRs were not conducted during the weekend, therefore food and drink eaten on Fridays and Saturdays was not recalled. Although the MPR method involved several prompts to avoid misreporting, misreporters have been estimated to be 26% of the cohort [28]. Even though the food groups used in the analysis contributed to most of the folate and vitamin B12 intake, other food sources might explain the remaining intake. Intakes of dietary folate equivalents (DFE) and of the crystalline form of vitamin B12 could not be determined because supplement use was collected qualitatively (type and brand but not frequency) and it was not certain which specific foods had been fortified during the dietary collection period (2006/2007). A general limitation of most dietary surveys, including ours, is that assessment of supplement usage may not be accurate by dietary intake records, dietary recalls and other questionnaires [51]. Furthermore, the irregular use of supplements by survey participants, including the alteration of usual patterns of supplement use during the period of dietary data collection, further adds bias to the estimation of true supplement use [51]. It is worth mentioning that the choice of vitamin B12 form used in supplements and fortified foods should also be taken into consideration because of concerns associated with cyanide/thiocyanate from cyanocobalamin [52].

Holotranscobalamin measures the vitamin's active form and because it might better reflect vitamin B12 status than plasma vitamin B12, its use might have yielded different results. There is currently no consensus on the biochemical threshold to use in order to define folate or vitamin B12 "inadequacy", especially in this population. Therefore, results from the binary logistic models might be different if different thresholds were used. Furthermore, atrophic gastritis impairs folate and vitamin B12 absorption. If available, the incidence of atrophic gastritis or a proxy measure, such as *Helicobacter pylori* infection, could have been used as an adjusting factor or to conduct a sensitivity analysis. The list of SNPs used is not exhaustive and other polymorphisms, such as some SNPs in the *TCN2* gene (e.g., rs731991) may influence the folate and vitamin B12 intake–status relationship [53].

5. Conclusions

In summary, almost one-fifth of the 85-year-old participants in the Newcastle 85+ Study had deficient plasma vitamin B12 concentrations but only a few individuals had deficient folate status, according to commonly used biochemical thresholds. Folate and vitamin B12 intakes were associated to RBC folate and plasma B12, respectively and folate intake from cereals and cereal products was strongly associated with RBC folate. This is possibly a consequence of voluntary folic acid fortification of breakfast cereals in the UK, and makes this food group an important source of folate for this population group. Estimates of the bioavailability of folate and vitamin B12 from total diets and from commonly consumed food groups in the very old should be taken into account when setting dietary guidelines.

Acknowledgments: The Newcastle 85+ Study has been funded by the Medical Research Council, Biotechnology and Biological Sciences Research Council and the Dunhill Medical Trust. The research was also supported by the National Institute for Health Research (NIHR) Newcastle Biomedical Research Centre, based at Newcastle upon Tyne Hospitals NHS Foundation Trust and Newcastle University. A.J.A. is funded by the NIHR as a Professor in translational research.

Author Contributions: N.M., T.R.H., C.J.S. and C.J. designed and conducted the study; N.M. analysed the data, performed statistical analyses and wrote the paper; A.J.A. collected the dietary data, C.M. analysed the plasma B12, RBC folate and conducted the genotyping work; and N.M. had primary responsibility for final content. All authors contributed to the interpretation of the findings, read, critically reviewed the paper, commented and approved the final manuscript.

References

1.   Locasale, J.W. Serine, glycine and the one-carbon cycle: Cancer metabolism in full circle. *Nat. Rev. Cancer* **2013**, *13*, 572–583. [CrossRef] [PubMed]

2.   Durga, J.; van Boxtel, M.P.; Schouten, E.G.; Kok, F.J.; Jolles, J.; Katan, M.B.; Verhoef, P. Effect of 3-year folic acid supplementation on cognitive function in older adults in the facit trial: A randomised, double blind, controlled trial. *Lancet* **2007**, *369*, 208–216. [CrossRef]

3.   Nurk, E.; Refsum, H.; Tell, G.S.; Engedal, K.; Vollset, S.E.; Ueland, P.M.; Nygaard, H.A.; Smith, A.D. Plasma total homocysteine and memory in the elderly: The hordaland homocysteine study. *Ann. Neurol.* **2005**, *58*, 847–857. [CrossRef] [PubMed]

4.   Kado, D.M.; Karlamangla, A.S.; Huang, M.H.; Troen, A.; Rowe, J.W.; Selhub, J.; Seeman, T.E. Homocysteine versus the vitamins folate, B6, and B12 as predictors of cognitive function and decline in older high-functioning adults: Macarthur studies of successful aging. *Am. J. Med.* **2005**, *118*, 161–167. [CrossRef] [PubMed]

5.   Saposnik, G.; Ray, J.G.; Sheridan, P.; McQueen, M.; Lonn, E. Homocysteine-lowering therapy and stroke risk, severity, and disability: Additional findings from the hope 2 trial. *Stroke* **2009**, *40*, 1365–1372. [CrossRef] [PubMed]

6.   Spence, J.D. Metabolic vitamin B12 deficiency: A missed opportunity to prevent dementia and stroke. *Nutr. Res.* **2016**, *36*, 109–116. [CrossRef] [PubMed]

7.   Fratoni, V.; Brandi, M.L. B vitamins, homocysteine and bone health. *Nutrients* **2015**, *7*, 2176–2192. [CrossRef] [PubMed]

8.   Yang, J.; Hu, X.; Zhang, Q.; Cao, H.; Wang, J.; Liu, B. Homocysteine level and risk of fracture: A meta-analysis and systematic review. *Bone* **2012**, *51*, 376–382. [CrossRef] [PubMed]

9.   Ericson, U.; Sonestedt, E.; Gullberg, B.; Olsson, H.; Wirfalt, E. High folate intake is associated with lower breast cancer incidence in postmenopausal women in the malmo diet and cancer cohort. *Am. J. Clin. Nutr.* **2007**, *86*, 434–443. [PubMed]

10.   Ter Borg, S.; Verlaan, S.; Hemsworth, J.; Mijnarends, D.M.; Schols, J.M.; Luiking, Y.C.; de Groot, L.C. Micronutrient intakes and potential inadequacies of community-dwelling older adults: A systematic review. *Br. J. Nutr.* **2015**, *113*, 1195–1206. [CrossRef] [PubMed]

11.   Bates, B.; Lennox, A.; Prentice, A.; Bates, C.; Page, P.; Nicholson, S.; Swan, G. National Diet and Nutrition Survey Years 1–4 (Combined) (2008/2009-2010/2012)-Appendices and Tables. Available online: https://www.gov.uk/government/statistics/national-diet-and-nutrition-survey-results-from-years-1-to-

4-combined-of-the-rolling-programme-for-2008-and-2009-to-2011-and-2012 (accessed on 15 August 2015).

12. Johnson, M.A. If high folic acid aggravates vitamin B12 deficiency what should be done about it? *Nutr. Rev.* **2007**, *65*, 451–458. [CrossRef] [PubMed]

13. Hughes, C.F.; Ward, M.; Hoey, L.; McNulty, H. Vitamin B12 and ageing: Current issues and interaction with folate. *Ann. Clin. Biochem.* **2013**, *50*, 315–329. [CrossRef] [PubMed]

14. Zinck, J.W.; de Groh, M.; MacFarlane, A.J. Genetic modifiers of folate, vitamin B-12, and homocysteine status in a cross-sectional study of the Canadian population. *Am. J. Clin. Nutr.* **2015**, *101*, 1295–1304. [CrossRef] [PubMed]

15. Kwan, L.L.; Bermudez, O.I.; Tucker, K.L. Low vitamin B-12 intake and status are more prevalent in Hispanic older adults of Caribbean origin than in neighborhood-matched non-hispanic whites. *J. Nutr.* **2002**, *132*, 2059–2064. [PubMed]

16. Bor, M.V.; Lydeking-Olsen, E.; Moller, J.; Nexo, E. A daily intake of approximately 6 microg vitamin B-12 appears to saturate all the vitamin B-12-related variables in danish postmenopausal women. *Am. J. Clin. Nutr.* **2006**, *83*, 52–58. [PubMed]

17. Powers, H.J.; Hill, M.H.; Welfare, M.; Spiers, A.; Bal, W.; Russell, J.; Duckworth, Y.; Gibney, E.; Williams, E.A.; Mathers, J.C. Responses of biomarkers of folate and riboflavin status to folate and riboflavin supplementation in healthy and colorectal polyp patients (the fab2 study). *Cancer Epidemiol. Biomark. Prev.* **2007**, *16*, 2128–2135. [CrossRef] [PubMed]

18. Bates, C.J.; Schneede, J.; Mishra, G.; Prentice, A.; Mansoor, M.A. Relationship between methylmalonic acid, homocysteine, vitamin B12 intake and status and socio-economic indices, in a subset of participants in the british national diet and nutrition survey of people aged 65 y and over. *Eur. J. Clin. Nutr.* **2003**, *57*, 349–357. [CrossRef] [PubMed]

19. Brouwer-Brolsma, E.M.; Dhonukshe-Rutten, R.A.; van Wijngaarden, J.P.; Zwaluw, N.L.; Velde, N.; de Groot, L.C. Dietary sources of vitamin B-12 and their association with vitamin B-12 status markers in healthy older adults in the B-proof study. *Nutrients* **2015**, *7*, 7781–7797. [CrossRef] [PubMed]

20. Howard, J.M.; Azen, C.; Jacobsen, D.W.; Green, R.; Carmel, R. Dietary intake of cobalamin in elderly people who have abnormal serum cobalamin, methylmalonic acid and homocysteine levels. *Eur. J. Clin. Nutr.* **1998**, *52*, 582–587. [CrossRef] [PubMed]

21. Yang, L.K.; Wong, K.C.; Wu, M.Y.; Liao, S.L.; Kuo, C.S.; Huang, R.F. Correlations between folate, B12, homocysteine levels, and radiological markers of neuropathology in elderly post-stroke patients. *J. Am. Coll. Nutr.* **2007**, *26*, 272–278. [CrossRef] [PubMed]

22. Van Guelpen, B.; Hultdin, J.; Johansson, I.; Stegmayr, B.; Hallmans, G.; Nilsson, T.K.; Weinehall, L.; Witthoft, C.; Palmqvist, R.; Winkvist, A. Folate, vitamin B12, and risk of ischemic and hemorrhagic stroke: A prospective, nested case-referent study of plasma concentrations and dietary intake. *Stroke* **2005**, *36*, 1426–1431. [CrossRef] [PubMed]

23. EFSA NDA Panel (EFSA Panel on Dietetic Products Nutrition and Allergies). Scientific opinion on dietary reference values for folate. *EFSA J.* **2015**, *12*, 3893.

24. EFSA NDA Panel (EFSA Panel on Dietetic Products Nutrition and Allergies). Scientific opinion on dietary reference values for cobalamin (vitamin B12). *EFSA J.* **2015**, *13*, 4150.

25. Collerton, J.; Davies, K.; Jagger, C.; Kingston, A.; Bond, J.; Eccles, M.P.; Robinson, L.A.; Martin-Ruiz, C.; von Zglinicki, T.; James, O.F.; et al. Health and disease in 85 year olds: Baseline findings from the newcastle 85+ cohort study. *BMJ* **2009**, *339*, b4904. [CrossRef] [PubMed]

26. Hill, T.R.; Mendonça, N.; Granic, A.; Siervo, M.; Jagger, C.; Seal, C.J.; Kerse, N.; Wham, C.; Adamson, A.J.; Mathers, J.C. What do we know about the nutritional status of the very old? Insights from three cohorts of advanced age from the UK and New Zealand. *Proc. Nutr. Soc.* **2016**, *75*, 420–430. [CrossRef] [PubMed]

27. Davies, K.; Kingston, A.; Robinson, L.; Hughes, J.; Hunt, J.M.; Barker, S.A.H.; Edwards, J.; Collerton, J.; Jagger, C.; Kirkwood, T.B.L. Improving retention of very old participants in longitudinal research: Experiences from the newcastle 85+ study. *PLoS ONE* **2014**, *9*, e108370. [CrossRef] [PubMed]

28. Mendonça, N.; Hill, T.R.; Granic, A.; Mathers, J.C.; Wrieden, W.; Siervo, M.; Seal, C.; Jagger, C.; Adamson, A.J. Macronutrient intake and food sources in the very old: Analysis of the Newcastle 85+ study. *Br. J. Nutr.* **2016**, *115*, 2170–2180. [CrossRef] [PubMed]

29. Food Standards Agency. *Mccance and Widdowson's the Composition of Foods*, 6th ed.; Royal Society of Chemistry: Cambridge, UK, 2002.

30. Mendonça, N.; Hill, T.R.; Granic, A.; Mathers, J.C.; Wrieden, W.; Siervo, M.; Seal, C.; Jagger, C.; Adamson, A.J. Micronutrient intake and food sources in the very old: Analysis of the Newcastle 85+ study. *Br. J. Nutr.* **2016**, *116*, 751–761. [CrossRef] [PubMed]

31. Martin-Ruiz, C.; Jagger, C.; Kingston, A.; Collerton, J.; Catt, M.; Davies, K.; Dunn, M.; Hilkens, C.; Keavney, B.; Pearce, S.H.S.; et al. Assessment of a large panel of candidate biomarkers of ageing in the newcastle 85+ study. *Mech. Ageing Dev.* **2011**, *132*, 496–502. [CrossRef] [PubMed]

32. Deelen, J.; Beekman, M.; Uh, H.W.; Broer, L.; Ayers, K.L.; Tan, Q.; Kamatani, Y.; Bennet, A.M.; Tamm, R.; Trompet, S.; et al. Genome-wide association meta-analysis of human longevity identifies a novel locus conferring survival beyond 90 years of age. *Hum. Mol. Genet.* **2014**, *23*, 4420–4432. [CrossRef] [PubMed]

33. Department of Health: Committee on Medical Aspects of Food Policy (COMA). *Report on Health and Social Subjects 41: Dietary Reference Values for Food Energy and Nutrients for the United Kingdom*; Department of Health: Committee on Medical Aspects of Food Policy: London, UK, 1991.

34. Vogiatzoglou, A.; Oulhaj, A.; Smith, A.D.; Nurk, E.; Drevon, C.A.; Ueland, P.M.; Vollset, S.E.; Tell, G.S.; Refsum, H. Determinants of plasma methylmalonic acid in a large population: Implications for assessment of vitamin B12 status. *Clin. Chem.* **2009**, *55*, 2198–2206. [CrossRef] [PubMed]

35. Bang, H.; Mazumdar, M.; Spence, J.D. Tutorial in biostatistics: Analyzing associations between total plasma homocysteine and B vitamins using optimal categorization and segmented regression. *Neuroepidemiology* **2006**, *27*, 188–200. [CrossRef] [PubMed]

36. The 1000 Genomes Project Consortium. 1000 Genomes Project Phase 3. Available online: http://browser.1000genomes.org/Homo_sapiens/Variation/Population?r=1:11855878-11856878;v= rs1801133;vdb=variation;vf=1230309 (accessed on 10 December 2015).

37. Pfeiffer, C.M.; Hughes, J.P.; Lacher, D.A.; Bailey, R.L.; Berry, R.J.; Zhang, M.; Yetley, E.A.; Rader, J.I.; Sempos, C.T.; Johnson, C.L. Estimation of trends in serum and RBC folate in the U.S. Population from pre- to postfortification using assay-adjusted data from the NHANES 1988–2010. *J. Nutr.* **2012**, *142*, 886–893. [CrossRef] [PubMed]

38. Institute of Medicine (US) Food and Nutrition Board. *Dietary Reference Intakes for Thiamin, Riboflavin, Niacin, Vitamin B6, Folate, Vitamin B12, Pantothenic acid, Biotin, and Choline*; National Academy Press: Washington, DC, USA, 1998.

39. Bailey, R.L.; Fulgoni, V.L.; Keast, D.R.; Dwyer, J.T. Examination of vitamin intakes among us adults by dietary supplement use. *J. Acad. Nutr. Diet.* **2012**, *112*, 657–663.e4. [CrossRef] [PubMed]

40. Yang, Q.; Cogswell, M.E.; Hamner, H.C.; Carriquiry, A.; Bailey, L.B.; Pfeiffer, C.M.; Berry, R.J. Folic acid source, usual intake, and folate and vitamin B-12 status in us adults: National health and nutrition examination survey (NHANES) 2003–2006. *Am. J. Clin. Nutr.* **2010**, *91*, 64–72. [CrossRef] [PubMed]

41. Caudill, M.A. Folate bioavailability: Implications for establishing dietary recommendations and optimizing status. *Am. J. Clin. Nutr.* **2010**, *91*, 1455S–1460S. [CrossRef] [PubMed]

42. Brouwer, I.A.; van Dusseldorp, M.; West, C.E.; Steegers-Theunissen, R.P. Bioavailability and bioefficacy of folate and folic acid in man. *Nutr. Res. Rev.* **2001**, *14*, 267–294. [CrossRef] [PubMed]

43. Hoey, L.; McNulty, H.; Askin, N.; Dunne, A.; Ward, M.; Pentieva, K.; Strain, J.; Molloy, A.M.; Flynn, C.A.; Scott, J.M. Effect of a voluntary food fortification policy on folate, related B vitamin status, and homocysteine in healthy adults. *Am. J. Clin. Nutr.* **2007**, *86*, 1405–1413. [PubMed]

44. Doscherholmen, A.; McMahon, J.; Ripley, D. Vitamin B12 assimilation from chicken meat. *Am. J. Clin. Nutr.* **1978**, *31*, 825–830. [PubMed]

45. Heyssel, R.M.; Bozian, R.C.; Darby, W.J.; Bell, M.C. Vitamin B12 turnover in man. The assimilation of vitamin B12 from natural foodstuff by man and estimates of minimal daily dietary requirements. *Am. J. Clin. Nutr.* **1966**, *18*, 176–184. [PubMed]

46. Vogiatzoglou, A.; Smith, A.D.; Nurk, E.; Berstad, P.; Drevon, C.A.; Ueland, P.M.; Vollset, S.E.; Tell, G.S.; Refsum, H. Dietary sources of vitamin B-12 and their association with plasma vitamin B-12 concentrations in the general population: The hordaland homocysteine study. *Am. J. Clin. Nutr.* **2009**, *89*, 1078–1087. [CrossRef] [PubMed]

47. Suter, P.M.; Golner, B.B.; Goldin, B.R.; Morrow, F.D.; Russell, R.M. Reversal of protein-bound vitamin B12 malabsorption with antibiotics in atrophic gastritis. *Gastroenterology* **1991**, *101*, 1039–1045. [CrossRef]

48. Russell, R.M.; Baik, H.; Kehayias, J.J. Older men and women efficiently absorb vitamin B-12 from milk and fortified bread. *J. Nutr.* **2001**, *131*, 291–293. [PubMed]

49. Tanaka, T.; Scheet, P.; Giusti, B.; Bandinelli, S.; Piras, M.G.; Usala, G.; Lai, S.; Mulas, A.; Corsi, A.M.; Vestrini, A.; et al. Genome-wide association study of vitamin B6, vitamin B12, folate, and homocysteine blood concentrations. *Am. J. Hum. Genet.* **2009**, *84*, 477–482. [CrossRef] [PubMed]

50. Hazra, A.; Kraft, P.; Selhub, J.; Giovannucci, E.L.; Thomas, G.; Hoover, R.N.; Chanock, S.J.; Hunter, D.J. Common variants of FUT2 are associated with plasma vitamin B12 levels. *Nat. Genet.* **2008**, *40*, 1160–1162. [CrossRef] [PubMed]

51. Bates, C.J.; Prentice, A.; van der Pols, J.C.; Walmsley, C.; Pentieva, K.D.; Finch, S.; Smithers, G.; Clarke, P.C. Estimation of the use of dietary supplements in the national diet and nutrition survey: People aged 65 years and over. An observed paradox and a recommendation. *Eur. J. Clin. Nutr.* **1998**, *52*, 917–923. [CrossRef] [PubMed]

52. Hasuike, Y.; Nakanishi, T.; Moriguchi, R.; Otaki, Y.; Nanami, M.; Hama, Y.; Naka, M.; Miyagawa, K.; Izumi, M.; Takamitsu, Y. Accumulation of cyanide and thiocyanate in haemodialysis patients. *Nephrol. Dial. Transplant.* **2004**, *19*, 1474–1479. [CrossRef] [PubMed]

53. Castro, R.; Barroso, M.; Rocha, M.; Esse, R.; Ramos, R.; Ravasco, P.; Rivera, I.; de Almeida, I.T. The TCN2 776CNG polymorphism correlates with vitamin B (12) cellular delivery in healthy adult populations. *Clin. Biochem.* **2010**, *43*, 645–649. [CrossRef] [PubMed]

13

Nutrition, One-Carbon Metabolism and Neural Tube Defects

Kelei Li [1], **Mark L. Wahlqvist** [2,3] and **Duo Li** [1,3,]*

[1] Department of Food Science and Nutrition, Zhejiang University, Hangzhou 310058, China; wfujfqcc@sina.com
[2] Fuli Institute, Zhejiang University, Hangzhou 310058, China; mark.wahlqvist@gmail.com
[3] Monash Asia Institute and Departments of Medicine and of Nutrition and Dietetics, Monash University, Melbourne 3006, Australia
* Correspondence: duoli@zju.edu.cn

Abstract: Neural tube defects (NTDs) are a group of severe congenital malformations, induced by the combined effects of genes and the environment. The most valuable finding so far has been the protective effect of folic acid supplementation against NTDs. However, many women do not take folic acid supplements until they are pregnant, which is too late to prevent NTDs effectively. Long-term intake of folic acid–fortified food is a good choice to solve this problem, and mandatory folic acid fortification should be further promoted, especially in Europe, Asia and Africa. Vitamin B2, vitamin B-6, vitamin B-12, choline, betaine and n-3 polyunsaturated fatty acids (PUFAs) can also reduce the NTD risk by interacting with the one-carbon metabolism pathway. This suggest that multivitamin B combined with choline, betaine and n-3 PUFAs supplementation may have a better protective effect against NTDs than folic acid alone. Genetic polymorphisms involved in one-carbon metabolism are associated with NTD risk, and gene screening for women of childbearing age prior to pregnancy may help prevent NTDs induced by the risk allele. In addition, the consumption of alcohol, tea and coffee, and low intakes of fruit and vegetable are also associated with the increased risk of NTDs, and should be avoided by women of childbearing age.

Keywords: folate; neural tube defects; vitamin B; choline; betaine; one-carbon metabolism; tea; alcohol; coffee

1. Introduction

Neural tube defects (NTDs) are a group of severe congenital malformations. It is estimated that approximately one out of 1000 newborns present with this type of defect [1]. The development and closure of neural tube happen during normal embryogenesis between the 18th and 28th days after fertilization. Failure of the neural tube to close in embryonic development results in NTDs [2]. The etiology of NTDs is still unknown. One possible reason may be the disturbance of the one-carbon metabolism pathway [3,4]. However, there are also folate-resistant NTDs, indicating that folate deficiency is not the unique reason for NTDs, and other potential pathogeneses may also responsible for NTDs. The deficiency of other nutritional factors involved in one-carbon metabolism, such as vitamin B-2, B-6, B-12, choline, betaine, and n-3 polyunsaturated fatty acids, may be also associated with NTDs. Genetic factors are another important cause of NTDs. Many loci on genes have been identified as associated with the risk of NTDs, especially on genes involved in the one-carbon metabolism pathway, such as methylenetetrahydrofolate reductase (*MTHFR*) and 5-methyltetrahydrofolate-homocysteine methyltransferase (*MTR*) [5,6].

In this study, we review the research progress on the effect of nutritional factors and genes involved in the one-carbon metabolism pathway on NTDs. This should provide a basis for better nutritional approaches to NTD prevention.

2. B-Vitamins, One-Carbon Metabolism and NTDs

2.1. Folate

Folate, also known as vitamin B-9, plays an important role in the homocysteine (Hcy) metabolism, one-carbon pathway and DNA synthesis (Figure 1). In 1991, the Medical Research Council Vitamin Study Research Group conducted a large-scale randomized controlled trial (RCT) with 1817 women from 33 centers in seven countries to assess the effect of folic acid on the reoccurrence of neural tube defects and found that 4 mg folic acid supplementation per day lowered the risk of NTDs by 72% compared with the control group (without folic acid supplementation) [7]. Another important RCT was conducted by Czeizel et al. in Hungarian women without a history of NTD-affected pregnancy [3]. In that study, no NTD cases occurred in 2104 women who received multivitamins containing 0.8 mg folic acid per day, while six NTD cases occurred in 2052 women who received only trace elements and vitamin C. In 1999, Berry et al. conducted a cohort intervention study in an area of China with high rates of neural tube defects (the northern region) and one with low rates (the southern region), and found that preconceptional supplementation (starting supplementation before the last menstrual period before conception and stopping at the end of the first trimester) of 400 µg folic acid (a synthetic form of folate) per day reduced the NTD risk by 85% in the northern subgroup of 31,960 women and by 40% in the southern subgroup of 215,871 women [4]. These results of intervention studies have provided the most persuasive evidence for the protective effect of folic acid against NTDs.

In 1995, a case-control study by Daly first reported a dose-response relationship between the red blood cell folate concentration of mothers and the risk of NTDs, and that a red blood cell folate concentration ≥906 nmol/L (400 ng/mL) can provide optimal protection against NTDs [8]. In 2014, Crider et al. analyzed data from two intervention studies in Chinese women (400 µg folic acid per day from preconception through the end of the first trimester) by a Bayesian model, and found a dose-response relationship between maternal red blood cell folate and the risk of NTDs: a folate concentration >1000 nmol/L substantially reduced the risk of NTDs [5]. This was consistent with the result of Daly's study. Based on these results, in 2015 the World Health Organization (WHO) recommended a threshold value of the maternal red blood cell folate concentration of 906 nmol/L (400 ng/mL) to prevent NTDs. Folic acid supplementation is a solution for the insufficient dietary intake of folate. A daily intake of 0.4 mg (at least one month before conception through the first three months of conception) folic acid is recommended by the Centers for Disease Control and Prevention for women who do not have a history of a previous NTD-affected pregnancy; this dose can prevent 50% of NTDs [9]. As for women who have had a previous NTD-affected pregnancy, the dose of folic acid is increased to 4 mg per day (at least one month before pregnancy through the first three months of pregnancy) [9]. Although recommendations for preconceptional folic acid supplementation have existed for decades, only a small number of women were actually supplemented with folic acid before conception [10]. Most women started folic acid supplementation when they knew they were pregnant, and this was often too late for the effective prevention of NTDs [11]. Long-term intake of folic acid–fortified foods should complement preconceptional folic acid supplementation. Arth et al. reported that mandatory folic acid fortification of wheat and maize flour prevented 13.2% folic acid–preventable NTDs (35,500 of approximately 268,700 global cases) in 58 countries [12]. Seventy-eight countries have fortified flour with folic acid mandatorily, while most countries in Asia, Europe and Africa do not mandate folic acid fortification [13]. Khoshnood et al. conducted an observational study to assess the long-term trend in NTD prevalence in 19 European countries and found that, without mandatory folic acid fortification, the long-existent recommendation for preconceptional folic acid supplementation and voluntary folic acid fortification did not significantly decrease the prevalence of NTDs [14]. In 2016, an intervention study in 16,648 women in Shanxi,

China (one of the most NTD-affected regions, with a 13.8‰ to 19.9‰ prevalence), found that folic acid–fortified flour decreased the NTD burden by 58.5%, which has informed the future implementation of mandatory folic acid fortification in China [15]. Further promotion of mandatory folic acid fortification is needed to prevent NTDs.

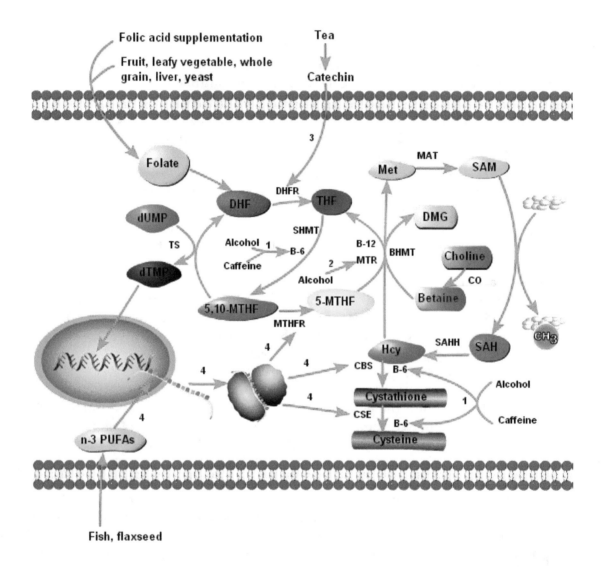

Figure 1. B vitamins and other dietary factors interact with the one-carbon metabolism to influence the development of NTDs. 1, alcohol and caffeine lower vitamin B-6, and thus disturb vitamin B-6–dependent one-carbon metabolism pathways; 2, alcohol reduces the activity of *MTR*, leading to increased Hcy and reduced SAM; 3, catechins in tea reduce the activity of *DHFR*, and hinder the synthesis of THF; 4, *n*-3 PUFAs increase the mRNA expression of enzymes involved in one-carbon metabolism, such as *MTHFR*, *CBS*, and *CSE*. Abbreviations: DHF, dihydrofolate; THF, tetrahydrofolate; 5,10-MTHF, 5,10-methylenetetrahydrofolate; 5-MTHF, 5-methyltetrahydrofolate; dUMP, deoxyuridine monophosphate; dTMP, thymidinemonophosphate; Hcy, homocysteine; Met, methionine; SAM, S-adenosylmethionine; SAH, S-adenosylhomocysteine; DMG, dimethylglycine; *DHFR*, dihydrofolate reductase; *SHMT*, serine hydroxymethyltransferase; *MTHFR*, methylenetetrahydrofolate reductase; *MTR*, 5-methyltetrahydrofolate-homocysteine methyltransferase; *TS*, thymidylate synthase; *BHMT*, betaine-homocysteine methyltransferase; *MAT*, methionine adenosyltransferase; *SAHH*, S-adenosylhomocysteine hydrolase; *CBS*, cystathionine-beta-synthase; *CSE*, cystathionine-gamma-lyase.

Several genes involved in the folate-dependent one-carbon metabolism have been shown to be associated with the risk of NTDs. One of the most important is the gene encoding *MTHFR*, an enzyme that catalyzes the conversion of 5,10-methylenetetrahydrofolate (5,10-MTHF) to 5-methyltetrahydrofolate (5-MTHF) and provides the methyl group needed for remethylation of Hcy to form methionine (Met) (Figure 1) [16]. The T allele of *MTHFR* 677C>T is associated with an increased risk of NTDs in the western population [17–19]. Similar observations are made in Chinese mothers even when they supplement with folic acid [5,16,20]. Two considerations may help explain this association between *MTHFR* 677C>T and NTDs. On the one hand, the TT genotype of *MTHFR* 677C>T can attenuate the plasma and red blood cell (RBC) folate response to folic acid supplementation [21]. In addition, previous studies have reported that the T allele carriers of *MTHFR* 677C>T had lower folate concentrations than non-carriers [18,22]. On the other hand, the *MTHFR* 677C>T mutation is associated with reduced *MTHFR* activity [18,23]. *MTHFR* 1298A>C is yet another mutation associated with decreased *MTHFR* activity [23]. However, the link between *MTHFR* 1298A>C and NTDs remains controversial: one study in Italy reported that the C allele of *MTHFR* 1298A>C was associated with a higher risk of NTDs [24], several other studies found no significant association between *MTHFR* 1298A>C and NTDs [6,25–27], while one study in China even found that the C allele of *MTHFR* 1298A>C had a protective role against NTDs [28].

In addition to *MTHFR*, other genes involved in the folate metabolism have been demonstrated to influence the development of NTDs in the Chinese. *MTR* is an enzyme that catalyzes the remethylation of Hcy to Met and is dependent on the provision of methyl groups from 5-MTHF (Figure 1). The mutation of *MTR* is associated with the increased risk of NTDs [6,19,29,30]. Solute carrier family 19 member 1 (*SCF19M1*) can transport folate into cells. The mutation of *SCF19M1* is associated with increased NTD risk even when mothers are supplemented with folic acid [6]. In addition, mutations on *BHMT* [6,19,31], *CBS* [19,32], *MTRR* [19,33,34], *MTHFD1* [19,35–41], *MTHFD2* [19], *SHMT1* [36], *FOLH1* [42], *RFC1* [43,44], *SARDH* [45], *PEMT* [40], *GART* [40] and *TYMS* [19,36] have also been reported to be associated with the risk of NTDs.

2.2. Vitamins B-2, B-6 and B-12

Vitamin B-12 is the cofactor of *MTR* (Figure 1). Additionally, B-12 deficiency is associated with elevated Hcy [46,47]. In case-control studies, vitamin B-12 status has been found to be protective against NTDs in the Chinese [47,48]. According to a study in 1170 women in northwest China, the prevalence of vitamin B-12 deficiency was 45% [49], indicating that vitamin B-12 supplementation maybe also be needed to prevent NTDs in China. The negative association between vitamin B-12 and the risk of NTDs is also observed in other populations [50–52], and remains significant even in folic acid–fortified populations [53,54]. Transcobalamin II (*TCN2*) is a carrier protein that can bind vitamin B12. The mutation of *TCN2* is associated with an increased NTD risk even when mothers are supplemented with folate [6]. *CUBN* is a gene that encodes the intestinal receptor responsible for the uptake of the vitamin B12–intrinsic factor complex. The mutation of *CUBN* is also associated with the risk of NTDs [40,55]. This genetic evidence also demonstrates the role of vitamin B-12 in the development of NTDs.

Besides folate and vitamin B-12, vitamin B-2 and B-6 are also important enzyme cofactors involved in the one-carbon metabolism. The conversion of 5,10-MTHF to 5-MTHF is catalyzed by *MTHFR* and depends on FADH2, the hydroquinone form of flavin adenine dinucleotide (FAD) (a derivative of vitamin B-2). Hustad et al., in a cross-sectional study, found that plasma vitamin B-2 was negatively associated with Hcy [56]. An intervention study by McNulty et al. in healthy adults found that vitamin B-2 supplementation lowered the concentration of Hcy only in subjects with a TT genotype of *MTHFR* 677C>T, but there was no effect in CC or CT genotypes [57]. In addition, vitamin B-2 can interact with folate to modulate Hcy concentrations. One intervention study found that folic acid supplementation (400 μg/day) had a greater Hcy-lowering effect in subjects with a high plasma level of vitamin B-2, and this effect was unrelated to *MTHFR* 677C>T polymorphism [58]. Several intervention studies have found that preconceptional multivitamin supplementation (including vitamin B-2 and several other vitamins such as folic acid, vitamin B-6, vitamin B-12, vitamin E, thiamin, vitamin A, vitamin D, nicotinamide, and ascorbic acid) could reduce the risk of NTDs [3,59]. Vitamin B-6 is the cofactor for betaine-Hcy methyltransferase (*BHMT*) (an enzyme that catalyzes the remethylation of Hcy to Met with betaine providing the methyl needed), cystathionine-beta-synthase (*CBS*) (an enzyme that catalyzes the reaction from Hcy to cystathionine) and cystathionine-gamma-lyase (*CSE*) (an enzyme that catalyzes the reaction from cystathionine to cysteine) (Figure 1). Vitamin B-6 deficiency is also associated with increased Hcy [46]. A French case-control study found that maternal plasma vitamin B-6 was negatively associated with NTD risk [33]. Thus, supplementation of vitamin B-2, vitamin B-6 and vitamin B-12 together with folic acid may have a better protective effect against NTDs than folic acid supplementation alone. However, this still needs to be demonstrated by well-designed intervention studies.

2.3. Potential Adverse Effects of B Vitamins

Despite the beneficial effect for NTD prevention, observational studies showed that very high doses of folic acid supplementation during conception also have several adverse effects. However, the evidence is still inconsistent. Observational studies showed that folic acid supplementation during conception was associated with the increased risk of wheezing in children through 18 months of age (dose was not reported) [60] and the increased risk of infant asthma (>72,000 µg·day) [61]. Evidence from observational studies showed that folic acid supplementation was associated with the increased risk of infant clefts (dose was not reported) [62] and spontaneous preterm delivery (mean dose (interquartile range): 313 (167–558) µg/day) [63]. Valera-Gran et al. found that high folic acid supplementation for mothers during conception (>5000 µg/day) had a detrimental effect on the psychomotor development of children [64]. However, Tolarova et al. found that preconceptional supplementation of 10 mg/day folic acid plus multivitamins significantly reduced the risk of infant clefts [65]. One population-based cohort study in China found that preconceptional folic acid supplementation (400 µg/day) significantly reduced the risk of spontaneous preterm delivery [66]. McGarel et al. reported that folic acid supplementation had a beneficial effect on brain development and cognitive performance [67]. The FDA's safe upper limit of folic acid is 1000 µg [68]. Folic acid is the synthetic form of folate. Before entry into the circulation system, folic acid undergoes reduction (by DHFR) and methylation to 5-MTHF, the circulating form of folic acid. However, when folic acid supplementation exceeds a certain dose, other transport mechanisms, such as passive diffusion, will complement the normal absorption mechanism, and thus unaltered folic acid enters the circulation system [69]. That is unmetabolized folic acid. One acute study found that folic acid supplementation of more than 800 µg/day can cause unmetabolized folic acid accumulation in the serum, but when the dose was no more than 400 µg/day, the unmetabolized folic acid in the serum was undetectable [69]. A prospective study of pregnant Canadian women found that unmetabolized folic acid was detectable in more than 90% of maternal and cord plasma samples, which may be a result of excess folic acid supplementation [70]. One RCT found that folic acid supplementation with a dose of 400 µg/day during conception had no significant influence on the unmetabolized folic acid concentration in maternal plasma or newborn cord blood plasma [71]. Therefore, a dose of 400 µg/day is safer than 1000 µg/day for folic acid supplementation.

Bailey reported that a higher vitamin B-6 intake (>1.85 mg/day) of mothers during the last six months of pregnancy was associated with a higher risk of childhood lymphoblastic leukemia [72]. However, one case-control study found that the per 1 mg increase of preconceptional vitamin B-6 intake from food and supplements was associated with a 11% decreased risk of childhood acute lymphoblastic leukemia. As suggested by US authorities, the level of vitamin B-6 with no observed adverse effect is set at 200 mg per day while the safe upper limit is at 100 mg per day [73]. Supplementation of vitamins B-2 and B-12 has not been associated with any adverse effects. Additionally, there is still insufficient evidence to set safe upper intake levels for vitamin B-2 and vitamin B-12 [74].

3. Choline, Betaine, One-Carbon Metabolism and NTDs

Choline is a nutrient associated with NTDs. Food sources of choline are principally those rich in lecithin (phosphatidylcholine) such as eggs and soy beans [75]. Betaine, which may be derived from choline, is found mostly in green leafy vegetables and beets (root vegetables). Choline can be synthesized in vivo by the methylation of phosphatidylethanolamine (PE) to phosphatidylcholine (PC) [76]. However, its biosynthesis is limited and dietary intake of choline is necessary [76]. Choline can be metabolized to betaine, catalyzed by choline oxidase (Figure 1). Similar to 5-MTHF, betaine can also provide the methyl needed in the remethylation of Hcy to Met, a reaction catalyzed by *BHMT* (Figure 1). The mutation of *BHMT* has been demonstrated to be associated with the risk of NTDs [6,19,31]. The ability of betaine supplementation to lower Hcy has been reported in the Netherlands [77]. Abnormal choline metabolism can lead to NTDs in the mouse [78]. An observational study found that preconceptional dietary intake of choline and betaine was negatively associated with the risk of fetal NTDs independent of folate intake in Americans [79].

However, choline and betaine intake can adversely affect serum lipid concentrations, such as increase total serum cholesterol, low density lipoprotein (LDL), high density lipoprotein (HDL) and triacylglycerol. Through the gut microbiome and trimethylamine production, they can also increase the risk of atherosclerotic vascular disease [80]. The safe upper level of choline may be 3500 mg/day for people with an age $\geq$19 years [81]. The safe upper level of betaine is unknown.

4. Other Dietary Factors Interact with the One-Carbon Metabolism to Influence the Development of NTDs

A case-control study has found that preconceptional tea consumption increases the risk of NTDs in Shanxi, China [82]. Similar findings have been observed in a case-control study in Atlanta [83]. In another case-control study conducted in the US, tea consumption was not associated with the risk of NTDs; however, when subjects were divided into subgroups according to the dose of folic acid intake, tea consumption was associated with an increased risk of NTDs in subjects with a folic acid intake >400 μg, and the authors suggested that tea consumption might interact with the folate metabolism pathway to influence the occurrence of NTDs [84]. The effects of tea consumption on the blood folate level are controversial [85,86]. One study has reported a lowering effect of tea consumption on blood folate [86]. A related case-control study found an association between the polymorphisms of catechol-*O*-methyltransferase (*COMT*) (encoding the enzyme that catalyzes the methylation of catecholamines with S-adenosylmethionine (SAM), a methyl donor) and the risk of NTDs in the Chinese: the mutant homozygotes of rs73,785 or rs4633 had a higher risk of NTDs than the wild homozygotes did, while the heterozygotes of rs4680 had a lower risk of NTDs than the wild homozygotes did, and the rs4680 genotype interacted with tea drinking to alter the risk of NTDs [87]. The effect of tea drinking on the development of NTDs can be explained by an inhibitory effect of tea catechins on dihydrofolatereductase [88]. Dihydrofolatereductase (*DHFR*) is an enzyme that catalyzes the conversion of dihydrofolate (DHF) to tetrahydrofolate (THF), the active form of folate. THF plays an important role in homocysteine metabolism and thymidine monophosphate (dTMP) synthesis. In summary, tea catechins inhibit the activity of *DHFR*, thus blocking DNA synthesis and homocysteine clearance, and this may help explain the association between tea consumption and the risk of NTDs (Figure 1).

One case-control study in Italians found that alcohol, low fruit and vegetable intake, and coffee were associated with an increased risk of NTDs [89]. Alcohol consumption is associated with lower blood folate as well as pyridoxal 5′-phosphate (the active form of vitamin B-6) and higher Hcy [90]. Animal studies showed that alcohol consumption can reduce the level of SAM (the major methyl donor) [91,92] and the activity of *MTR* (the enzyme catalyzing the remethylation of Hcy to Met) (Figure 1) [93]. Fruit and vegetables are rich in folate, and thus a low intake of these foods may be associated with inadequate folate intake (Figure 1). In pregnant Japanese women, it has been found that caffeine intake is associated with elevated Hcy only in subjects with a high intake of vitamin B-6 [94].

The positive association of caffeine with the level of Hcy and the risk of NTDs can be attributed to it having a similar chemical structure to theophylline, which can decrease pyridoxal 5′-phosphate (the active form of vitamin B-6) by acting as an inhibitor of pyridoxal kinase (Figure 1) [95,96].

In addition, n-3 PUFAs can lower Hcy [97–100], and upregulate the expression of several enzymes involved in the one-carbon metabolism, such as *MTHFR*, *CBS*, and *CSE* (Figure 1) [101]. Our unpublished case-control study in the Chinese has found that placental C18:3n-3, C20:5n-3 and C22:5n-3 are negatively associated with fetal NTD occurrence. The meta-analysis indicates that n-3 PUFAs combined with vitamin B supplementation have a greater Hcy-lowering effect than n-3 PUFAs alone [100]. However, there has been a concern that high-dose n-3 PUFA supplementation might induce bleeding [102]. However, there is little evidence to support this [103–105]. Previous studies showed that marine-derived n-3 PUFAs supplementation can promote LDL oxidation [106], but this is still controversial [107].

5. Perspective and Prospects

Although preconceptional folic acid supplementation has been recommended for decades, its overall ability to reduce the prevalence of NTDs is limited. Many women do not take a folic acid supplement until they are pregnant, which is too late for the effective prevention of NTDs. Long-term intake of folic acid–fortified foods should complement preconceptional folic acid supplementation. However, mandatory folic acid fortification is still not universally in place in Europe, Asia or Africa. However, folate-resistant NTDs exist, so there are other reasons for NTDs other than folate deficiency. In recent years, studies have indicated that the low intake and status of vitamin B-2, B-6, B-12, choline, betaine or n-3 PUFAs, and the consumption of alcohol, tea, or coffee are also associated with an increased risk of NTDs. Further cohort and intervention studies are needed to demonstrate whether multivitamin B (folate, vitamin B-2, B-6, B-12) combined with choline, betaine and n-3 PUFAs, or simply a biodiverse diet, has a better protective effect against NTDs than folic acid alone. In addition, genetic factors play an important role in the development of NTDs. There are many genetic variants involved in the one-carbon metabolism demonstrated to be associated with the risk of NTDs. Some variants can increase the risk of NTDs regardless of folic acid supplementation. Therefore, gene screening of women of childbearing age prior to pregnancy could enhance efforts to prevent NTDs.

6. Conclusions

Further cohort and intervention studies are needed to demonstrate whether multivitamin B (folate, vitamin B-2, B-6, B-12) combined with choline, betaine and n-3 PUFAs supplementation, or a biodiverse diet, has a better protective effect against NTDs than folic acid alone. Mandatory folic acid fortification and nutrition education, targeted at women in the reproductive age group, should be promoted and gene screening for women of childbearing age prior to pregnancy should be made available to prevent NTDs. These strategies would help decrease the burden of this oppressive health problem, especially in high-risk populations.

Acknowledgments: This study was funded by National Natural Science Foundation of China (NSFC, No. J20121077); by the Ph.D. Programs of the Foundation of Ministry of Education of China (J20130084); and by the National Basic Research Program of China (973 Program: 2015CB553600).

Author Contributions: D.L. and M.L.W. conceived this paper; K.L. wrote the paper; D.L. and M.L.W. revised the paper.

References

1.   Mitchell, L.E. Epidemiology of Neural Tube Defects. In *American Journal of Medical Genetics Part C: Seminars in Medical Genetics, 2005*; Wiley Online Library: Hoboken, NJ, USA, 2005; pp. 88–94.

2. Detrait, E.R.; George, T.M.; Etchevers, H.C.; Gilbert, J.R.; Vekemans, M.; Speer, M.C. Human neural tube defects: Developmental biology, epidemiology, and genetics. *Neurotoxicol. Teratol.* **2005**, *27*, 515–524. [CrossRef] [PubMed]

3. Czeizel, A.E.; Dudas, I. Prevention of the first occurrence of neural-tube defects by periconceptional vitamin supplementation. *N. Engl. J. Med.* **1992**, *327*, 1832–1835. [CrossRef] [PubMed]

4. Berry, R.J.; Li, Z.; Erickson, J.D.; Li, S.; Moore, C.A.; Wang, H.; Mulinare, J.; Zhao, P.; Wong, L.Y.; Gindler, J.; et al. Prevention of neural-tube defects with folic acid in China. China-U.S. Collaborative project for neural tube defect prevention. *N. Engl. J. Med.* **1999**, *341*, 1485–1490. [CrossRef] [PubMed]

5. Crider, K.S.; Devine, O.; Hao, L.; Dowling, N.F.; Li, S.; Molloy, A.M.; Li, Z.; Zhu, J.; Berry, R.J. Population red blood cell folate concentrations for prevention of neural tube defects: Bayesian model. *BMJ* **2014**, *29*, g4554. [CrossRef] [PubMed]

6. Liu, J.; Qi, J.; Yu, X.; Zhu, J.; Zhang, L.; Ning, Q.; Luo, X. Investigations of single nucleotide polymorphisms in folate pathway genes in Chinese families with neural tube defects. *J. Neurol. Sci.* **2014**, *337*, 61–66. [CrossRef] [PubMed]

7. MRC Vitamin Study Research Group. Prevention of neural tube defects: Results of the medical research council vitamin study. Mrc vitamin study research group. *Lancet* **1991**, *338*, 131–137.

8. Daly, L.E.; Kirke, P.N.; Molloy, A.; Weir, D.G.; Scott, J.M. Folate levels and neural tube defects. Implications for prevention. *JAMA* **1995**, *274*, 1698–1702. [CrossRef] [PubMed]

9. Centers for Disease Control and Prevention. Recommendations for the use of folic acid to reduce the number of cases of spina bifida and other neural tube defects. *MMWR Recomm. Rep.* **1992**, *41*, 1–7.

10. Bestwick, J.P.; Huttly, W.J.; Morris, J.K.; Wald, N.J. Prevention of neural tube defects: A cross-sectional study of the uptake of folic acid supplementation in nearly half a million women. *PLoS ONE* **2014**, *9*. [CrossRef] [PubMed]

11. Ren, A.G. Prevention of neural tube defects with folic acid: The Chinese experience. *World J. Clin. Pediatr.* **2015**, *4*, 41–44. [CrossRef] [PubMed]

12. Arth, A.; Kancherla, V.; Pachon, H.; Zimmerman, S.; Johnson, Q.; Oakley, G.P., Jr. A 2015 global update on folic acid-preventable spina bifida and anencephaly. *Birth Defects Res. A Clin. Mol. Teratol.* **2016**, *106*, 520–529. [CrossRef] [PubMed]

13. Santos, L.M.; Lecca, R.C.; Cortez-Escalante, J.J.; Sanchez, M.N.; Rodrigues, H.G. Prevention of neural tube defects by the fortification of flour with folic acid: A population-based retrospective study in brazil. *Bull. World Health Organ.* **2016**, *94*, 22–29. [CrossRef] [PubMed]

14. Khoshnood, B.; Loane, M.; de Walle, H.; Arriola, L.; Addor, M.C.; Barisic, I.; Beres, J.; Bianchi, F.; Dias, C.; Draper, E.; et al. Long term trends in prevalence of neural tube defects in europe: Population based study. *BMJ* **2015**, *24*, h5949. [CrossRef] [PubMed]

15. Wang, H.; De Steur, H.; Chen, G.; Zhang, X.; Pei, L.; Gellynck, X.; Zheng, X. Effectiveness of folic acid fortified flour for prevention of neural tube defects in a high risk region. *Nutrients* **2016**, *8*, 152. [CrossRef] [PubMed]

16. Liu, Z.Z.; Zhang, J.T.; Liu, D.; Hao, Y.H.; Chang, B.M.; Xie, J.; Li, P.Z. Interaction between maternal 5,10-methylenetetrahydrofolate reductase c677t and methionine synthase a2756g gene variants to increase the risk of fetal neural tube defects in a Shanxi han population. *Chin. Med. J.* **2013**, *126*, 865–869. [PubMed]

17. Morales de Machin, A.; Mendez, K.; Solis, E.; Borjas de Borjas, L.; Bracho, A.; Hernandez, M.L.; Negron, A.; Delgado, W.; Sanchez, Y. c677t polymorphism of the methylentetrahydrofolate reductase gene in mothers of children affected with neural tube defects. *Investig. Clin.* **2015**, *56*, 284–295.

18. Van der Put, N.M.; Steegers-Theunissen, R.P.; Frosst, P.; Trijbels, F.J.; Eskes, T.K.; van den Heuvel, L.P.; Mariman, E.C.; den Heyer, M.; Rozen, R.; Blom, H.J. Mutated methylenetetrahydrofolate reductase as a risk factor for spina bifida. *Lancet* **1995**, *346*, 1070–1071. [CrossRef]

19. Shaw, G.M.; Lu, W.; Zhu, H.; Yang, W.; Briggs, F.B.; Carmichael, S.L.; Barcellos, L.F.; Lammer, E.J.; Finnell, R.H. 118 snps of folate-related genes and risks of spina bifida and conotruncal heart defects. *BMC Med. Genet.* **2009**, *10*, 1471–2350. [CrossRef] [PubMed]

20. Yan, L.; Zhao, L.; Long, Y.; Zou, P.; Ji, G.; Gu, A.; Zhao, P. Association of the maternal mthfr c677t polymorphism with susceptibility to neural tube defects in offsprings: Evidence from 25 case-control studies. *PLoS ONE* **2012**, *7*, 3. [CrossRef] [PubMed]

21. Crider, K.S.; Zhu, J.H.; Hao, L.; Yang, Q.H.; Yang, T.P.; Gindler, J.; Maneval, D.R.; Quinlivan, E.P.; Li, Z.; Bailey, L.B.; et al. Mthfr 677c→t genotype is associated with folate and homocysteine concentrations in

a large, population-based, double-blind trial of folic acid supplementation. *Am. J. Clin. Nutr.* **2011**, *93*, 1365–1372. [CrossRef] [PubMed]

22. Tsang, B.L.; Devine, O.J.; Cordero, A.M.; Marchetta, C.M.; Mulinare, J.; Mersereau, P.; Guo, J.; Qi, Y.P.; Berry, R.J.; Rosenthal, J.; et al. Assessing the association between the methylenetetrahydrofolate reductase (mthfr) 677c>t polymorphism and blood folate concentrations: A systematic review and meta-analysis of trials and observational studies. *Am. J. Clin. Nutr.* **2015**, *101*, 1286–1294. [CrossRef] [PubMed]

23. Van der Put, N.M.; Gabreels, F.; Stevens, E.M.; Smeitink, J.A.; Trijbels, F.J.; Eskes, T.K.; van den Heuvel, L.P.; Blom, H.J. A second common mutation in the methylenetetrahydrofolate reductase gene: An additional risk factor for neural-tube defects? *Am. J. Hum. Genet.* **1998**, *62*, 1044–1051. [CrossRef] [PubMed]

24. De Marco, P.; Calevo, M.G.; Moroni, A.; Arata, L.; Merello, E.; Finnell, R.H.; Zhu, H.; Andreussi, L.; Cama, A.; Capra, V. Study of mthfr and ms polymorphisms as risk factors for ntd in the italian population. *J. Hum. Genet.* **2002**, *47*, 319–324. [CrossRef] [PubMed]

25. Stegmann, K.; Ziegler, A.; Ngo, E.T.; Kohlschmidt, N.; Schroter, B.; Ermert, A.; Koch, M.C. Linkage disequilibrium of mthfr genotypes 677c/t-1298a/c in the german population and association studies in probands with neural tube defects(ntd). *Am. J. Med. Genet.* **1999**, *87*, 23–29. [CrossRef]

26. Barber, R.; Shalat, S.; Hendricks, K.; Joggerst, B.; Larsen, R.; Suarez, L.; Finnell, R. Investigation of folate pathway gene polymorphisms and the incidence of neural tube defects in a texas hispanic population. *Mol. Genet. Metab.* **2000**, *70*, 45–52. [CrossRef] [PubMed]

27. Volcik, K.A.; Blanton, S.H.; Tyerman, G.H.; Jong, S.T.; Rott, E.J.; Page, T.Z.; Romaine, N.K.; Northrup, H. Methylenetetrahydrofolate reductase and spina bifida: Evaluation of level of defect and maternal genotypic risk in hispanics. *Am. J. Med. Genet.* **2000**, *95*, 21–27. [CrossRef]

28. Wang, Y.; Liu, Y.; Ji, W.; Qin, H.; Wu, H.; Xu, D.; Turtuohut, T.; Wang, Z. Variants in mthfr gene and neural tube defects susceptibility in China. *Metab. Brain Dis.* **2015**, *30*, 1017–1026. [CrossRef] [PubMed]

29. Wang, Y.; Liu, Y.; Ji, W.; Qin, H.; Wu, H.; Xu, D.; Tukebai, T.; Wang, Z. Analysis of mtr and mtrr polymorphisms for neural tube defects risk association. *Medicine* **2015**, *94*, 1367. [CrossRef] [PubMed]

30. Sliwerska, E.; Szpecht-Potocka, A. Mutations of MTHFR, MTR, MTRR genes as high risk factors for neural tube defects. *Med. Wieku Rozwoj* **2002**, *6*, 371–382. [PubMed]

31. Boyles, A.L.; Billups, A.V.; Deak, K.L.; Siegel, D.G.; Mehltretter, L.; Slifer, S.H.; Bassuk, A.G.; Kessler, J.A.; Reed, M.C.; Nijhout, H.F.; et al. Neural tube defects and folate pathway genes: Family-based association tests of gene-gene and gene-environment interactions. *Environ. Health Perspect.* **2006**, *114*, 1547–1552. [CrossRef] [PubMed]

32. Richter, B.; Stegmann, K.; Roper, B.; Boddeker, I.; Ngo, E.T.; Koch, M.C. Interaction of folate and homocysteine pathway genotypes evaluated in susceptibility to neural tube defects (ntd) in a german population. *J. Hum. Genet.* **2001**, *46*, 105–109. [CrossRef] [PubMed]

33. Candito, M.; Rivet, R.; Herbeth, B.; Boisson, C.; Rudigoz, R.C.; Luton, D.; Journel, H.; Oury, J.F.; Roux, F.; Saura, R.; et al. Nutritional and genetic determinants of vitamin B and homocysteine metabolisms in neural tube defects: A multicenter case-control study. *Am. J. Med. Genet. A* **2008**, *1*, 1128–1133. [CrossRef] [PubMed]

34. Yadav, U.; Kumar, P.; Yadav, S.K.; Mishra, O.P.; Rai, V. Polymorphisms in folate metabolism genes as maternal risk factor for neural tube defects: An updated meta-analysis. *Metab. Brain Dis.* **2015**, *30*, 7–24. [CrossRef] [PubMed]

35. De Marco, P.; Merello, E.; Calevo, M.G.; Mascelli, S.; Raso, A.; Cama, A.; Capra, V. Evaluation of a methylenetetrahydrofolate-dehydrogenase 1958g>a polymorphism for neural tube defect risk. *J. Hum. Genet.* **2006**, *51*, 98–103. [CrossRef] [PubMed]

36. Etheredge, A.J.; Finnell, R.H.; Carmichael, S.L.; Lammer, E.J.; Zhu, H.; Mitchell, L.E.; Shaw, G.M. Maternal and infant gene-folate interactions and the risk of neural tube defects. *Am. J. Med. Genet. A* **2012**, *10*, 17. [CrossRef] [PubMed]

37. Jiang, J.; Zhang, Y.; Wei, L.; Sun, Z.; Liu, Z. Association between mthfd1 g1958a polymorphism and neural tube defects susceptibility: A meta-analysis. *PLoS ONE* **2014**, *9*. [CrossRef] [PubMed]

38. Meng, J.; Han, L.; Zhuang, B. Association between mthfd1 polymorphisms and neural tube defect susceptibility. *J. Neurol. Sci.* **2015**, *348*, 188–194. [CrossRef] [PubMed]

39. Parle-McDermott, A.; Pangilinan, F.; O'Brien, K.K.; Mills, J.L.; Magee, A.M.; Troendle, J.; Sutton, M.; Scott, J.M.; Kirke, P.N.; Molloy, A.M.; et al. A common variant in mthfd1l is associated with neural tube defects and mrna splicing efficiency. *Hum. Mutat.* **2009**, *30*, 1650–1656. [CrossRef] [PubMed]

40. Pangilinan, F.; Molloy, A.M.; Mills, J.L.; Troendle, J.F.; Parle-McDermott, A.; Signore, C.; O'Leary, V.B.; Chines, P.; Seay, J.M.; Geiler-Samerotte, K.; et al. Evaluation of common genetic variants in 82 candidate genes as risk factors for neural tube defects. *BMC Med. Genet.* **2012**, *13*, 62. [CrossRef] [PubMed]

41. Wu, J.; Bao, Y.; Lu, X.; Wu, L.; Zhang, T.; Guo, J.; Yang, J. Polymorphisms in mthfd1 gene and susceptibility to neural tube defects: A case-control study in a Chinese han population with relatively low folate levels. *Med. Sci. Monit.* **2015**, *21*, 2630–2637. [CrossRef] [PubMed]

42. Guo, J.; Xie, H.; Wang, J.; Zhao, H.; Wang, F.; Liu, C.; Wang, L.; Lu, X.; Bao, Y.; Zou, J.; et al. The maternal folate hydrolase gene polymorphism is associated with neural tube defects in a high-risk Chinese population. *Genes Nutr.* **2013**, *8*, 191–197. [CrossRef] [PubMed]

43. Pei, L.J.; Zhu, H.P.; Li, Z.W.; Zhang, W.; Ren, A.G.; Zhu, J.H.; Li, Z. Interaction between maternal periconceptional supplementation of folic acid and reduced folate carrier gene polymorphism of neural tube defects. *Zhonghua Yi Xue Yi Chuan Xue Za Zhi* **2005**, *22*, 284–287. [PubMed]

44. Zhang, T.; Lou, J.; Zhong, R.; Wu, J.; Zou, L.; Sun, Y.; Lu, X.; Liu, L.; Miao, X.; Xiong, G. Genetic variants in the folate pathway and the risk of neural tube defects: A meta-analysis of the published literature. *PLoS ONE* **2013**, *8*, e59570. [CrossRef] [PubMed]

45. Piao, W.; Guo, J.; Bao, Y.; Wang, F.; Zhang, T.; Huo, J.; Zhang, K. Analysis of polymorphisms of genes associated with folate-mediated one-carbon metabolism and neural tube defects in Chinese han population. *Birth Defects Res. A Clin. Mol. Teratol.* **2016**, *106*, 232–239. [CrossRef] [PubMed]

46. Hao, L.; Ma, J.; Zhu, J.; Stampfer, M.J.; Tian, Y.; Willett, W.C.; Li, Z. High prevalence of hyperhomocysteinemia in Chinese adults is associated with low folate, vitamin B-12, and vitamin B-6 status. *J. Nutr.* **2007**, *137*, 407–413. [PubMed]

47. Gu, Q.; Li, Y.; Cui, Z.L.; Luo, X.P. Homocysteine, folate, vitamin B12 and B6 in mothers of children with neural tube defects in Xinjiang, China. *Acta Paediatr.* **2012**, *101*, 1651–2227. [CrossRef] [PubMed]

48. Zhang, T.; Xin, R.; Gu, X.; Wang, F.; Pei, L.; Lin, L.; Chen, G.; Wu, J.; Zheng, X. Maternal serum vitamin B12, folate and homocysteine and the risk of neural tube defects in the offspring in a high-risk area of China. *Public Health Nutr.* **2009**, *12*, 680–686. [CrossRef] [PubMed]

49. Dang, S.; Yan, H.; Zeng, L.; Wang, Q.; Li, Q.; Xiao, S.; Fan, X. The status of vitamin B12 and folate among Chinese women: A population-based cross-sectional study in northwest China. *PLoS ONE* **2014**, *9*. [CrossRef] [PubMed]

50. Gaber, K.R.; Farag, M.K.; Soliman, S.E.; El-Bassyouni, H.T.; El-Kamah, G. Maternal vitamin B12 and the risk of fetal neural tube defects in egyptian patients. *Clin. Lab.* **2007**, *53*, 69–75. [PubMed]

51. Molloy, A.M.; Kirke, P.N.; Troendle, J.F.; Burke, H.; Sutton, M.; Brody, L.C.; Scott, J.M.; Mills, J.L. Maternal vitamin B12 status and risk of neural tube defects in a population with high neural tube defect prevalence and no folic acid fortification. *Pediatrics* **2009**, *123*, 917–923. [CrossRef] [PubMed]

52. Nasri, K.; Ben Fradj, M.K.; Touati, A.; Aloui, M.; Ben Jemaa, N.; Masmoudi, A.; Elmay, M.V.; Omar, S.; Feki, M.; Kaabechi, N.; et al. Association of maternal homocysteine and vitamins status with the risk of neural tube defects in tunisia: A case-control study. *Birth Defects Res. A Clin. Mol. Teratol.* **2015**, *103*, 1011–1020. [CrossRef] [PubMed]

53. Ray, J.G.; Wyatt, P.R.; Thompson, M.D.; Vermeulen, M.J.; Meier, C.; Wong, P.Y.; Farrell, S.A.; Cole, D.E. Vitamin B12 and the risk of neural tube defects in a folic-acid-fortified population. *Epidemiology* **2007**, *18*, 362–366. [CrossRef] [PubMed]

54. Thompson, M.D.; Cole, D.E.; Ray, J.G. Vitamin B-12 and neural tube defects: The canadian experience. *Am. J. Clin. Nutr.* **2009**, *89*, 30. [CrossRef] [PubMed]

55. Franke, B.; Vermeulen, S.H.; Steegers-Theunissen, R.P.; Coenen, M.J.; Schijvenaars, M.M.; Scheffer, H.; den Heijer, M.; Blom, H.J. An association study of 45 folate-related genes in spina bifida: Involvement of cubilin (cubn) and trna aspartic acid methyltransferase 1 (trdmt1). *Birth Defects Res. A Clin. Mol. Teratol.* **2009**, *85*, 216–226. [CrossRef] [PubMed]

56. Hustad, S.; Ueland, P.M.; Vollset, S.E.; Zhang, Y.; Bjorke-Monsen, A.L.; Schneede, J. Riboflavin as a determinant of plasma total homocysteine: Effect modification by the methylenetetrahydrofolate reductase c677t polymorphism. *Clin. Chem.* **2000**, *46*, 1065–1071. [PubMed]

57. McNulty, H.; Dowey le, R.C.; Strain, J.J.; Dunne, A.; Ward, M.; Molloy, A.M.; McAnena, L.B.; Hughes, J.P.; Hannon-Fletcher, M.; Scott, J.M. Riboflavin lowers homocysteine in individuals homozygous for the mthfr 677c→t polymorphism. *Circulation* **2006**, *113*, 74–80. [CrossRef] [PubMed]

58. Moat, S.J.; Ashfield-Watt, P.A.; Powers, H.J.; Newcombe, R.G.; McDowell, I.F. Effect of riboflavin status on the homocysteine-lowering effect of folate in relation to the mthfr (c677t) genotype. *Clin. Chem.* **2003**, *49*, 295–302. [CrossRef] [PubMed]

59. Smithells, R.W.; Sheppard, S.; Schorah, C.J.; Seller, M.J.; Nevin, N.C.; Harris, R.; Read, A.P.; Fielding, D.W. Apparent prevention of neural tube defects by periconceptional vitamin supplementation. *Arch. Dis. Child.* **1981**, *56*, 911–918. [CrossRef] [PubMed]

60. Haberg, S.E.; London, S.J.; Stigum, H.; Nafstad, P.; Nystad, W. Folic acid supplements in pregnancy and early childhood respiratory health. *Arch. Dis. Child.* **2009**, *94*, 180–184. [CrossRef] [PubMed]

61. Yang, L.; Jiang, L.; Bi, M.; Jia, X.; Wang, Y.; He, C.; Yao, Y.; Wang, J.; Wang, Z. High dose of maternal folic acid supplementation is associated to infant asthma. *Food Chem. Toxicol.* **2015**, *75*, 88–93. [CrossRef] [PubMed]

62. Rozendaal, A.M.; van Essen, A.J.; te Meerman, G.J.; Bakker, M.K.; van der Biezen, J.J.; Goorhuis-Brouwer, S.M.; Vermeij-Keers, C.; de Walle, H.E. Periconceptional folic acid associated with an increased risk of oral clefts relative to non-folate related malformations in the northern netherlands: A population based case-control study. *Eur. J. Epidemiol.* **2013**, *28*, 875–887. [CrossRef] [PubMed]

63. Sengpiel, V.; Bacelis, J.; Myhre, R.; Myking, S.; Devold Pay, A.S.; Haugen, M.; Brantsaeter, A.L.; Meltzer, H.M.; Nilsen, R.M.; Magnus, P.; et al. Folic acid supplementation, dietary folate intake during pregnancy and risk for spontaneous preterm delivery: A prospective observational cohort study. *BMC Pregnancy Childbirth* **2014**, *14*, 014–0375. [CrossRef] [PubMed]

64. Valera-Gran, D.; Garcia de la Hera, M.; Navarrete-Munoz, E.M.; Fernandez-Somoano, A.; Tardon, A.; Julvez, J.; Forns, J.; Lertxundi, N.; Ibarluzea, J.M.; Murcia, M.; et al. Folic acid supplements during pregnancy and child psychomotor development after the first year of life. *JAMA Pediatr.* **2014**, *168*, 3. [CrossRef] [PubMed]

65. Tolarova, M.; Harris, J. Reduced recurrence of orofacial clefts after periconceptional supplementation with high-dose folic acid and multivitamins. *Teratology* **1995**, *51*, 71–78. [CrossRef] [PubMed]

66. Li, Z.; Ye, R.; Zhang, L.; Li, H.; Liu, J.; Ren, A. Periconceptional folic acid supplementation and the risk of preterm births in China: A large prospective cohort study. *Int. J. Epidemiol.* **2014**, *43*, 1132–1139. [CrossRef] [PubMed]

67. McGarel, C.; Pentieva, K.; Strain, J.J.; McNulty, H. Emerging roles for folate and related B-vitamins in brain health across the lifecycle. *Proc. Nutr. Soc.* **2015**, *74*, 46–55. [CrossRef] [PubMed]

68. Quinlivan, E.P.; Gregory, J.F., 3rd. Effect of food fortification on folic acid intake in the united states. *Am. J. Clin. Nutr.* **2003**, *77*, 221–225. [PubMed]

69. Kelly, P.; McPartlin, J.; Goggins, M.; Weir, D.G.; Scott, J.M. Unmetabolized folic acid in serum: Acute studies in subjects consuming fortified food and supplements. *Am. J. Clin. Nutr.* **1997**, *65*, 1790–1795. [PubMed]

70. Plumptre, L.; Masih, S.P.; Ly, A.; Aufreiter, S.; Sohn, K.J.; Croxford, R.; Lausman, A.Y.; Berger, H.; O'Connor, D.L.; Kim, Y.I. High concentrations of folate and unmetabolized folic acid in a cohort of pregnant canadian women and umbilical cord blood. *Am. J. Clin. Nutr.* **2015**, *102*, 848–857. [CrossRef] [PubMed]

71. Pentieva, K.; Selhub, J.; Paul, L.; Molloy, A.M.; McNulty, B.; Ward, M.; Marshall, B.; Dornan, J.; Reilly, R.; Parle-McDermott, A.; et al. Evidence from a randomized trial that exposure to supplemental folic acid at recommended levels during pregnancy does not lead to increased unmetabolized folic acid concentrations in maternal or cord blood. *J. Nutr.* **2016**, *146*, 494–500. [CrossRef] [PubMed]

72. Bailey, H.D.; Miller, M.; Langridge, A.; de Klerk, N.H.; van Bockxmeer, F.M.; Attia, J.; Scott, R.J.; Armstrong, B.K.; Milne, E. Maternal dietary intake of folate and vitamins B6 and B12 during pregnancy and the risk of childhood acute lymphoblastic leukemia. *Nutr. Cancer* **2012**, *64*, 1122–1130. [CrossRef] [PubMed]

73. Katan, M.B. How much vitamin B6 is toxic? *Ned. Tijdschr. Geneeskd.* **2005**, *149*, 2545–2546. [PubMed]

74. Rogovik, A.L.; Vohra, S.; Goldman, R.D. Safety considerations and potential interactions of vitamins: Should vitamins be considered drugs? *Ann. Pharmacother.* **2010**, *44*, 311–324. [CrossRef] [PubMed]

75. Chu, D.-M.; Wahlqvist, M.L.; Chang, H.-Y.; Yeh, N.-H. Choline and betaine food sources and intakes in taiwanese. *Asia Pac. J. Clin. Nutr.* **2012**, *21*, 547–557. [PubMed]

76. Zeisel, S.H.; da Costa, K.A. Choline: An essential nutrient for public health. *Nutr. Rev.* **2009**, *67*, 615–623. [CrossRef] [PubMed]

77. Steenge, G.R.; Verhoef, P.; Katan, M.B. Betaine supplementation lowers plasma homocysteine in healthy men and women. *J. Nutr.* **2003**, *133*, 1291–1295. [PubMed]

78. Fisher, M.C.; Zeisel, S.H.; Mar, M.H.; Sadler, T.W. Perturbations in choline metabolism cause neural tube defects in mouse embryos in vitro. *FASEB J.* **2002**, *16*, 619–621. [CrossRef] [PubMed]

79. Shaw, G.M.; Carmichael, S.L.; Yang, W.; Selvin, S.; Schaffer, D.M. Periconceptional dietary intake of choline and betaine and neural tube defects in offspring. *Am. J. Epidemiol.* **2004**, *160*, 102–109. [CrossRef] [PubMed]

80. Wang, Z.; Klipfell, E.; Bennett, B.J.; Koeth, R.; Levison, B.S.; Dugar, B.; Feldstein, A.E.; Britt, E.B.; Fu, X.; Chung, Y.M.; et al. Gut flora metabolism of phosphatidylcholine promotes cardiovascular disease. *Nature* **2011**, *472*, 57–63. [CrossRef] [PubMed]

81. Sanders, L.M.; Zeisel, S.H. Choline: Dietary requirements and role in brain development. *Nutr. Today* **2007**, *42*, 181–186. [CrossRef] [PubMed]

82. Ye, R.; Ren, A.; Zhang, L.; Li, Z.; Liu, J.; Pei, L.; Zheng, X. Tea drinking as a risk factor for neural tube defects in northern China. *Epidemiology* **2011**, *22*, 491–496. [CrossRef] [PubMed]

83. Correa, A.; Stolley, A.; Liu, Y. Prenatal tea consumption and risks of anencephaly and spina bifida. *Ann. Epidemiol.* **2000**, *10*, 476–477. [CrossRef]

84. Yazdy, M.M.; Tinker, S.C.; Mitchell, A.A.; Demmer, L.A.; Werler, M.M. Maternal tea consumption during early pregnancy and the risk of spina bifida. *Birth Defects Res. Part A Clin. Mol. Teratol.* **2012**, *94*, 756–761. [CrossRef] [PubMed]

85. Augustin, K.; Frank, J.; Augustin, S.; Langguth, P.; Ohrvik, V.; Witthoft, C.M.; Rimbach, G.; Wolffram, S. Greeen tea extracts lower serum folates in rats at very high dietary concentrations only and do not affect plasma folates in a human pilot study. *J. Physiol. Pharmacol.* **2009**, *60*, 103–108. [PubMed]

86. Shiraishi, M.; Haruna, M.; Matsuzaki, M.; Ota, E.; Murayama, R.; Murashima, S. Association between the serum folate levels and tea consumption during pregnancy. *Biosci. Trends* **2010**, *4*, 225–230. [PubMed]

87. Liu, J.; Wang, L.; Fu, Y.; Li, Z.; Zhang, Y.; Zhang, L.; Jin, L.; Ye, R.; Ren, A. Association between maternal comt gene polymorphisms and fetal neural tube defects risk in a Chinese population. *Birth Defects Res. A Clin. Mol. Teratol.* **2014**, *100*, 22–29. [CrossRef] [PubMed]

88. Navarro-Peran, E.; Cabezas-Herrera, J.; Campo, L.S.; Rodriguez-Lopez, J.N. Effects of folate cycle disruption by the green tea polyphenol epigallocatechin-3-gallate. *Int. J. Biochem. Cell Biol.* **2007**, *39*, 2215–2225. [CrossRef] [PubMed]

89. De Marco, P.; Merello, E.; Calevo, M.G.; Mascelli, S.; Pastorino, D.; Crocetti, L.; De Biasio, P.; Piatelli, G.; Cama, A.; Capra, V. Maternal periconceptional factors affect the risk of spina bifida-affected pregnancies: An italian case-control study. *Childs Nerv. Syst.* **2011**, *27*, 1073–1081. [CrossRef] [PubMed]

90. Cravo, M.L.; Gloria, L.M.; Selhub, J.; Nadeau, M.R.; Camilo, M.E.; Resende, M.P.; Cardoso, J.N.; Leitao, C.N.; Mira, F.C. Hyperhomocysteinemia in chronic alcoholism: Correlation with folate, vitamin B-12, and vitamin B-6 status. *Am. J. Clin. Nutr.* **1996**, *63*, 220–224. [PubMed]

91. Stickel, F.; Choi, S.W.; Kim, Y.I.; Bagley, P.J.; Seitz, H.K.; Russell, R.M.; Selhub, J.; Mason, J.B. Effect of chronic alcohol consumption on total plasma homocysteine level in rats. *Alcohol. Clin. Exp. Res.* **2000**, *24*, 259–264. [CrossRef] [PubMed]

92. Murillo-Fuentes, M.L.; Artillo, R.; Ubeda, N.; Varela-Moreiras, G.; Murillo, M.L.; Carreras, O. Hepatic s-adenosylmethionine after maternal alcohol exposure on offspring rats. *Addict. Biol.* **2005**, *10*, 139–144. [CrossRef] [PubMed]

93. Barak, A.J.; Beckenhauer, H.C.; Junnila, M.; Tuma, D.J. Dietary betaine promotes generation of hepatic s-adenosylmethionine and protects the liver from ethanol-induced fatty infiltration. *Alcohol. Clin. Exp. Res.* **1993**, *17*, 552–555. [CrossRef] [PubMed]

94. Shiraishi, M.; Haruna, M.; Matsuzaki, M.; Ota, E.; Murayama, R.; Sasaki, S.; Yeo, S.; Murashima, S. Relationship between plasma total homocysteine level and dietary caffeine and vitamin B6 intakes in pregnant women. *Nurs. Health Sci.* **2014**, *16*, 164–170. [CrossRef] [PubMed]

95. Ubbink, J.B.; Delport, R.; Becker, P.J.; Bissbort, S. Evidence of a theophylline-induced vitamin B6 deficiency caused by noncompetitive inhibition of pyridoxal kinase. *J. Lab. Clin. Med.* **1989**, *113*, 15–22. [PubMed]

96. Ubbink, J.B.; Delport, R.; Bissbort, S.; Vermaak, W.J.; Becker, P.J. Relationship between vitamin B-6 status and elevated pyridoxal kinase levels induced by theophylline therapy in humans. *J. Nutr.* **1990**, *120*, 1352–1359. [PubMed]

97. Huang, T.; Li, K.; Asimi, S.; Chen, Q.; Li, D. Effect of vitamin B-12 and *n*-3 polyunsaturated fatty acids on plasma homocysteine, ferritin, c-reaction protein, and other cardiovascular risk factors: A randomized controlled trial. *Asia Pac. J. Clin. Nutr.* **2015**, *24*, 403–411. [PubMed]

98. Huang, T.; Yu, X.; Shou, T.; Wahlqvist, M.L.; Li, D. Associations of plasma phospholipid fatty acids with plasma homocysteine in Chinese vegetarians. *Br. J. Nutr.* **2013**, *109*, 1688–1694. [CrossRef] [PubMed]

99. Huang, T.; Asimi, S.; Lou, D.; Li, D. Plasma phospholipid polyunsaturated fatty acids and homocysteine in Chinese type 2 diabetes patients. *Asia Pac. J. Clin. Nutr.* **2012**, *21*, 394–399. [PubMed]

100. Dawson, S.L.; Bowe, S.J.; Crowe, T.C. A combination of omega-3 fatty acids, folic acid and b-group vitamins is superior at lowering homocysteine than omega-3 alone: A meta-analysis. *Nutr. Res.* **2016**, *36*, 499–508. [CrossRef] [PubMed]

101. Huang, T.; Hu, X.; Khan, N.; Yang, J.; Li, D. Effect of polyunsaturated fatty acids on homocysteine metabolism through regulating the gene expressions involved in methionine metabolism. *Sci. World J.* **2013**, *23*, 931626. [CrossRef] [PubMed]

102. Detopoulou, P.; Papamikos, V. Gastrointestinal bleeding after high intake of omega-3 fatty acids, cortisone and antibiotic therapy: A case study. *Int. J. Sport Nutr. Exerc. Metab.* **2014**, *24*, 253–257. [CrossRef] [PubMed]

103. Wachira, J.K.; Larson, M.K.; Harris, W.S. *N*-3 fatty acids affect haemostasis but do not increase the risk of bleeding: Clinical observations and mechanistic insights. *Br. J. Nutr.* **2014**, *111*, 1652–1662. [CrossRef] [PubMed]

104. Meredith, D.S.; Kepler, C.K.; Huang, R.C.; Hirsch, B.; Nguyen, J.; Farmer, J.C.; Girardi, F.P.; O'Leary, P.F.; Cammisa, F.P. The effect of omega-3 fatty-acid supplements on perioperative bleeding following posterior spinal arthrodesis. *Eur. Spine J.* **2012**, *21*, 2659–2663. [CrossRef] [PubMed]

105. Salisbury, A.C.; Harris, W.S.; Amin, A.P.; Reid, K.J.; O'Keefe, J.H., Jr.; Spertus, J.A. Relation between red blood cell omega-3 fatty acid index and bleeding during acute myocardial infarction. *Am. J. Cardiol.* **2012**, *109*, 13–18. [CrossRef] [PubMed]

106. Finnegan, Y.E.; Minihane, A.M.; Leigh-Firbank, E.C.; Kew, S.; Meijer, G.W.; Muggli, R.; Calder, P.C.; Williams, C.M. Plant- and marine-derived *n*-3 polyunsaturated fatty acids have differential effects on fasting and postprandial blood lipid concentrations and on the susceptibility of ldl to oxidative modification in moderately hyperlipidemic subjects. *Am. J. Clin. Nutr.* **2003**, *77*, 783–795. [PubMed]

107. Mori, T.A.; Woodman, R.J.; Burke, V.; Puddey, I.B.; Croft, K.D.; Beilin, L.J. Effect of eicosapentaenoic acid and docosahexaenoic acid on oxidative stress and inflammatory markers in treated-hypertensive type 2 diabetic subjects. *Free Radic. Biol. Med.* **2003**, *35*, 772–781. [CrossRef]

14

Nutrients in Energy and One-Carbon Metabolism: Learning from Metformin Users

Fedra Luciano-Mateo [1], Anna Hernández-Aguilera [1], Noemi Cabre [1], Jordi Camps [1], Salvador Fernández-Arroyo [1,2], Jose Lopez-Miranda [3], Javier A. Menendez [2,4,*] and Jorge Joven [1,5,*]

[1] Unitat de Recerca Biomèdica, Hospital Universitari Sant Joan, Institut d'Investigació Sanitària Pere Virgili, Universitat Rovira i Virgili, 43201 Reus, Spain; fedra.luciano@gmail.com (F.L.-M.); anna.hernandeza@gmail.com (A.H.-A.); noemi.cabre@gmail.com (N.C.); jcamps@grupsagessa.com (J.C.); salvador.fernandez@iispv.cat (S.F.-A.)
[2] Molecular Oncology Group, Girona Biomedical Research Institute (IDIBGI), 17190 Girona, Spain
[3] CIBER Fisiopatología Obesidad y Nutrición (CIBEROBN), Instituto de Salud Carlos III, 28029 Madrid, Spain; jlopezmir@uco.es
[4] ProCURE (Program against Cancer Therapeutic Resistance), Metabolism and Cancer Group, Catalan Institute of Oncology, 17190 Girona, Spain
[5] The Campus of International Excellence Southern Catalonia, 43003 Tarragona, Spain
* Correspondence: jmenendez@idibgi.org (J.A.M.); jorge.joven@urv.cat (J.J.)

Abstract: Metabolic vulnerability is associated with age-related diseases and concomitant co-morbidities, which include obesity, diabetes, atherosclerosis and cancer. Most of the health problems we face today come from excessive intake of nutrients and drugs mimicking dietary effects and dietary restriction are the most successful manipulations targeting age-related pathways. Phenotypic heterogeneity and individual response to metabolic stressors are closely related food intake. Understanding the complexity of the relationship between dietary provision and metabolic consequences in the long term might provide clinical strategies to improve healthspan. New aspects of metformin activity provide a link to many of the overlapping factors, especially the way in which organismal bioenergetics remodel one-carbon metabolism. Metformin not only inhibits mitochondrial complex 1, modulating the metabolic response to nutrient intake, but also alters one-carbon metabolic pathways. Here, we discuss findings on the mechanism(s) of action of metformin with the potential for therapeutic interpretations.

Keywords: diabetes mellitus; energy intake; epigenetics; folic acid; food-drug interactions; food source; obesity; vitamins B

---

1. Introduction

Food restriction extends health and lifespan in some models [1], but what nutrients should be restricted and to what extent? Qualitative changes in the provision of dietary macronutrients induce metabolic and endocrine adaptations that are clinically relevant to the nutritional status of both, patients with low food availability and those with a persistent intake of excessive amounts of food [2]. In particular, the relationship between energy and one-carbon (1C) metabolism is extremely sensitive to food intake [3–6]. We envision that the inclusion of metformin in current strategies promoting metabolic fitness [7] is in accordance with the clinical response to dietary environment in disease states and the beneficial effects in metabolically vulnerable cells [8–11]. That is, it is important to revise what we can learn from metformin users and which are the potential implications. Metformin, as a calorie-restriction mimetic drug affecting mitochondrial function, integrates metabolic signals and the direct effect on folate metabolism may provide therapeutic clues [12–15]. We highlight the effects of metformin on signaling pathways associated with some of the hallmarks of aging and the likely beneficial effects in the pathogenesis of comorbidities associated with metabolic diseases (Figure 1). Whether metformin can be safely used with these new indications remains to be established.

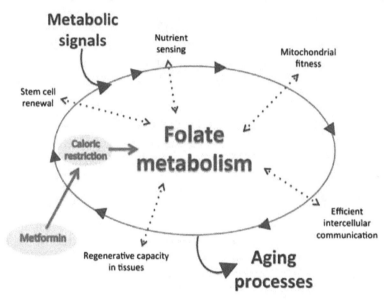

Figure 1. The effect of metformin on signaling pathways associated with nutrient excess. These effects are likely regulated by folate metabolism and represent direct effects on some of the hallmarks of tissue aging. It remains to be determined whether metformin can safely slow the development of age-related comorbidities in metabolic diseases.

Metformin is currently used exclusively in the treatment of type 2 diabetes mellitus (T2DM), but there is potential for additional indications in obesity, inflammatory disorders, cardiovascular diseases and cancer. For instance, in obese patients without diabetes, the weight loss effects of metformin are not inferior to those of a recently approved drug for obesity [16] and the antenatal administration of metformin during pregnancy reduces maternal weight gain without effects on neonatal outcomes [17–19]. Moreover, the Diabetes Prevention Program has found beneficial effects in diabetes prevention and a durable weight loss attributable to metformin [20–22]. Cardiovascular benefits are also likely, and, when compared to sulfonylurea or insulin therapy, metformin monotherapy is associated with a higher reduction in cardiovascular events [23,24]. In addition, the anti-inflammatory actions of metformin can be separated from its metabolic effects, and there is ongoing research assessing the role of metformin in the prevention and recurrence of breast cancer [25,26].

All these effects are crucial in preventing disease and promoting health. We discuss here the metabolic alterations connecting the metformin response and the function of essential nutrients, which emphasize that careful attention to diet might shape clinical strategies [27]. Our arguments are framed in the relationship between energy and one-carbon metabolism, reinforced by the mechanisms of action proposed for metformin.

2. One-Carbon Metabolism: Inputs and Outputs

Folate coenzymes play a crucial role in health and disease and are present in virtually all organisms and cell types. Moreover, although controversial, some dietary arguments support the addition of folic acid or related compounds to common foods [28–30]. In humans, dietary folic acid is reduced to 7,8-dihydrofolate (DHF) and then to 5,6,7,8-tetrahydrofolate (THF) by dihydrofolate reductase (DHFR), initiating the folate cycle. Biochemical reactions converge here, using the ability of THF to carry 1C units in different oxidation states. Folate coenzymes contain poly-γ-glutamate tails attached to a p-aminobenzoic acid moiety by the activity of folylpolyglutamate synthetase (FPGS), an essential enzyme that regulates the distribution of different folate forms in cellular compartments and specific actions in cell proliferation pathways [31,32]. Serine, glycine and methionine are readily provided in the diet. Serine is oxidized in the mitochondria and transferred to THF by serine hydroxyl-methyl-transferase (SHMT), resulting in glycine and 5,10-methylene-THF (CH2-THF). Glycine may be incorporated directly into purine nucleotide bases or glutathione (GSH) and CH2-THF can be converted to 5-methyl-THF in a reaction catalyzed by methylenetetrahydrofolate reductase (MTHFR) or 10-formyl-THF according to cellular needs. Of note, serine and glycine may be synthesized de novo through glycolysis, aldol cleavage (from threonine, in some cells) or reactions involving demethylation (from choline, betaine, dimethylglycine and sarcosine) [31,32].

The folate cycle, closely linked to the methionine cycle, regulates the availability of methyl groups (CH3) through the sequential conversion of methionine to S-adenosylmethionine (SAM), S-adenosylhomocysteine (SAH) and homocysteine. Conversely, in the presence of 5-methyl-THF (5-mTHF) and methionine synthase, which requires vitamin B12 (cobalamin), methionine can be regenerated. Transmethylation reactions and intermediate metabolites are crucial to the synthesis of high-energy molecules, structural macromolecules, thymidine, and purines and to the maintenance of the cellular redox state and the transsulfuration pathway [33,34]. Dietary vitamins also communicate bioenergetics and 1C metabolism. For instance, the conversion of homocysteine to cysteine (transsulfuration pathway) and the synthesis of glutathione require vitamin B6 (pyridoxine) and vitamin B12 is essential (via the mitochondrial enzyme methylmalonyl-CoA mutase) to form succinyl-CoA, a key substrate of the citric acid cycle (Figure 2).

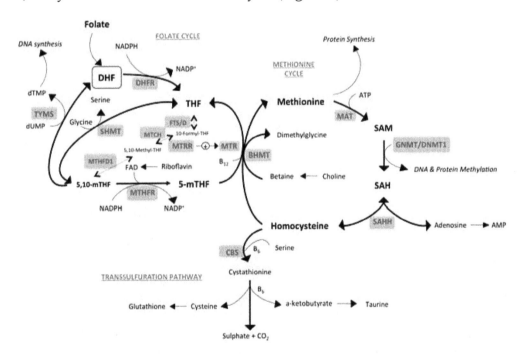

Figure 2. Metabolic pathways indicating the close dietary dependence in the folate cycle, methionine cycle and transsulfuration pathways. The role of B vitamins is paramount in regulating the expected complexities in relevant enzymes and circulating levels of metabolites. BHMT, betaine-homocysteine S-methyltransferase; CBS, cystathionine beta-synthase; DHFR, dihydrofolate reductase; DNMT, DNA methyltransferase; FAD, flavin adenine dinucleotide; GNMT, glycine N-methyltransferase; MAT, aminomethyltransferase; MTHFR, methylenetetrahydrofolate reductase; MTR, methyltransferase; SAH, S-adenosylhomocysteine; SAHH, S-adenosylhomocysteine hydrolase; SAM, S-adenosylmethionine; SHMT, serine hydroxymethyltransferase; THF, tetrahydrofolate; TYMS, thymidylate synthase; UDP, uridine diphosphate.

The cellular functions that depend on these micronutrients illustrate how important careful dietary intake is to avoid deficiencies and how difficult it is to establish clinically based data to be used in both the management of disease states and drug treatments. It may appear paradoxical, but diseases associated with excessive food intake may present deleterious effects that could result from excess in micronutrients [30]. The challenge is to achieve an adequate nutrient balance in the different groups within the general population. In this context, several complexities at the organismal level may be illustrative. For instance, the hepatic effects of diets deficient in choline and methionine are practically indistinguishable from those observed with methionine rich, high-fat, high-energy diets. In contrast, the balanced provision of methionine increases healthy lifespan in experimental models [35–37]. These nutritional observations exemplify the close dependence among regulatory pathways in energy and one-carbon metabolism and the critical importance of the equilibrium between inputs and outputs (Figures 2 and 3).

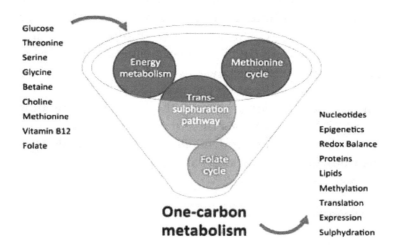

Figure 3. Schematic representation summarizing the importance of appropriate equilibrium in inputs and outputs of one-carbon metabolism. Excessive intake of a given nutrient influences the availability of other nutrients and can perturb metabolism with deleterious consequences. Understanding the events linking metabolism and diet-dependent pathways may provide crucial insight into their role in health and disease.

3. The Lack of Redundancy between Cytoplasmatic and Mitochondrial One-Carbon Metabolism Affects Tissue-Specific Responses to Nutrients

Deficient or excessive intake of nutrients causes changes in the mitochondrial electron transport chain that model the organismal response to the environment. In human cells, the specific forms of folate cofactors and the extent of polyglutamylation differ in cytosolic and mitochondrial pools. Curiously, 1C metabolism is compartmentalized, and mechanisms controlling the flux of components through these compartments are strictly regulated ([38] and references therein). Whether mitochondrial dysfunction is a cause or a consequence of disease remains debatable, but it appears that mitochondria receive monoglutamate THF, which is polyglutamylated, charged with 1C units, and later released to the cytosol [39,40], ensuring the correct function of cellular 1C metabolism.

Energy and one-carbon metabolism jointly integrate the cellular nutrient status. Reactions of glycine and serine are particularly important connecting nutrition, 1C metabolism and the effects of biguanides, as demonstrated in experimental models of glycine auxotrophy. Data in these models indicate that the cytoplasmic serine hydroxymethyltransferase (SHMT) isozyme is not essential, but glycine biosynthesis requires a different mitochondrial isozyme, which is not reversed by external addition of nutrients [41]. Moreover, in the absence of cytoplasmic SHMT, serine donates 1C units and formate flows normally to the cytoplasmic THF pool through the activity of mitochondrial methylene tetrahydrofolate dehydrogenase (MTHFD), a trifunctional folate-dependent enzyme with activity as a CH2-THF dehydrogenase, CH+-THF cyclohydrolase and 10-formyl-THF synthetase. Mice without these mitochondrial isozymes (MTHFD2/MTHFD2L) are not viable [42–44]. In addition, glycine is broken down by the exclusively mitochondrial glycine cleavage system (GCS) and in this reaction direction, the electrons are delivered to complex I of the mitochondrial respiratory chain [45]. Metformin affects mitochondrial biology at this point, but information on compensatory pathways is limited [8,31].

Understanding the transport processes between compartments and how these differences in cytoplasm and mitochondria control metabolic processes might provide a rationale for treating metabolic abnormalities. The strictly mitochondrial GCS activities support a model of multiple carrier-facilitated diffusion of metabolites between cytosol and mitochondria [30]. Because there is no methionine adenosyltransferase (MAT) activity in mitochondria, putative carriers are also necessary for the constant transport of SAM from the cytosol to the mitochondria [46]. The relationship between compartments might also explain the metabolism of choline, which is obtained primarily as phosphatidylcholine in the diet. In the liver, choline is a major source of methyl groups through conversion to betaine (N,N,N-trimethylglycine). The cytosolic betaine hydroxymethyltransferase (BHMT) generates methionine and N,N-dimethylglycine (DMG), but DMG absolutely requires the activity of mitochondrial dehydrogenase (DMGDH) to act as a 1C donor in mitochondria. Similarly, sarcosine (N-methylglycine) can be a 1C donor in the cytoplasm, but in the mitochondria, it requires sarcosine dehydrogenase (SDH) [47].

Collectively, these multiple regulatory steps indicate essential mechanisms for preventing disease. Experiments with genetically engineered mice, examining each step, are of limited value to understand human disease [48], but in humans there are associations between genetic variants and several diseases [49–54]. Similarly, available data suggest that mitochondrial 1C metabolism is critical for metabolic adaptations and cell survival in cancer and T cell-mediated (immune) pathologies [55–57]. T cell activation does not increase the expression of proteins related to glycolysis, pentose phosphate pathway or oxidative phosphorylation. In contrast, T cell activation produces new and specialized mitochondria characterized by the massive induction of enzymes involved in folate-mediated 1C metabolism [55], indicating that the mitochondrial and cytosolic pathways for generating and processing 1C units are not redundant. That is, cytosolic 1C metabolism is insufficient to support T cell proliferation, cancer cell immortality and excessive metabolic impact when mitochondrial 1C metabolism is impaired [31,58–62] (Figure 4).

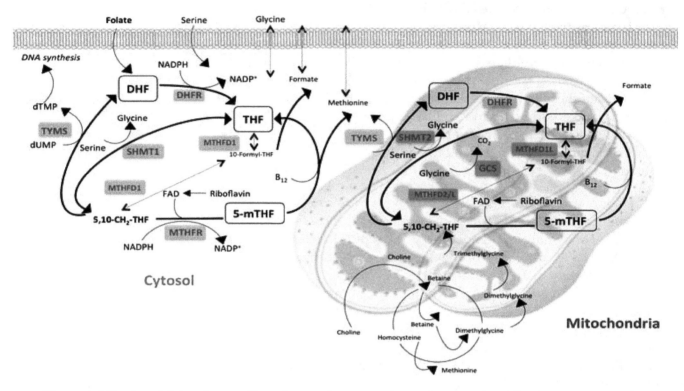

Figure 4. Mitochondrial and cytosolic pathways for generating and processing 1C units are separated but not redundant and depend on extracellular provision. Metabolically active cells may survive deficiencies in cytosolic isozymes but require the correct function of mitochondrial isozymes (marked in red). GCS, glycine cleavage system.

Mechanisms affecting energy and 1C metabolism are likely linked to cellular biosynthesis, redox maintenance and epigenetic status. Accurate information on the activities of the aforementioned enzymes in complex diseases might provide clues regarding how nutritional status or dietary and pharmacologic manipulations affect physiological regulation with evident therapeutic opportunities.

4. The Importance of Drugs and Diets That Modulate Mitochondrial Activity

Mitochondrial function, epigenetic signals and nutrient-sensing pathways are likely combined to promote health at both the cellular and the organismal levels [63,64]. Drugs and dietary regimens that directly modulate mitochondrial activity are promising [65].

Mitochondria are not only providers of energy but also of signaling units, and the existence of mitochondrial-derived peptides (MDPs) suggest the new concept of the existence of mitochondrial hormones and metabolic regulators [66–68]. Similar to metformin [12,69], targets of these MDPs include one-carbon metabolism, thiosulfate sulfurtransferase and AMP-activated protein kinase (AMPK), critical links between nutrients and health. Nutrient sensing is important for the distribution of energy, and changes in food intake alter metabolic strategies [70,71]. Notably, metformin activates AMPK, inducing changes in bioactive metabolites connected to transcriptional regulators through as yet undefined mechanisms [72,73] but probably including an interplay among food intake, metabolism and mTOR signaling in clinically relevant settings [74,75].

In particular, metabolic aspects in cancer are now a renewed source of potential therapeutic targets. Cells depleted of mitochondrial DNA identify metabolic vulnerabilities and illustrate that 1C metabolism, serine biosynthesis and transsulfuration are sensitive to mitochondrial dysfunction and stress [76]. Similarly, cancer cells without the ability to catalyze the conversion of isocitrate to α-ketoglutarate reveal that perturbing mitochondrial metabolism with metformin may help to kill cancer cells [77]. The challenge is to learn how to use cell- and tissue-specific variations in the mitochondrial management of 1C donors and how to interpret the clinical response to manipulations in nutrient availability. Several lines of evidence indicate that crosstalk between epigenetic signals and cellular metabolism may be a clinically useful field of research because it represents a mechanism to convert dietary-induced metabolic changes into stable patterns of altered gene expression [78–81].

5. Is Gene Expression Reprogrammed in Response to Metabolic and Dietary Stimuli Affecting One-Carbon Metabolism?

Whether epigenetic mechanisms are causally coupled to changes in metabolic phenotypes is a question posed by epidemiological studies examining extreme nutritional changes during fetal development [82–85]. It is not surprising, however, to find contradictory data because exposure windows and conditions are not controlled in documented "experiments" on long-term famine [82–84]. These studies do not reveal the contribution of specific nutrients, but studies in other cohorts associate defects in energy and one-carbon metabolism in pregnant women with future risk in offspring ([85] and references therein). Taken together, these data indicate that epigenetic modulation of metabolic pathways may promote adverse phenotypes in later life [86,87].

In the current context of excessive food intake, it is urgent to understand the potential implications of modifying epigenetic marks by nutrition and whether diet-induced changes in metabolic or phenotypic traits may affect future generations. Nutritional, pharmacological and metabolic signals induce epigenetic drift (i.e., metabolic states correlated with chromatin states), and several epigenetic marks influence the expression of neighboring genes through generations. It is apparently the feedback or combination among different epigenetic mechanisms that dynamically configures the chromatin landscape throughout life [88,89] but DNA methylation alone has strong mechanistic support to explain modifications by dietary changes. DNA methylation and certain metabolites generated by mitochondrial respiration interact with transcription factors, suggesting metabolo-epigenetic links between energy and one-carbon metabolism [90–92]. It is plausible that cellular transcriptional machinery and chromatin-associated proteins integrate inputs derived from food as part of the response of living organisms to continuous fluctuations in the availability of energy substrates.

Alterations in genes that encode enzymes affecting chromatin regulation, such as kinases, acetyltransferases, demethylases and methyltransferases, are common in dietary-related diseases [93]. These enzymes use cellular metabolites as sources of phosphate, acetyl or methyl groups, and interpret the metabolic state of a specific cell. For instance, the levels of SAM, a methyl donor, SAH and threonine alter methylation status through pathways involving acetyl-coA metabolism, and specific dietary restrictions cause transcriptional and metabolic responses [94,95]. We recently provided an example of how metformin-driven reduction of acetyl-CoA is sufficient to correct histone H3 acetylation, indicating that metformin regulates mitonuclear communication and the cellular epigenetic landscape. These data may result in knowledge that can be applied to metabolo-epigenetic strategies for prevention or therapy [96]. Future research will ascertain how dietary manipulations and synthetic epigenetic modifiers contribute to DNA methylation and how plastic the genome is to dietary changes. It is also important to establish what magnitude of metabolic stimuli is required to produce appreciable changes and whether epigenetic changes can be reversed.

6. The Ability of Metformin to Target One-Carbon Metabolism: Perspectives in Clinical Practice Outcomes

The dietary inputs associated with the folate and methionine cycles support cellular integrity and health, but there is some risk in manipulating bioactive elements in the absence of well-proven associations between consumption and disease. This probably explains why nutritional manipulation is not incorporated into clinical practice against cancer, but we should not forget that the action of B vitamins led to the discovery of folate antagonists as a major class of cancer chemotherapy agents [97] and that restriction in some nutrients negatively affect tumor formation in mice [98].

The multi-faceted activity of metformin and its likely interconnected mechanisms of action are relevant to potential applications in diseases characterized by mitochondrial dysfunction, gene deregulation and failure in metabolic homeostasis [99–103]. The global metabolic impact of metformin and the generated energetic stress suggest a strong association with the overall management of food intake. Metformin stimulates glucose uptake by muscle, inhibits hepatic gluconeogenesis and stimulates AMPK through effects in NADH ubiquinone oxidoreductase, the first component of the electron transport chain. Other putative actions with dietary associations include AMPK-independent signaling through glucagon-dependent cyclic AMP and the inhibition of mitochondrial glycerophosphate dehydrogenase [103–105]. These findings on metformin action suggest an approach for treating metabolic diseases not restricted to the field of diabetes.

It could be argued that drugs reducing insulin levels may reduce cancer risk, and drugs that increase circulating insulin may increase cancer risk, but the effects of metformin in cancer cells seem specific, preventing the boost in glycolytic intermediates, decreasing citric acid cycle intermediates, and depleting the cellular glutathione content [106]. Moreover, metformin impairs one-carbon metabolism in a manner similar to drugs that target folate-related enzymes and have long been used to treat inflammatory diseases and cancer [8,12,106–109]. Efforts to clinically address this issue remain incomplete and difficult to interpret because heterogeneity in metformin response is considerable and only partially explained by genetic and nutritional factors. Metformin pharmacodynamics and pharmacokinetics have been reviewed recently ([110] and references therein). Current formulations have a bioavailability of ~50% (approximately 40% is absorbed in the duodenum and proximal jejunum, and ~10% in the ileum and colon). Unabsorbed drug is eliminated in the feces, and metformin circulates in the plasma unbound and without transformation until cleared by the kidneys. Metformin is a hydrophilic molecule requiring specific mechanisms of transport, primarily organic cation transporters (OCT). Briefly, plasma membrane monoamine transporter (PMAT) and OCT3 contribute to gastrointestinal uptake, and OCT1 may be responsible for transport into the interstitial fluid of the intestine. OCT1, OCT3 and multidrug and toxin extrusion proteins (MATE) are expressed on the basolateral membrane of hepatocytes. In the kidney, metformin is taken up into renal epithelial cells by OCT2 and excreted into the urine via MATE1 and MATE2. OCT1 and PMAT may contribute to metformin reabsorption. Genetic variants of these and other transporters may be important to explain the therapeutic action of metformin, the high inter-individual variability in gastrointestinal tolerance and drug–drug interactions [111–114]. It would be useful to ascertain whether these genetic variants could have predictive value in patients before they take the drug [115], but genetics alone frequently fail to explain phenotypes. In this context, we foresee that considering metformin for non-diabetic indications is an example of the value of applying metabolomics to useful clinical research. The next task is connecting energy and one-carbon metabolism to physiology, describing heterogeneous phenotypes and defining the role of nutrition in the response to drug treatment.

7. The One-Carbon Cycle in Metformin Users and Potential Adverse Effects

We believe that metformin is best described as an "antimetabolite" drug, and, as such, several deleterious effects might be expected among long-term metformin users. Trials to ascertain these effects are scarce, and data are frequently contradictory, but people at risk of deficiency in one-carbon-related metabolites include vegans, vegetarians, pregnant women, breastfeeding women, the elderly and patients with anemia or poor renal function [116].

There is no evidence of risk in humans from taking metformin during pregnancy, but this issue requires attention [17]. Folate deficiency in metformin users is rare, but a decrease in serum and red blood cell (RBC) folate concentration is common [117]. It is difficult to ascertain the effect of folate fortification in some foods due to discrepancies in results [118] and the lack of data regarding folate bioavailability in metformin users [34,119]. Favoring the consumption of foods that are endogenously high in folates is probably reminiscent of decades using folates with cytotoxic agents, but this empirical practice requires caution. For instance, lessons from a prospective study in rural India indicate that normal/high folate concentrations associated with deficiencies in vitamin B12, attributable to a lacto-vegetarian diet combined with folic acid supplementation, may be associated with a higher risk of insulin resistance in the offspring [120]. This is relevant because metformin might facilitate the mechanism known as "methyl folate trap", which acts on the regulation of the methionine/folate cycle and cysteine oxidation [121]. According to this concept, although only demonstrated in pernicious anemia, the cell would mistakenly interpret vitamin B12 deficiency as a lack of methionine, and will divert the remaining folate away from DNA biosynthesis towards the methylation of homocysteine to methionine, building up 5 methyl THF that the cell will not be able to use [121].

The relationship between vitamin B12 deficiency and metformin treatment has been studied since the beginning of the 1970s with some clinical confusion likely related to the extreme heterogeneity among studies [122–124]. Among metformin users, a slight reduction in serum vitamin B12 concentrations is common, but some studies have reported contradictory results indicating that metformin has no effect or even might improve vitamin B12 metabolism [125–127]. No mechanism has been proposed and the issue requires further research but there is probably no clinical relevance in these observations as discussed below. Moreover, the possible benefits of vitamin B12 supplements in metformin users have not been assayed and the notion of causality is complicated because diabetes and obesity are also associated with vitamin B12 reductions [128].

Metformin does not significantly increase blood lactate levels, but we are probably depriving some patients from potential benefits based on the putative risk of lactic acidosis [129]. After 70 years of real-world clinical experience, the incidence of lactic acidosis is mostly based in anecdotal reports. However, caution is important in individuals with reduced metformin clearance (i.e., poor renal function), reduced lactate clearance (i.e., impaired hepatic metabolism), and/or increased lactate production (i.e., sepsis or reduced tissue perfusion). Advanced age may also increase risk because of age-related decline in renal function and increased risk for acute renal failure (i.e., dehydration), drug–drug interactions and other medical conditions. Moreover, elderly patients with type 2 diabetes are independently at greater risk for hyperlactatemia and have a reduced threshold for the development of lactic acidosis in response to a secondary event [130].

The most frequent adverse effects are gastrointestinal in nature: diarrhea, nausea, and to a lesser extent, vomiting, flatulence or heartburn. Of note, in randomized controlled trials, similar effects are found in the placebo group, indicating potential bias [131]. Those patients without preexisting gastrointestinal conditions are apparently free of these effects, but it is not uncommon that some patients decline using metformin [112,113]. Metformin response and tolerance are intrinsically associated with the gut and the intake of nutrients [132]. Metformin could increase serum glucagon-like peptide 1 concentration by increasing its secretion from L cells, distributed throughout the intestine, and/or by reducing its breakdown by dipeptidyl peptidase-4 in the intestinal mucosa and portal system [133]. Curiously, serotonin and histamine release from the intestine are associated with similar effects (nausea, vomiting, increased gut motility and diarrhea). It is possible that metformin inhibits diamine oxidase, which is highly expressed in enterocytes and responsible for the metabolism of these gut peptides [134]. Metformin might also disrupt the enterohepatic circulation of bile salts, predominantly through reduced ileal absorption and osmotic effects facilitating diarrhea [135]. Finally, the gut microbiome is considered an environmental factor contributing to the development of metabolic diseases and a possible target of metformin. A reduction in butyrate-producing bacteria and an increase in opportunistic pathogens are common in type 2 diabetes and could potentially influence gastrointestinal tolerance [136–138].

8. Measuring the Impact of Folate-Related Deficiencies in the Clinical Setting: Potential for Targeted Metabolomics

Results from immunoassays in clinical laboratories are difficult to interpret and limited by the availability of reagents and automated biochemistry platforms. Methodological constraints, confounding factors, and poor inter-laboratory reproducibility are common pitfalls [139–141].

Consequently, the picture obtained when exploring folate metabolism is partial at best. For instance, total circulating B12 in serum is unreliable in some clinical conditions and practically useless as a method to detect true, functional B12 deficiency [142]. Most (80%) of B12 is bound in serum to haptocorrin, and a variable proportion (5%–20%) is bound to transcobalamin II and ready for tissue uptake (holotranscobalamin). Measuring in the same batch serum holotranscobalamin, homocysteine and/or methylmalonic acid can mitigate limitations [125,143]. Some pitfalls were made evident in a large cohort of participants enrolled in the REasons for Geographic and Racial Differences in Stroke (REGARDS) study [144]. The proportion of participants with low serum B12 concentration was exactly the same (2%; not clinically evident) in participants without diabetes and in long-term metformin users with diabetes. However, serum B12 concentrations were lower in metformin users than in those who did not use metformin. Curiously, metformin users were less likely to have taken multivitamins (6–25 μg of vitamin B12 per dose), and multivitamin users had a significantly higher serum B12 concentration compared to those who did not take multivitamins [144]. A longitudinal study to assess the impact of metformin is warranted, but it appears that laboratory biomarkers do not add significantly to clinical decisions and that dietary advice might contribute to better management of metformin users [145].

Similarly, measurement of serum folate with standard immunoassays is accompanied by possible errors in interpretation. For instance, obesity appears to be associated with decreased serum (measuring recent folate intake) but also with increased RBC folate (measuring a long term intake) concentrations compared with lean subjects. The association is plausible but the presence of obesity-associated metabolic disturbances hampers further interpretations [146]. It was recently clarified that folate measurements in serum and in RBC display similar performance in assessing folate status [147]. The use of both measures generates higher and unnecessary costs, but the RBC folate assay is less likely to provide falsely normal levels attributable to dietary behavior or recent supplements [147]. The observation that metformin is associated with a slight, but sometimes significant, raise in homocysteine and/or decrease in folate needs careful consideration, but there is no sufficient evidence to recommend folic acid supplements to metformin users [148,149].

It remains unknown how nutritional manipulations may affect the complex relationships among metabolites involved in the 1C cycle, but studies in women with seasonal variations in nutrient intake highlight the need to measure all metabolites and cofactors [150,151]. Analytical platforms should provide measurements of different folate species, especially 5-methyltetrahydrofolate as the active 1C donor [150,151]. Specifically, it is important to confirm data suggesting that levels of maternal one-carbon metabolites at conception influence DNA methylation in the early embryo and that offspring methylation correlates with the paternal somatic methylation pattern [152]. This effort implies better tools for measuring intermediate metabolites either side of the involved reactions [153,154]. Targeted metabolomics may help in pursuing a better interpretation. In this context, ultra-high pressure liquid chromatography coupled to an electrospray ionization source and a triple-quadrupole mass spectrometer is an affordable choice to quantitatively examine the methionine/folate bi-cyclic 1C metabolome [155]. This method has been used to explore the activation of methylogenesis in some models. This essential function of 1C metabolism provides a labile pool of methyl groups required for successfully establishing and maintaining the DNA methylation imprint [155]. A similar approach has been used to explore energy metabolism with a simple and rapid method based on gas chromatography coupled to quadrupole time-of-flight mass spectrometry and an electron impact source [156]. The accurate and simultaneous measurement of selected metabolites facilitates the understanding of metabolic responses to changing environmental factors and has the potential for searching quantitative biomarkers of disease and signals indicating the ability of drugs to restore cellular homeostasis [157]. In addition, this analytical approach may serve to assess the expected toxicity in potential applications for metformin employed in oncology at doses notably higher than those used chronically in the management of diabetes [8].

9. Conclusions

Metformin users may provide data on the effect of nutrients in health and disease. There is growing evidence demonstrating the multiple protective effects of metformin against obesity-associated diseases, a major challenge to global public health. Some findings support the idea that metformin mediates the mitochondrial response to excessive food intake and the effect of different micronutrients. In particular, the mechanism of action of metformin involves effects on both energy and one-carbon metabolism and suggests novel strategies that involve the combination of lifestyle modification with pharmacotherapy. The concept is more important in individuals whose risk factors are not reduced by dietary interventions and dietary regimens in metformin users may provide valuable information. We envision that several analytical approaches in the field of metabolomics can provide diagnostic indicators on multiple metabolic aspects and may ascertain the effects of nutrient intake. Accordingly, it is especially relevant to assess the role of significant nutrients, such as serine, glycine, methionine, folic acid or other B vitamins, affecting one-carbon metabolism. Efforts to repurpose metformin, the first choice as an oral treatment of type 2 diabetes, as an antimetabolite drug, reinforce the interest in understanding food and drug interactions and the expected toxic effects caused by a change in dose range.

Acknowledgments: We apologize to the many researchers whose valuable contributions we were unable to cite or discuss. Current work in our laboratories is supported by grants from the Plan Nacional de I+D+I, Spain, Instituto de Salud Carlos III (Grant PI15/00285 co-founded by the European Regional Development Fund (FEDER)) to J.J., and the Ministerio de Ciencia e Innovación (Grant SAF2016-80639) to J.M. We also acknowledge the support by the Agència de Gestió d'Ajuts Universitaris i de Recerca (AGAUR) (Grants 2014 SGR1227 and 2014 SGR229), and the Fundació La Marató de TV3. The American Journal Experts provided assistance in English editing.

Author Contributions: J.J., J.A.M. and J.L.-M. designed the concept. F.L.-M., A.H.-A. and N.C. conducted the search and retrieved articles from the literature. J.J. and J.A.M. wrote the manuscript and supervised review development. J.C., J.L.-M. and S.F.-A. wrote key sections. All authors critically reviewed the manuscript and approved the final version.

References

1. Mirzaei, H.; Di Biase, S.; Longo, V.D. Dietary Interventions, Cardiovascular Aging, and Disease: Animal Models and Human Studies. *Circ. Res.* **2016**, *118*, 1612–1625. [CrossRef] [PubMed]
2. Hall, K.D.; Bemis, T.; Brychta, R.; Chen, K.Y.; Courville, A.; Crayner, E.J.; Goodwin, S.; Guo, J.; Howard, L.; Knuth, N.D.; et al. Calorie for Calorie, Dietary Fat Restriction Results in More Body Fat Loss than Carbohydrate Restriction in People with Obesity. *Cell Metab.* **2015**, *22*, 427–436. [CrossRef]
3. Kim, W.; Woo, H.D.; Lee, J.; Choi, I.J.; Kim, Y.W.; Sung, J.; Kim, J. Dietary folate, one-carbon metabolism-related genes, and gastric cancer risk in Korea. *Mol. Nutr. Food Res.* **2016**, *60*, 337–345. [CrossRef] [PubMed]
4. Martínez-Reyes, I.; Chandel, N.S. Mitochondrial one-carbon metabolism maintains redox balance during hypoxia. *Cancer Discov.* **2014**, *4*, 1371–1373. [CrossRef] [PubMed]
5. Duncan, T.M.; Reed, M.C.; Nijhout, H.F. A population model of folate-mediated one-carbon metabolism. *Nutrients* **2013**, *5*, 2457–2474. [CrossRef] [PubMed]
6. Bailey, L.B.; Stover, P.J.; McNulty, H.; Fenech, M.F.; Gregory, J.F.; Mills, J.L.; Pfeiffer, C.M.; Fazili, Z.; Zhang, M.; Ueland, P.M.; et al. Biomarkers of Nutrition for Development. *J. Nutr.* **2015**, *145*, 1636S–1680S. [CrossRef] [PubMed]
7. López-Otín, C.; Galluzzi, L.; Freije, J.M.; Madeo, F.; Kroemer, G. Metabolic Control of Longevity. *Cell* **2016**, *166*, 802–821. [CrossRef] [PubMed]
8. Menendez, J.A.; Quirantes-Piné, R.; Rodríguez-Gallego, E.; Cufí, S.; Corominas-Faja, B.; Cuyàs, E.; Bosch-Barrera, J.; Martin-Castillo, B.; Segura-Carretero, A.; Joven, J. Oncobiguanides: Paracelsus' law and nonconventional routes for administering diabetobiguanides for cancer treatment. *Oncotarget* **2014**, *5*, 2344–2348. [CrossRef] [PubMed]
9. Pollak, M. Potential applications for biguanides in oncology. *J. Clin. Investig.* **2013**, *123*, 3693–3700. [CrossRef]

10. Coperchini, F.; Leporati, P.; Rotondi, M.; Chiovato, L. Expanding the therapeutic spectrum of metformin: From diabetes to cancer. *J. Endocrinol. Investig.* **2015**, *38*, 1047–1055. [CrossRef] [PubMed]

11. Pryor, R.; Cabreiro, F. Repurposing metformin: An old drug with new tricks in its binding pockets. *Biochem. J.* **2015**, *471*, 307–322. [CrossRef] [PubMed]

12. Corominas-Faja, B.; Quirantes-Pine, R.; Oliveras-Ferraros, C.; Vazquez-Martin, A.; Cufi, S.; Martin-Castillo, B.; Micol, V.; Joven, J.; Segura-Carretero, A.; Menendez, J.A. Metabolomic fingerprint reveals that metformin impairs one-carbon metabolism in a manner similar to the antifolate class of chemotherapy drugs. *Aging* **2012**, *4*, 480–498. [CrossRef] [PubMed]

13. Novelle, M.G.; Ali, A.; Diéguez, C.; Bernier, M.; de Cabo, R. Metformin: A Hopeful Promise in Aging Research. *Cold Spring Harb. Perspect. Med.* **2016**, *6*, a025932. [CrossRef] [PubMed]

14. Carmona, J.J.; Michan, S. Biology of Healthy Aging and Longevity. *Rev. Investig. Clin.* **2016**, *68*, 7–16.

15. Cabreiro, F.; Au, C.; Leung, K.Y.; Vergara-Irigaray, N.; Cochemé, H.M.; Noori, T.; Weinkove, D.; Schuster, E.; Greene, N.D.; Gems, D. Metformin retards aging in *C. elegans* by altering microbial folate and methionine metabolism. *Cell* **2013**, *153*, 228–239. [CrossRef] [PubMed]

16. Domecq, J.P.; Prutsky, G.; Leppin, A.; Sonbol, M.B.; Altayar, O.; Undavalli, C.; Wang, Z.; Elraiyah, T.; Brito, J.P.; Mauck, K.F.; et al. Clinical review: Drugs commonly associated with weight change: A systematic review and meta-analysis. *J. Clin. Endocrinol. Metab.* **2015**, *100*, 363–370. [CrossRef] [PubMed]

17. Syngelaki, A.; Nicolaides, K.H.; Balani, J.; Hyer, S.; Akolekar, R.; Kotecha, R.; Pastides, A.; Shehata, H. Metformin versus Placebo in Obese Pregnant Women without Diabetes Mellitus. *N. Engl. J. Med.* **2016**, *374*, 434–443. [CrossRef] [PubMed]

18. Cassina, M.; Donà, M.; Di Gianantonio, E.; Litta, P.; Clementi, M. First-trimester exposure to metformin and risk of birth defects: A systematic review and meta-analysis. *Hum. Reprod. Update* **2014**, *20*, 656–669. [CrossRef] [PubMed]

19. Legro, R.S.; Arslanian, S.A.; Ehrmann, D.A.; Hoeger, K.M.; Murad, M.H.; Pasquali, R.; Welt, C.K. Diagnosis and treatment of polycystic ovary syndrome: An Endocrine Society clinical practice guideline. *J. Clin. Endocrinol. Metab.* **2013**, *98*, 4565–4592. [CrossRef] [PubMed]

20. Knowler, W.C.; Fowler, S.E.; Hamman, R.F.; Christophi, C.A.; Hoffman, H.J.; Brenneman, A.T.; Brenneman, A.T.; Brown-Friday, J.O.; Goldberg, R.; Venditti, E.; et al. 10-year follow-up of diabetes incidence and weight loss in the Diabetes Prevention Program Outcomes Study. *Lancet* **2009**, *374*, 1677–1686. [PubMed]

21. Hostalek, U.; Gwilt, M.; Hildemann, S. Therapeutic Use of Metformin in Prediabetes and Diabetes Prevention. *Drugs* **2015**, *75*, 1071–1094. [CrossRef] [PubMed]

22. Igel, L.I.; Sinha, A.; Saunders, K.H.; Apovian, C.M.; Vojta, D.; Aronne, L.J. Metformin: An Old Therapy that Deserves a New Indication for the Treatment of Obesity. *Curr. Atheroscler. Rep.* **2016**, *18*, 16. [CrossRef] [PubMed]

23. Lamanna, C.; Monami, M.; Marchionni, N.; Mannucci, E. Effect of metformin on cardiovascular events and mortality: A meta-analysis of randomized clinical trials. *Diabetes Obes. Metab.* **2011**, *13*, 221–228. [CrossRef] [PubMed]

24. DeFronzo, R.A.; Goodman, A.M. Efficacy of metformin in patients with non-insulin-dependent diabetes mellitus. The Multicenter Metformin Study Group. *N. Engl. J. Med.* **1995**, *333*, 541–549. [CrossRef] [PubMed]

25. Cameron, A.R.; Morrison, V.L.; Levin, D.; Mohan, M.; Forteath, C.; Beall, C.; McNeilly, A.D.; Balfour, D.J.; Savinko, T.; Wong, A.K.; et al. Anti-Inflammatory Effects of Metformin Irrespective of Diabetes Status. *Circ. Res.* **2016**, *119*, 652–665. [CrossRef] [PubMed]

26. Goodwin, P.J. Obesity and Breast Cancer Outcomes: How Much Evidence Is Needed to Change Practice? *J. Clin. Oncol.* **2016**, *34*, 646–648. [CrossRef] [PubMed]

27. Barzilai, N.; Crandall, J.P.; Kritchevsky, S.B.; Espeland, M.A. Metformin as a Tool to Target Aging. *Cell Metab.* **2016**, *23*, 1060–1065. [CrossRef] [PubMed]

28. Allen, L.H. Current Information Gaps in Micronutrient Research, Programs and Policy: How Can We Fill Them? *World Rev. Nutr. Diet* **2016**, *115*, 109–117. [PubMed]

29. Bruins, M.J.; Kupka, R.; Zimmermann, M.B.; Lietz, G.; Engle-Stone, R.; Kraemer, K. Maximizing the benefits and minimizing the risks of intervention programs to address micronutrient malnutrition: Symposium report. *Matern. Child Nutr.* **2016**, *12*, 940–948. [CrossRef] [PubMed]

30. Patel, K.R.; Sobczyńska-Malefora, A. The adverse effects of an excessive folic acid intake. *Eur. J. Clin. Nutr.* **2016**. [CrossRef] [PubMed]

31. Locasale, J.W. Serine, glycine and one-carbon units: Cancer metabolism in full circle. *Nat. Rev. Cancer* **2013**, *13*, 572–583. [CrossRef] [PubMed]

32. Mattaini, K.R.; Sullivan, M.R.; Vander Heiden, M.G. The importance of serine metabolism in cancer. *J. Cell Biol.* **2016**, *214*, 249–257. [CrossRef] [PubMed]

33. Kopp, M.; Morisset, R.; Koehler, P.; Rychlik, M. Stable Isotope Dilution Assays for Clinical Analyses of Folates and Other One-Carbon Metabolites: Application to Folate-Deficiency Studies. *PLoS ONE* **2016**, *11*, E0156610. [CrossRef] [PubMed]

34. Mönch, S.; Netzel, M.; Netzel, G.; Ott, U.; Frank, T.; Rychlik, M. Folate bioavailability from foods rich in folates assessed in a short term human study using stable isotope dilution assays. *Food Funct.* **2015**, *6*, 242–248. [CrossRef] [PubMed]

35. Mato, J.M.; Martinez-Chantar, M.L.; Lu, S.C. Methionine metabolism and liver disease. *Annu. Rev. Nutr.* **2008**, *28*, 273–293. [CrossRef] [PubMed]

36. Pacana, T.; Cazanave, S.; Verdianelli, A.; Patel, V.; Min, H.K.; Mirshahi, F.; Quinlivan, E.; Sanyal, A.J. Dysregulated Hepatic Methionine Metabolism Drives Homocysteine Elevation in Diet-Induced Nonalcoholic Fatty Liver Disease. *PLoS ONE* **2015**, *10*, E0136822. [CrossRef] [PubMed]

37. Lee, B.C.; Kaya, A.; Gladyshev, V.N. Methionine restriction and life-span control. *Ann. N. Y. Acad. Sci.* **2016**, *1363*, 116–124. [CrossRef] [PubMed]

38. Tibbetts, A.S.; Appling, D.R. Compartmentalization of Mammalian folate-mediated one-carbon metabolism. *Annu. Rev. Nutr.* **2010**, *30*, 57–81. [CrossRef] [PubMed]

39. Lin, B.F.; Huang, R.F.; Shane, B. Regulation of folate and one-carbon metabolism in mammalian cells. III. Role of mitochondrial folylpoly-gamma-glutamate synthetase. *J. Biol. Chem.* **1993**, *268*, 21674–21679. [PubMed]

40. Lawrence, S.A.; Titus, S.A.; Ferguson, J.; Heineman, A.L.; Taylor, S.M.; Moran, R.G. Mammalian mitochondrial and cytosolic folylpolyglutamate synthetase maintain the subcellular compartmentalization of folates. *J. Biol. Chem.* **2014**, *289*, 29386–29396. [CrossRef] [PubMed]

41. McCarthy, E.A.; Titus, S.A.; Taylor, S.M.; Jackson-Cook, C.; Moran, R.G. A mutation inactivating the mitochondrial inner membrane folate transporter creates a glycine requirement for survival of Chinese hamster cells. *J. Biol. Chem.* **2004**, *279*, 33829–33836. [CrossRef] [PubMed]

42. Christensen, K.E.; Patel, H.; Kuzmanov, U.; Mejia, N.R.; MacKenzie, R.E. Disruption of the mthfd1 gene reveals a monofunctional 10-formyltetrahydrofolate synthetase in mammalian mitochondria. *J. Biol. Chem.* **2005**, *280*, 7597–7602. [CrossRef] [PubMed]

43. Field, M.S.; Kamynina, E.; Stover, P.J. MTHFD1 regulates nuclear de novo thymidylate biosynthesis and genome stability. *Biochimie* **2016**, *126*, 27–30. [CrossRef] [PubMed]

44. Giardina, G.; Brunotti, P.; Fiascarelli, A.; Cicalini, A.; Costa, M.G.; Buckle, A.M.; di Salvo, M.L.; Giorgi, A.; Marani, M.; Paone, A.; et al. How pyridoxal 5′-phosphate differentially regulates human cytosolic and mitochondrial serine hydroxymethyltransferase oligomeric state. *FEBS J.* **2015**, *282*, 1225–1241. [CrossRef] [PubMed]

45. Hampson, R.K.; Barron, L.L.; Olson, M.S. Regulation of the glycine cleavage system in isolated rat liver mitochondria. *J. Biol. Chem.* **1983**, *258*, 2993–2999. [PubMed]

46. Horne, D.W.; Holloway, R.S.; Wagner, C. Transport of S-adenosylmethionine in isolated rat liver mitochondria. *Arch. Biochem. Biophys.* **1997**, *343*, 201–206. [CrossRef] [PubMed]

47. O'Donoghue, N.; Sweeney, T.; Donagh, R.; Clarke, K.J.; Porter, R.K. Control of choline oxidation in rat kidney mitochondria. *Biochim. Biophys. Acta* **2009**, *1787*, 1135–1139. [CrossRef] [PubMed]

48. Peng, L.; Dreumont, N.; Coelho, D.; Guéant, J.L.; Arnold, C. Genetic animal models to decipher the pathogenic effects of vitamin B12 and folate deficiency. *Biochimie* **2016**, *126*, 43–51. [CrossRef] [PubMed]

49. Cheng, T.Y.; Makar, K.W.; Neuhouser, M.L.; Miller, J.W.; Song, X.; Brown, E.C.; Beresford, S.A.; Zheng, Y.; Poole, E.M.; Galbraith, R.L.; et al. Folate-mediated one-carbon metabolism genes and interactions with nutritional factors on colorectal cancer risk: Women's Health Initiative Observational Study. *Cancer* **2015**, *121*, 3684–3691. [CrossRef] [PubMed]

50. Pangilinan, F.; Molloy, A.M.; Mills, J.L.; Troendle, J.F.; Parle-McDermott, A.; Kay, D.M.; Browne, M.L.; McGrath, E.C.; Abaan, H.O.; Sutton, M.; et al. Replication and exploratory analysis of 24 candidate risk polymorphisms for neural tube defects. *BMC Med. Genet.* **2014**, *15*, 102. [CrossRef] [PubMed]

51. Krishna, S.M.; Dear, A.; Craig, J.M.; Norman, P.E.; Golledge, J. The potential role of homocysteine mediated DNA methylation and associated epigenetic changes in abdominal aortic aneurysm formation. *Atherosclerosis* **2013**, *228*, 295–305. [CrossRef] [PubMed]

52. De Vilbiss, E.A.; Gardner, R.M.; Newschaffer, C.J.; Lee, B.K. Maternal folate status as a risk factor for autism spectrum disorders: A review of existing evidence. *Br. J. Nutr.* **2015**, *114*, 663–672. [CrossRef] [PubMed]

53. Martorell, L.; Segués, T.; Folch, G.; Valero, J.; Joven, J.; Labad, A.; Vilella, E. New variants in the mitochondrial genomes of schizophrenic patients. *Eur. J. Hum. Genet.* **2006**, *14*, 520–528. [CrossRef] [PubMed]

54. Vilella, E.; Virgos, C.; Murphy, M.; Martorell, L.; Valero, J.; Simó, J.M.; Joven, J.; Fernández-Ballart, J.; Labad, A. Further evidence that hyperhomocysteinemia and methylenetetrahydrofolate reductase C677T and A1289C polymorphisms are not risk factors for schizophrenia. *Prog. Neuropsychopharmacol. Biol. Psychiatry* **2005**, *29*, 1169–1174. [CrossRef] [PubMed]

55. Ron-Harel, N.; Santos, D.; Ghergurovich, J.M.; Sage, P.T.; Reddy, A.; Lovitch, S.B.; Dephoure, N.; Satterstrom, F.K.; Sheffer, M.; Spinelli, J.B.; et al. Mitochondrial Biogenesis and Proteome Remodeling Promote One-Carbon Metabolism for T Cell Activation. *Cell Metab.* **2016**, *24*, 104–117. [CrossRef] [PubMed]

56. DeBerardinis, R.J.; Lum, J.J.; Hatzivassiliou, G.; Thompson, C.B. The biology of cancer: Metabolic reprogramming fuels cell growth and proliferation. *Cell Metab.* **2008**, *7*, 11–20. [CrossRef] [PubMed]

57. Sullivan, L.B.; Gui, D.Y.; Hosios, A.M.; Bush, L.N.; Freinkman, E.; Vander Heiden, M.G. Supporting aspartate biosynthesis is an essential function of respiration in proliferating cells. *Cell* **2015**, *162*, 552–563. [CrossRef] [PubMed]

58. Fan, J.; Ye, J.; Kamphorst, J.J.; Shlomi, T.; Thompson, C.B.; Rabinowitz, J.D. Quantitative flux analysis reveals folate-dependent NADPH production. *Nature* **2014**, *510*, 298–302. [CrossRef] [PubMed]

59. Ye, J.; Fan, J.; Venneti, S.; Wan, Y.W.; Pawel, B.R.; Zhang, J.; Finley, L.W.; Lu, C.; Lindsten, T.; Cross, J.R. Serine catabolism regulates mitochondrial redox control during hypoxia. *Cancer Discov.* **2014**, *4*, 1406–1417. [CrossRef] [PubMed]

60. Piskounova, E.; Agathocleous, M.; Murphy, M.M.; Hu, Z.; Huddlestun, S.E.; Zhao, Z.; Leitch, A.M.; Johnson, T.M.; DeBerardinis, R.J.; Morrison, S.J. Oxidative stress inhibits distant metastasis by human melanoma cells. *Nature* **2015**, *527*, 186–191. [CrossRef] [PubMed]

61. Jain, M.; Nilsson, R.; Sharma, S.; Madhusudhan, N.; Kitami, T.; Souza, A.L.; Kafri, R.; Kirschner, M.W.; Clish, C.B.; Mootha, V.K. Metabolite profiling identifies a key role for glycine in rapid cancer cell proliferation. *Science* **2012**, *336*, 1040–1044. [CrossRef] [PubMed]

62. Maddocks, O.D.; Berkers, C.R.; Mason, S.M.; Zheng, L.; Blyth, K.; Gottlieb, E.; Vousden, K.H. Serine starvation induces stress and p53-dependent metabolic remodelling in cancer cells. *Nature* **2013**, *493*, 542–546. [CrossRef] [PubMed]

63. Finkel, T. The metabolic regulation of aging. *Nat. Med.* **2015**, *21*, 1416–1423. [CrossRef] [PubMed]

64. Sena, L.A.; Chandel, N.S. Physiological roles of mitochondrial reactive oxygen species. *Mol. Cell* **2012**, *48*, 158–167. [CrossRef] [PubMed]

65. Suliman, H.B.; Piantadosi, C.A. Mitochondrial Quality Control as a Therapeutic Target. *Pharmacol. Rev.* **2016**, *68*, 20–48. [CrossRef] [PubMed]

66. Guo, B.; Zhai, D.; Cabezas, E.; Welsh, K.; Nouraini, S.; Satterthwait, A.C.; Reed, J.C. Humanin peptide suppresses apoptosis by interfering with Bax activation. *Nature* **2003**, *423*, 456–461. [CrossRef] [PubMed]

67. Lee, C.; Zeng, J.; Drew, B.G.; Sallam, T.; Martin-Montalvo, A.; Wan, J.; Kim, S.J.; Mehta, H.; Hevener, A.L.; de Cabo, R.; et al. The mitochondrial-derived peptide MOTS-c promotes metabolic homeostasis and reduces obesity and insulin resistance. *Cell Metab.* **2015**, *21*, 443–454. [CrossRef] [PubMed]

68. Quirós, P.M.; Mottis, A.; Auwerx, J. Mitonuclear communication in homeostasis and stress. *Nat. Rev. Mol. Cell Biol.* **2016**, *17*, 213–226. [CrossRef] [PubMed]

69. Morton, N.M.; Beltram, J.; Carter, R.N.; Michailidou, Z.; Gorjanc, G.; McFadden, C.; Barrios-Llerena, M.E.; Rodriguez-Cuenca, S.; Gibbins, M.T.; Aird, R.E.; et al. Genetic identification of thiosulfate sulfurtransferase as an adipocyte-expressed antidiabetic target in mice selected for leanness. *Nat. Med.* **2016**, *22*, 771–779. [CrossRef] [PubMed]

70. Fitzgibbons, T.P.; Czech, M.P. Emerging evidence for beneficial macrophage functions in atherosclerosis and obesity-induced insulin resistance. *J. Mol. Med.* **2016**, *94*, 267–275. [CrossRef] [PubMed]

71. Hardie, D.G.; Schaffer, B.E.; Brunet, A. AMPK: An Energy-Sensing Pathway with Multiple Inputs and Outputs. *Trends Cell Biol.* **2016**, *26*, 190–201. [CrossRef] [PubMed]

72. Beltrán-Debón, R.; Rodríguez-Gallego, E.; Fernández-Arroyo, S.; Senan-Campos, O.; Massucci, F.A.; Hernández-Aguilera, A.; Sales-Pardo, M.; Guimerà, R.; Camps, J.; Menendez, J.A.; et al. The acute impact of polyphenols from Hibiscus sabdariffa in metabolic homeostasis: An approach combining metabolomics and gene-expression analyses. *Food Funct.* **2015**, *6*, 2957–2966. [CrossRef] [PubMed]

73. Liu, C.; Wu, J.; Zhu, J.; Kuei, C.; Yu, J.; Shelton, J.; Sutton, S.W.; Li, X.; Yun, S.J.; Mirzadegan, T.; et al. Lactate inhibits lipolysis in fat cells through activation of an orphan G-protein-coupled receptor, GPR81. *J. Biol. Chem.* **2009**, *284*, 2811–2822. [CrossRef] [PubMed]

74. Haas, R.; Cucchi, D.; Smith, J.; Pucino, V.; Macdougall, C.E.; Mauro, C. Intermediates of Metabolism: From Bystanders to Signalling Molecules. *Trends Biochem. Sci.* **2016**, *41*, 460–471. [CrossRef] [PubMed]

75. Jha, A.K.; Huang, S.C.; Sergushichev, A.; Lampropoulou, V.; Ivanova, Y.; Loginicheva, E.; Chmielewski, K.; Stewart, K.M.; Ashall, J.; Everts, B.; et al. Network integration of parallel metabolic and transcriptional data reveals metabolic modules that regulate macrophage polarization. *Immunity* **2015**, *42*, 419–430. [CrossRef] [PubMed]

76. Bao, X.R.; Ong, S.E.; Goldberger, O.; Peng, J.; Sharma, R.; Thompson, D.A.; Vafai, S.B.; Cox, A.G.; Marutani, E.; Ichinose, F.; et al. Mitochondrial dysfunction remodels one-carbon metabolism in human cells. *eLife* **2016**, *5*, E10575. [CrossRef] [PubMed]

77. Cuyàs, E.; Fernández-Arroyo, S.; Corominas-Faja, B.; Rodríguez-Gallego, E.; Bosch-Barrera, J.; Martin-Castillo, B.; de Llorens, R.; Joven, J.; Menendez, J.A. Oncometabolic mutation IDH1 R132H confers a metformin-hypersensitive phenotype. *Oncotarget* **2015**, *6*, 12279–12296. [CrossRef] [PubMed]

78. Katada, S.; Imhof, A.; Sassone-Corsi, P. Connecting threads: Epigenetics and metabolism. *Cell* **2012**, *148*, 24–28. [CrossRef] [PubMed]

79. Huypens, P.; Sass, S.; Wu, M.; Dyckhoff, D.; Tschöp, M.; Theis, F.; Marschall, S.; Hrabe de Angelis, M.; Beckers, J. Epigenetic germline inheritance of diet-induced obesity and insulin resistance. *Nat. Genet.* **2016**, *48*, 497–499. [CrossRef] [PubMed]

80. Öst, A.; Lempradl, A.; Casas, E.; Weigert, M.; Tiko, T.; Deniz, M.; Pantano, L.; Boenisch, U.; Itskow, P.M.; Stoeckius, M.; et al. Paternal diet defines offspring chromatin state and intergenerational obesity. *Cell* **2014**, *159*, 1352–1364. [CrossRef] [PubMed]

81. Foster, G.D.; Wyatt, H.R.; Hill, J.O.; Makris, A.P.; Rosenbaum, D.L.; Brill, C.; Stein, R.I.; Mohammed, B.S.; Miller, B.; Rader, D.J.; et al. Weight and metabolic outcomes after 2 years on a low-carbohydrate versus low-fat diet: A randomized trial. *Ann. Intern. Med.* **2010**, *153*, 147–157. [CrossRef] [PubMed]

82. Painter, R.C.; Roseboom, T.J.; Bleker, O.P. Prenatal exposure to the Dutch famine and disease in later life: An overview. *Reprod. Toxicol.* **2005**, *20*, 345–352. [CrossRef] [PubMed]

83. Li, Y.; He, Y.; Qi, L.; Jaddoe, V.W.; Feskens, E.J.; Yang, X.; Ma, G.; Hu, F.N. Exposure to the Chinese famine in early life and the risk of hyperglycemia and type 2 diabetes in adulthood. *Diabetes* **2010**, *59*, 2400–2406. [CrossRef] [PubMed]

84. Stanner, S.A.; Bulmer, K.; Andrès, C.; Lantseva, O.E.; Borodina, V.; Poteen, V.V.; Yudkin, J.S. Does malnutrition in utero determine diabetes and coronary heart disease in adulthood? Results from the Leningrad siege study, a cross sectional study. *BMJ* **1997**, *315*, 1342–1348. [CrossRef] [PubMed]

85. Finer, S.; Saravanan, P.; Hitman, G.; Yajnik, C. The role of the one-carbon cycle in the developmental origins of Type 2 diabetes and obesity. *Diabet. Med.* **2014**, *31*, 263–272. [CrossRef] [PubMed]

86. Tobi, E.W.; Goeman, J.J.; Monajemi, R.; Gu, H.; Putter, H.; Zhang, Y.; Slieker, R.C.; Stok, A.P.; Thijssen, P.E.; Müller, F.; et al. DNA methylation signatures link prenatal famine exposure to growth and metabolism. *Nat. Commun.* **2014**, *5*, 5592. [CrossRef] [PubMed]

87. Hernández-Aguilera, A.; Fernández-Arroyo, S.; Cuyàs, E.; Luciano-Mateo, F.; Cabre, N.; Camps, J.; Lopez-Miranda, J.; Menendez, J.A.; Joven, J. Epigenetics and nutrition-related epidemics of metabolic diseases: Current perspectives and challenges. *Food. Chem. Toxicol.* **2016**, *96*, 191–204. [CrossRef] [PubMed]

88. Klosin, A.; Lehner, B. Mechanisms, timescales and principles of trans-generational epigenetic inheritance in animals. *Curr. Opin. Genet. Dev.* **2016**, *36*, 41–49. [CrossRef] [PubMed]

89. Fontana, L.; Partridge, L. Promoting health and longevity through diet: From model organisms to humans. *Cell* **2015**, *161*, 106–118. [CrossRef] [PubMed]

90. Martinez-Outschoorn, U.E.; Peiris-Pagés, M.; Pestell, R.G.; Sotgia, F.; Lisanti, M.P. Cancer metabolism: A therapeutic perspective. *Nat. Rev. Clin. Oncol.* **2016**. [CrossRef] [PubMed]

91. Maddocks, O.D.; Labuschagne, C.F.; Adams, P.D.; Vousden, K.H. Serine metabolism supports the methionine cycle and DNA/RNA methylation through de novo ATP Synthesis in Cancer Cells. *Mol. Cell* **2016**, *61*, 210–221. [CrossRef] [PubMed]

92. Mentch, S.J.; Locasale, J.W. One-carbon metabolism and epigenetics: Understanding the specificity. *Ann. N. Y. Acad. Sci.* **2016**, *1363*, 91–98. [CrossRef] [PubMed]

93. Dawson, M.A.; Kouzarides, T. Cancer epigenetics: From mechanism to therapy. *Cell* **2012**, *150*, 12–27. [CrossRef] [PubMed]

94. Fang, D.; Gan, H.; Lee, J.H.; Han, J.; Wang, Z.; Riester, S.M.; Jin, L.; Chen, J.; Zhou, H.; Wang, J.; et al. The histone H3.3K36M mutation reprograms the epigenome of chondroblastomas. *Science* **2016**, *352*, 1344–1348. [CrossRef] [PubMed]

95. Orgeron, M.L.; Stone, K.P.; Wanders, D.; Cortez, C.C.; Van, N.T.; Gettys, T.W. The impact of dietary methionine restriction on biomarkers of metabolic health. *Prog. Mol. Biol. Transl. Sci.* **2014**, *121*, 351–376. [PubMed]

96. Cuyàs, E.; Fernández-Arroyo, S.; Joven, J.; Menendez, J.A. Metformin targets histone acetylation in cancer-prone epithelial cells. *Cell Cycle* **2016**, *15*, 3413–3416. [CrossRef] [PubMed]

97. Farber, S.; Diamond, L.K. Temporary remissions in acute leukemia in children produced by folic acid antagonist, 4-aminopteroyl-glutamic acid. *N. Engl. J. Med.* **1948**, *238*, 787–793. [CrossRef] [PubMed]

98. Tannenbaum, A. The dependence of tumor formation on the composition of the calorie- restricted diet as well as on the degree of restriction. *Cancer Res.* **1945**, *5*, 616–625.

99. Heckman-Stoddard, B.M.; Gandini, S.; Puntoni, M.; Dunn, B.K.; De Censi, A.; Szabo, E. Repurposing old drugs to chemoprevention: The case of metformin. *Semin. Oncol.* **2016**, *43*, 123–133. [CrossRef] [PubMed]

100. Marini, C.; Bianchi, G.; Buschiazzo, A.; Ravera, S.; Martella, R.; Bottoni, G.; Petretto, A.; Emionite, L.; Monteverde, E.; Capitanio, S.; et al. Divergent targets of glycolysis and oxidative phosphorylation result in additive effects of metformin and starvation in colon and breast cancer. *Sci. Rep.* **2016**, *6*, 19569. [CrossRef] [PubMed]

101. Menendez, J.A.; Oliveras-Ferraros, C.; Cufí, S.; Corominas-Faja, B.; Joven, J.; Martin-Castillo, B. Vazquez-Martin, A. Metformin is synthetically lethal with glucose withdrawal in cancer cells. *Cell Cycle* **2012**, *11*, 2782–2792. [CrossRef] [PubMed]

102. Van Wijk, J.P.; de Koning, E.J.; Cabezas, M.C.; op't Roodt, J.; Joven, J.; Rabelink, T.J.; Hoepelman, A.I. Comparison of rosiglitazone and metformin for treating HIV lipodystrophy: A randomized trial. *Ann. Intern. Med.* **2005**, *143*, 337–346. [CrossRef] [PubMed]

103. Hawley, S.A.; Ross, F.A.; Chevtzoff, C.; Green, K.A.; Evans, A.; Fogarty, S.; Towler, M.C.; Brown, L.J.; Ogunbayo, O.A.; Evans, A.M.; et al. Use of cells expressing gamma subunit variants to identify diverse mechanisms of AMPK activation. *Cell Metab.* **2010**, *11*, 554–565. [CrossRef] [PubMed]

104. Zhou, G.; Myers, R.; Li, Y.; Chen, Y.; Shen, X.; Fenyk-Melody, J.; Wu, M.; Ventre, J.; Doebber, T.; Fujii, N.; et al. Role of AMP-activated protein kinase in mechanism of metformin action. *J. Clin. Investig.* **2001**, *108*, 1167–1174. [CrossRef] [PubMed]

105. Madiraju, A.K.; Erion, D.M.; Rahimi, Y.; Zhang, X.M.; Braddock, D.T.; Albright, R.A.; Prigaro, B.J.; Wood, J.L.; Bhanot, S.; MacDonald, M.J.; et al. Metformin suppresses gluconeogenesis by inhibiting mitochondrial glycerophosphate dehydrogenase. *Nature* **2014**, *510*, 542–546. [CrossRef] [PubMed]

106. Menendez, J.A.; Cufí, S.; Oliveras-Ferraros, C.; Martin-Castillo, B.; Joven, J.; Vellon, L.; Vazquez-Martín, A. Metformin and the ATM DNA damage response (DDR): Accelerating the onset of stress-induced senescence to boost protection against cancer. *Aging* **2011**, *3*, 1063–1077. [CrossRef] [PubMed]

107. Menendez, J.A.; Joven, J. One-carbon metabolism: An aging-cancer crossroad for the gerosuppressant metformin. *Aging* **2012**, *4*, 894–898. [CrossRef] [PubMed]

108. Menendez, J.A.; Martin-Castillo, B.; Joven, J. Metformin and cancer: Quo vadis et cui bono? *Oncotarget* **2016**. [CrossRef] [PubMed]

109. Municio, C.; Soler-Palacios, B.; Estrada-Capetillo, L.; Benguria, A.; Dopazo, A.; García-Lorenzo, E.; Fernández-Arroyo, S.; Joven, J.; Miranda-Carús, M.E.; González-Álvaro, I.; et al. Methotrexate selectively targets human proinflammatory macrophages through a thymidylate synthase/p53 axis. *Ann. Rheum. Dis.* **2016**, *75*, 2157–2165. [CrossRef] [PubMed]

110. Rena, G.; Pearson, E.R.; Sakamoto, K. Molecular mechanism of action of metformin: Old or new insights? *Diabetologia* **2013**, *56*, 1898–1906. [CrossRef] [PubMed]

111. Shu, Y.; Sheardown, S.A.; Brown, C.; Owen, R.P.; Zhang, S.; Castro, R.A.; Ianculescu, A.G.; Yue, L.; Lo, J.C.; Burchard, E.G.; et al. Effect of genetic variation in the organic cation transporter 1 (OCT1) on metformin action. *J. Clin. Investig.* **2007**, *117*, 1422–1431. [CrossRef] [PubMed]

112. Dujic, T.; Zhou, K.; Donnelly, L.A.; Tavendale, R.; Palmer, C.N.; Pearson, E.R. Association of organic cation transporter 1 with intolerance to metformin in type 2 diabetes: A GoDARTS study. *Diabetes* **2015**, *64*, 1786–1793. [CrossRef] [PubMed]

113. Dujic, T.; Causevic, A.; Bego, T.; Malenica, M.; Velija-Asimi, Z.; Pearson, E.R.; Semiz, S. Organic cation transporter 1 variants and gastrointestinal side effects of metformin in patients with type 2 diabetes. *Diabet. Med.* **2016**, *33*, 511–514. [CrossRef] [PubMed]

114. Zhou, K.; Bellenguez, C.; Spencer, C.C.; Bennett, A.J.; Coleman, R.L.; Tavendale, R.; Hawley, S.A.; Donnelly, L.A.; Schofield, C.; Groves, C.J.; et al. Common variants near ATM are associated with glycemic response to metformin in type 2 diabetes. *Nat. Genet.* **2011**, *43*, 117–120. [CrossRef] [PubMed]

115. Scheen, A.J. Personalising metformin therapy: A clinician's perspective. *Lancet Diabetes Endocrinol.* **2014**, *2*, 442–444. [CrossRef]

116. Ter Borg, S.; de Groot, L.C.; Mijnarends, D.M.; de Vries, J.H.; Verlaan, S.; Meijboom, S.; Luiking, Y.C.; Schols, J.M. Differences in Nutrient Intake and Biochemical Nutrient Status Between Sarcopenic and Nonsarcopenic Older Adults-Results From the Maastricht Sarcopenia Study. *J. Am. Med. Dir. Assoc.* **2016**, *17*, 393–401. [CrossRef] [PubMed]

117. Malaguarnera, G.; Gagliano, C.; Salomone, S.; Giordano, M.; Bucolo, C.; Pappalardo, A.; Drago, F.; Caraci, F.; Avitabile, T.; Motta, M. Folate status in type 2 diabetic patients with and without retinopathy. *Clin. Ophthalmol.* **2015**, *9*, 1437–1442. [CrossRef] [PubMed]

118. Mudryj, A.N.; de Groh, M.; Aukema, H.M.; Yu, N. Folate intakes from diet and supplements may place certain Canadians at risk for folic acid toxicity. *Br. J. Nutr.* **2016**, *116*, 1236–1245. [CrossRef] [PubMed]

119. Danenberg, P.V.; Gustavsson, B.; Johnston, P.; Lindberg, P.; Moser, R.; Odin, E.; Peters, G.J.; Petrelli, N. Folates as adjuvants to anticancer agents: Chemical rationale and mechanism of action. *Crit. Rev. Oncol. Hematol.* **2016**, *106*, 118–131. [CrossRef] [PubMed]

120. Yajnik, C.S.; Deshpande, S.S.; Jackson, A.A.; Refsum, H.; Rao, S.; Fisher, D.J.; Bhat, D.S.; Naik, S.S.; Coyaki, K.J.; Joglekar, C.V.; et al. Vitamin B12 and folate concentrations during pregnancy and insulin resistance in the offspring: The Pune Maternal Nutrition Study. *Diabetologia* **2008**, *51*, 29–38. [CrossRef] [PubMed]

121. Scott, J.M.; Weir, D.G. The methyl folate trap. A physiological response in man to prevent methyl group deficiency in kwashiorkor (methionine deficiency) and an explanation for folic-acid induced exacerbation of subacute combined degeneration in pernicious anaemia. *Lancet* **1981**, *2*, 337–340. [CrossRef]

122. Stowers, J.M.; Smith, O.A. Vitamin B12 and metformin. *BMJ* **1971**, *3*, 246–247. [CrossRef] [PubMed]

123. Ting, R.Z.; Szeto, C.C.; Chan, M.H.; Ma, K.K.; Chow, K.M. Risk factors of vitamin B12 deficiency in patients receiving metformin. *Arch. Intern. Med.* **2006**, *166*, 1975–1979. [CrossRef] [PubMed]

124. Liu, Q.; Li, S.; Quan, H.; Li, J. Vitamin B12 status in metformin treated patients: Systematic review. *PLoS ONE* **2014**, *9*, E100379. [CrossRef] [PubMed]

125. Obeid, R.; Jung, J.; Falk, J.; Herrmann, W.; Geisel, J.; Friesenhahn-Ochs, B.; Lammerts, F.; Fassbender, K.; Kostopoulos, P. Serum vitamin B12 not reflecting vitamin B12 status in patients with type 2 diabetes. *Biochimie* **2013**, *95*, 1056–1061. [CrossRef] [PubMed]

126. Greibe, E.; Trolle, B.; Bor, M.V.; Lauszus, F.F.; Nexo, E. Metformin lowers serum cobalamin without changing other markers of cobalamin status: A study on women with polycystic ovary syndrome. *Nutrients* **2013**, *5*, 2475–2482. [CrossRef] [PubMed]

127. Leung, S.; Mattman, A.; Snyder, F.; Kassam, R.; Meneilly, G.; Nexo, E. Metformin induces reductions in plasma cobalamin and haptocorrin bound cobalamin levels in elderly diabetic patients. *Clin. Biochem.* **2010**, *43*, 759–760. [CrossRef] [PubMed]

128. Ahmed, M.A. Metformin and Vitamin B12 Deficiency: Where Do We Stand? *J. Pharm. Pharm. Sci.* **2016**, *19*, 382–398. [CrossRef] [PubMed]

129. DeFronzo, R.; Fleming, G.A.; Chen, K.; Bicsak, T.A. Metformin-associated lactic acidosis: Current perspectives on causes and risk. *Metabolism* **2016**, *65*, 20–29. [CrossRef] [PubMed]

130. Pernicova, I.; Korbonits, M. Metformin—Mode of action and clinical implications for diabetes and cancer. *Nat. Rev. Endocrinol.* **2014**, *10*, 143–156. [CrossRef] [PubMed]

131. De Jager, J.; Kooy, A.; Lehert, P.; Wulffelé, M.G.; van der Kolk, J.; Bets, D.; Verburg, J.; Donker, A.J.; Stehouwer, C.D. Long term treatment with metformin in patients with type 2 diabetes and risk of vitamin B-12 deficiency: Randomised placebo controlled trial. *BMJ* **2010**, *340*, c2181. [CrossRef] [PubMed]

132. McCreight, L.J.; Bailey, C.J.; Pearson, E.R. Metformin and the gastrointestinal tract. *Diabetologia* **2016**, *59*, 426–435. [CrossRef] [PubMed]

133. Wu, T.; Thazhath, S.S.; Bound, M.J.; Jones, K.L.; Horowitz, M.; Rayner, C.K. Mechanism of increase in plasma intact GLP-1 by metformin in type 2 diabetes: Stimulation of GLP-1 secretion or reduction in plasma DPP-4 activity? *Diabetes Res. Clin. Pract.* **2014**, *106*, e3–e6. [CrossRef] [PubMed]

134. Yee, S.W.; Lin, L.; Merski, M.; Keiser, M.J.; Gupta, A.; Zhang, Y.; Chien, H.C.; Shoichet, B.K.; Giacomini, K.M. Prediction and validation of enzyme and transporter off-targets for metformin. *J. Pharmacokinet. Pharmacodyn.* **2015**, *42*, 463–475. [CrossRef] [PubMed]

135. Scarpello, J.H.; Hodgson, E.; Howlett, H.C. Effect of metformin on bile salt circulation and intestinal motility in type 2 diabetes mellitus. *Diabet. Med.* **1998**, *15*, 651–656. [CrossRef]

136. Forslund, K.; Hildebrand, F.; Nielsen, T.; Falony, G.; Le Chatelier, E.; Sunagawa, S.; Prifti, E.; Vieira-Silva, S.; Gudmundsdottir, V.; Krogh Pedersen, H.; et al. Disentangling type 2 diabetes and metformin treatment signatures in the human gut microbiota. *Nature* **2015**, *528*, 262–266. [CrossRef] [PubMed]

137. Burton, J.H.; Johnson, M.; Johnson, J.; Hsia, D.S.; Greenway, F.L.; Heiman, M.L. Addition of a gastrointestinal microbiome modulator to metformin improves metformin tolerance and fasting glucose levels. *J. Diabetes Sci. Technol.* **2015**, *9*, 808–814. [CrossRef] [PubMed]

138. Mardinoglu, A.; Boren, J.; Smith, U. Confounding Effects of Metformin on the Human Gut Microbiome in Type 2 Diabetes. *Cell Metab.* **2016**, *23*, 10–12. [CrossRef] [PubMed]

139. Bhalerao, K.D.; Lee, S.C.; Soboyejo, W.O.; Soboyejo, A.B. A folic acid-based functionalized surface for biosensor systems. *J. Mater. Sci. Mater. Med.* **2007**, *18*, 3–8. [CrossRef] [PubMed]

140. Armbruster, D.A.; Alexander, D.B. Sample to sample carryover: A source of analytical laboratory error and its relevance to integrated clinical chemistry/immunoassay systems. *Clin. Chim. Acta* **2006**, *373*, 37–43. [CrossRef] [PubMed]

141. Bertran, N.; Camps, J.; Fernández-Ballart, J.; Murphy, M.M.; Arija, V.; Ferré, N.; Tous, M.; Joven, J. Evaluation of a high-sensitivity turbidimetric immunoassay for serum C-reactive protein: Application to the study of longitudinal changes throughout normal pregnancy. *Clin. Chem. Lab. Med.* **2005**, *43*, 308–313. [CrossRef] [PubMed]

142. Wainwright, P.; Narayanan, S.; Cook, P. False-normal vitamin B12 results in a patient with pernicious anaemia. *Clin. Biochem.* **2015**, *48*, 1366–1377. [CrossRef] [PubMed]

143. Harrington, D.J. Holotranscobalamin: In the middle of difficultly lies opportunity. *Clin. Chem. Lab. Med.* **2016**, *54*, 1407–1409. [CrossRef] [PubMed]

144. Kancherla, V.; Garn, J.V.; Zakai, N.A.; Williamson, R.S.; Cashion, W.T.; Odewole, O.; Judd, S.E.; Oakley, G.P., Jr. Multivitamin Use and Serum Vitamin B12 Concentrations in Older-Adult Metformin Users in REGARDS, 2003–2007. *PLoS ONE* **2016**, *11*, E0160802. [CrossRef] [PubMed]

145. Russo, G.T.; Giandalia, A.; Romeo, E.L.; Scarcella, C.; Gambadoro, N.; Zingale, R.; Forte, F.; Perdichizzi, G.; Alibrandi, A.; Cucinotta, D. Diabetic neuropathy is not associated with homocysteine, folate, vitamin B12 levels, and MTHFR C677T mutation in type 2 diabetic outpatients taking metformin. *J. Endocrinol. Investig.* **2016**, *39*, 305–314. [CrossRef] [PubMed]

146. Bird, J.K.; Ronnenberg, A.G.; Choi, S.W.; Du, F.; Mason, J.B.; Liu, Z. Obesity is associated with increased red blood cell folate despite lower dietary intakes and serum concentrations. *J. Nutr.* **2015**, *145*, 79–86. [CrossRef] [PubMed]

147. Denimal, D.; Brindisi, M.C.; Lemaire, S.; Duvillard, L. Assessment of Folate Status in Obese Patients: Should We Measure Folate in Serum or in Red Blood Cells? *Obes. Surg.* **2016**. [CrossRef] [PubMed]

148. Yetley, E.A.; Johnson, C.L. Folate and vitamin B-12 biomarkers in NHANES: History of their measurement and use. *Am. J. Clin. Nutr.* **2011**, *94*, 322S–331S. [CrossRef] [PubMed]

149. Zhang, Q.; Li, S.; Li, L.; Li, Q.; Ren, K.; Sun, X.; Li, J. Metformin treatment and homocysteine: A systematic review and meta-analysis of randomized controlled trials. *Nutrients* **2016**, *8*, 798. [CrossRef] [PubMed]

150. Pfeiffer, C.M.; Sternberg, M.R.; Fazili, Z.; Lacher, D.A.; Zhang, M.; Johnson, C.L.; Hamner, H.C.; Bailey, R.L.; Rader, J.I.; Yamini, S. Folate status and concentrations of serum folate forms in the US population: National Health and Nutrition Examination Survey 2011–2012. *Br. J. Nutr.* **2015**, *113*, 1965–1977. [CrossRef] [PubMed]

151. Dominguez-Salas, P.; Moore, S.E.; Cole, D.; da Costa, K.A.; Cox, S.E.; Dyer, R.A.; Fuldord, A.J.; Innis, S.M.; Waterland, R.A.; Zeisel„ S.H.; et al. DNA methylation potential: Dietary intake and blood concentrations of one-carbon metabolites and cofactors in rural African women. *Am. J. Clin. Nutr.* **2013**, *97*, 1217–1227. [CrossRef] [PubMed]

152. Kühnen, P.; Handke, D.; Waterland, R.A.; Hennig, B.J.; Silver, M.; Fulford, A.J.; Dominguez-Salas, P.; Moore, S.E.; Prentice, A.M.; Spranger, J.; et al. Interindividual Variation in DNA Methylation at a Putative POMC Metastable Epiallele Is Associated with Obesity. *Cell Metab.* **2016**, *24*, 502–509. [CrossRef]

153. Eicher-Miller, H.A.; Fulgoni, V.L.; Keast, D.R. Processed Food Contributions to Energy and Nutrient Intake Differ among US Children by Race/Ethnicity. *Nutrients* **2015**, *7*, 10076–10088. [CrossRef] [PubMed]

154. Colditz, G.A. Overview of the epidemiology methods and applications: Strengths and limitations of observational study designs. *Crit. Rev. Food. Sci. Nutr.* **2010**, *50* (Suppl. 1), 10–12. [CrossRef] [PubMed]

155. Fernández-Arroyo, S.; Cuyàs, E.; Bosch-Barrera, J.; Alarcón, T.; Joven, J.; Menendez, J.A. Activation of the methylation cycle in cells reprogrammed into a stem cell-like state. *Oncoscience* **2016**, *2*, 958–967. [PubMed]

156. Riera-Borrull, M.; Rodríguez-Gallego, E.; Hernández-Aguilera, A.; Luciano, F.; Ras, R.; Cuyàs, E.; Camps, J.; Segura-Carretero, A.; Menendez, J.A.; Joven, J.; et al. Exploring the Process of Energy Generation in Pathophysiology by Targeted Metabolomics: Performance of a Simple and Quantitative Method. *J. Am. Soc. Mass. Spectrom.* **2016**, *27*, 168–177. [CrossRef] [PubMed]

157. Liu, X.; Romero, I.L.; Litchfield, L.M.; Lengyel, E.; Locasale, J.W. Metformin Targets Central Carbon Metabolism and Reveals Mitochondrial Requirements in Human Cancers. *Cell Metab.* **2016**. [CrossRef] [PubMed]

Permissions

All chapters in this book were first published by MDPI; hereby published with permission under the Creative Commons Attribution License or equivalent. Every chapter published in this book has been scrutinized by our experts. Their significance has been extensively debated. The topics covered herein carry significant findings which will fuel the growth of the discipline. They may even be implemented as practical applications or may be referred to as a beginning point for another development.

The contributors of this book come from diverse backgrounds, making this book a truly international effort. This book will bring forth new frontiers with its revolutionizing research information and detailed analysis of the nascent developments around the world.

We would like to thank all the contributing authors for lending their expertise to make the book truly unique. They have played a crucial role in the development of this book. Without their invaluable contributions this book wouldn't have been possible. They have made vital efforts to compile up to date information on the varied aspects of this subject to make this book a valuable addition to the collection of many professionals and students.

This book was conceptualized with the vision of imparting up-to-date information and advanced data in this field. To ensure the same, a matchless editorial board was set up. Every individual on the board went through rigorous rounds of assessment to prove their worth. After which they invested a large part of their time researching and compiling the most relevant data for our readers.

The editorial board has been involved in producing this book since its inception. They have spent rigorous hours researching and exploring the diverse topics which have resulted in the successful publishing of this book. They have passed on their knowledge of decades through this book. To expedite this challenging task, the publisher supported the team at every step. A small team of assistant editors was also appointed to further simplify the editing procedure and attain best results for the readers.

Apart from the editorial board, the designing team has also invested a significant amount of their time in understanding the subject and creating the most relevant covers. They scrutinized every image to scout for the most suitable representation of the subject and create an appropriate cover for the book.

The publishing team has been an ardent support to the editorial, designing and production team. Their endless efforts to recruit the best for this project, has resulted in the accomplishment of this book. They are a veteran in the field of academics and their pool of knowledge is as vast as their experience in printing. Their expertise and guidance has proved useful at every step. Their uncompromising quality standards have made this book an exceptional effort. Their encouragement from time to time has been an inspiration for everyone.

The publisher and the editorial board hope that this book will prove to be a valuable piece of knowledge for researchers, students, practitioners and scholars across the globe.

List of Contributors

Joshua M. Corbin
Department of Pathology, Oklahoma University Health Sciences Center, Oklahoma City, OK 73104, USA

Maria J. Ruiz-Echevarría
Department of Pathology, Oklahoma University Health Sciences Center and Stephenson Cancer Center, Oklahoma City, OK 73104, USA

Kassidy Burgess
College of Veterinary Medicine, Midwestern University, Glendale, AZ 85308, USA
Biomedical Sciences Program, Midwestern University, Glendale, AZ 85308, USA

Calli Bennett and Forrest Bethel
Biomedical Sciences Program, Midwestern University, Glendale, AZ 85308, USA
College of Osteopathic Medicine, Midwestern University, Glendale, AZ 85308, USA

Hannah Mosnier
School of Medicine, National University of Ireland Galway, H91 TK33, Ireland
College of Dental Medicine, Midwestern University, Glendale, AZ 85308, USA

Neha Kwatra
Biomedical Sciences Program, Midwestern University, Glendale, AZ 85308, USA
College of Dental Medicine, Midwestern University, Glendale, AZ 85308, USA

Nafisa M. Jadavji
College of Veterinary Medicine, Midwestern University, Glendale, AZ 85308, USA
Biomedical Sciences Program, Midwestern University, Glendale, AZ 85308, USA
Department of Neuroscience, Carleton University, Ottawa, ON K1S 5B6, Canada

Xiayu Wu, Weijiang Xu, Tao Zhou, Neng Cao, Juan Ni, Ziqing Liang and Xu Wang
School of Life Sciences, The Engineering Research Center of Sustainable Development and Utilization of Biomass Energy, Ministry of Education, Yunnan Normal University, Kunming 650500, Yunnan, China

Tianning Zou
Third Affiliated Hospital of Kunming Medical College, Kunming 650101, Yunnan, China

Michael Fenech
Genome Health and Personalized Nutrition, CSIRO Food and Nutrition, Adelaide SA 5000, Australia

Barbara Troesch, Peter Weber and M. Hasan Mohajeri
DSM Nutritional Products Ltd., Wurmisweg 576, Kaiseraugst 4303, Switzerland

Amy McMahon, Catherine F. Hughes, J. J. Strain and Mary Ward
Northern Ireland Centre for Food and Health, Ulster University, Coleraine BT52 1SA, UK

María Lourdes Samaniego-Vaesken, Elena Alonso-Aperte and Gregorio Varela-Moreiras
Department of Pharmaceutical and Health Sciences, Faculty of Pharmacy, CEU San Pablo University, Madrid 28668, Spain

Nithya Sukumar, Vinod Patel and Ponnusamy Saravanan
Warwick Medical School, University of Warwick, Coventry CV2 2DX, UK
Academic Department of Diabetes, Endocrinology and Metabolism, George Eliot Hospital, Nuneaton CV10 7DJ, UK

Hema Venkataraman
Warwick Medical School, University of Warwick, Coventry CV2 2DX, UK

Sean Wilson
Hull York Medical School, Hertford Building, University of Hull, Hull HU6 7RX, UK

Ilona Goljan and Selvin Selvamoni
Academic Department of Diabetes, Endocrinology and Metabolism, George Eliot Hospital, Nuneaton CV10 7DJ, UK

Chia-ling Ho and Teo A. W. Quay
Food Nutrition and Health, Faculty of Land and Food Systems, The University of British Columbia, 2205 East Mall, Vancouver, BC V6T 1Z4, Canada
Research Institute, British Columbia Children's Hospital, 950 West 28th Ave, Vancouver, BC V5Z 4H4, Canada

Anne M. Molloy
School of Medicine, Trinity College Dublin, Dublin 2, Ireland

Angela M. Devlin
Research Institute, British Columbia Children's Hospital, 950 West 28th Ave, Vancouver, BC V5Z 4H4, Canada
Department of Pediatrics, The University of British Columbia, 4480 Oak Street, Vancouver, BC V6H 3V4, Canada

Yvonne Lamers
Food Nutrition and Health, Faculty of Land and Food Systems, The University of British Columbia, 2205 East Mall, Vancouver, BC V6T 1Z4, Canada
Research Institute, British Columbia Children's Hospital, 950 West 28th Ave, Vancouver, BC V5Z 4H4, Canada
Fraser Health Authority, 10334 152A St, Surrey, BC V3R 7P8, Canada

Catherine F. Hughes, Mary Ward, Leane Hoey, Kristina Pentieva and Helene McNulty
Northern Ireland Centre for Food and Health, Ulster University, Cromore Road, Coleraine BT52 1SA, Northern Ireland, UK

Fergal Tracey
Causeway Hospital, Northern Health and Social Care Trust, Coleraine BT52 1HS, Northern Ireland, UK

Karen B. Kelly, John P. Kennelly, Randal Nelson, Kelly Leonard and Catherine J. Field
Department of Agricultural, Food & Nutritional Science, University of Alberta, Edmonton, AB T6G2P5, Canada

Marta Ordonez and Antonio Gomez-Muñoz
Department of Biochemistry and Molecular Biology, Faculty of Science and Technology, University of the Basque Country (UPV/EHU), Bilbao 48080, Spain

Sally Stabler
Department of Medicine, University of Colorado School of Medicine, Aurora, CO 80206, USA

René L. Jacobs
Department of Agricultural, Food & Nutritional Science, University of Alberta, Edmonton, AB T6G2P5, Canada
Department of Biochemistry, University of Alberta, Edmonton, AB T6G2R7, Canada

Danyel Bueno Dalto
Sherbrooke Research Centre, Agriculture and Agri-Food Canada, Sherbrooke, QC J1M 0C8, Canada
Department of Biology, Université de Sherbrooke, Sherbrooke, QC J1K 2R1, Canada

Jean-Jacques Matte
Sherbrooke Research Centre, Agriculture and Agri-Food Canada, Sherbrooke, QC J1M 0C8, Canada

Nuno Mendonça and Tom R. Hill
School of Agriculture Food and Rural Development, Newcastle University, Newcastle upon Tyne NE1 7RU, UK
Newcastle University Institute for Ageing, Newcastle University, Newcastle upon Tyne NE2 4AX, UK
Human Nutrition Research Centre, Newcastle University, Newcastle upon Tyne NE2 4HH, UK

John C. Mathers
Newcastle University Institute for Ageing, Newcastle University, Newcastle upon Tyne NE2 4AX, UK
Human Nutrition Research Centre, Newcastle University, Newcastle upon Tyne NE2 4HH, UK
Institute of Cellular Medicine, Newcastle upon Tyne NE2 4HH, UK

Ashley J. Adamson
Newcastle University Institute for Ageing, Newcastle University, Newcastle upon Tyne NE2 4AX, UK
Human Nutrition Research Centre, Newcastle University, Newcastle upon Tyne NE2 4HH, UK
Institute of Health and Society, Newcastle University, Newcastle upon Tyne NE2 5PL, UK

Carmen Martin-Ruiz
Newcastle University Institute for Ageing, Newcastle University, Newcastle upon Tyne NE2 4AX, UK

Chris J. Seal
School of Agriculture Food and Rural Development, Newcastle University, Newcastle upon Tyne NE1 7RU, UK
Human Nutrition Research Centre, Newcastle University, Newcastle upon Tyne NE2 4HH, UK

Carol Jagger
Newcastle University Institute for Ageing, Newcastle University, Newcastle upon Tyne NE2 4AX, UK
Institute of Health and Society, Newcastle University, Newcastle upon Tyne NE2 5PL, UK

Kelei Li
Department of Food Science and Nutrition, Zhejiang University, Hangzhou 310058, China

Mark L. Wahlqvist
Fuli Institute, Zhejiang University, Hangzhou 310058, China
Monash Asia Institute and Departments of Medicine and of Nutrition and Dietetics, Monash University, Melbourne 3006, Australia

Duo Li
Department of Food Science and Nutrition, Zhejiang University, Hangzhou 310058, China
Monash Asia Institute and Departments of Medicine and of Nutrition and Dietetics, Monash University, Melbourne 3006, Australia

Fedra Luciano-Mateo, Anna Hernández-Aguilera, Noemi Cabre and Jordi Camps
Unitat de Recerca Biomèdica, Hospital Universitari Sant Joan, Institut d'Investigació Sanitària Pere Virgili, Universitat Rovira i Virgili, 43201 Reus, Spain

Salvador Fernández-Arroyo
Unitat de Recerca Biomèdica, Hospital Universitari Sant Joan, Institut d'Investigació Sanitària Pere Virgili, Universitat Rovira i Virgili, 43201 Reus, Spain

Molecular Oncology Group, Girona Biomedical Research Institute (IDIBGI), 17190 Girona, Spain

Javier A. Menendez
Molecular Oncology Group, Girona Biomedical Research Institute (IDIBGI), 17190 Girona, Spain
ProCURE (Program against Cancer Therapeutic Resistance), Metabolism and Cancer Group, Catalan Institute of Oncology, 17190 Girona, Spain

Jorge Joven
Unitat de Recerca Biomèdica, Hospital Universitari Sant Joan, Institut d'Investigació Sanitària Pere Virgili, Universitat Rovira i Virgili, 43201 Reus, Spain
The Campus of International Excellence Southern Catalonia, 43003 Tarragona, Spain

Index

Printed in the USA
CPSIA information can be obtained
at www.ICGtesting.com
JSHW051402091023
49903JS00006B/242